Clinical Nephrology in Medical Practice

GAVIN J. BECKER
MD, FRACP
Nephrologist, Royal Melbourne Hospital, Victoria

JUDITH A. WHITWORTH
MD, FRACP, PhD
Professor of Medicine, Director of Nephrology
St George's Hospital, Kogarah, New South Wales

PRISCILLA KINCAID-SMITH
CBE, BSc, MD, FRCP, FRACP, DCP
Professor of Medicine, Director of Nephrology
Royal Melbourne Hospital, Victoria

OXFORD

BLACKWELL SCIENTIFIC PUBLICATIONS

LONDON   EDINBURGH   BOSTON

MELBOURNE   PARIS   BERLIN   VIENNA

© 1992 by
Blackwell Scientific Publications
Editorial Offices:
Osney Mead, Oxford OX2 0EL
25 John Street, London WC1N 2BL
23 Ainslie Place, Edinburgh EH3 6AJ
3 Cambridge Center, Cambridge
   Massachusetts 02142, USA
54 University Street, Carlton
   Victoria 3053, Australia

Other Editorial Offices:
Librairie Arnette SA
2, rue Casimir-Delavigne
75006 Paris
France

Blackwell Wissenschaft−Verlag
Meinekestrasse 4
D-1000 Berlin 15
Germany

Blackwell MZV
Feldgasse 13
A-1238 Wien
Austria

First published 1992

Set by Setrite, Hong Kong
Printed and bound in Great Britain
at the University Press,
Cambridge

DISTRIBUTORS

Marston Book Services Ltd
PO Box 87
Oxford OX2 0DT
(*Orders*: Tel: 0865 791155
          Fax: 0865 791927
          Telex: 837515)

USA
Blackwell Scientific
Publications, Inc.
3 Cambridge Center
Cambridge, MA 02142
(*Orders*: Tel: 800 759-6102)

Canada
Times Mirror Professional
Publishing, Ltd
5240 Finch Avenue East
Scarborough, Ontario M1S 5A2
(*Orders*: Tel: 416 298-1588)

Australia
Blackwell Scientific Publications
(Australia) Pty Ltd
54 University Street
Carlton, Victoria 3053
(*Orders*: Tel: 03 347-0300)

British Library
Cataloguing in Publication Data

Becker, Gavin J.
   Clinical nephrology in
   medical practice.
   I. Title II. Whitworth, Judith A.
   III. Kincaid-Smith, Priscilla
   616.61

   ISBN 0-632-03167-0

Contents

Preface

Our aim in writing this book was to produce a readable textbook of nephrology with an emphasis on clinical relevance. To keep it brief we have tended to be dogmatic. The book is intended for final year medical students, postgraduate trainees in medicine and renal nurses.

There are three sections, devoted to: renal structure and function, clinical presentation, and specific renal diseases. This results in a certain amount of repetition and some cross-referencing, however, it is hoped that the reader will find these divisions useful. Though the book can be read from front to back, we also hope that the reader who wishes to read only a specific topic will find the book adequate for such an approach.

In the first section renal anatomy and physiology is discussed, along with the clinical methods of assessment of structure and function. A final chapter covers the renal response to damage. The second section is a patient-oriented approach to renal disease, commencing with history taking and examination of the patient and the urine. We then discuss the approaches to the more common clinical syndromes with which patients with renal disease present. Specific renal diseases are covered in Section 3 which deals didactically with common diseases of the kidney. A traditional formal approach (definition, incidence, pathogenesis, pathology, clinical features, diagnosis, management) is used when appropriate. The final chapters deal with the special areas of drugs, pregnancy, dialysis and transplantation.

A list of further reading has been chosen with a bias towards recent publication, easy access and clinical relevance.

The list of people whose contributions could be acknowledged is virtually endless. First, and most importantly, we express thanks to our many colleagues and patients from whom we have learnt, and without whom this book could not exist. We would like to acknowledge specifically the help of Douglas Matthews for graphics and electron photomicrography, and Professor Bill Hare who supplied critical X-rays. Ian Birchall showed his usual artistry in the cutting and staining of renal biopsy material. The manuscript was prepared by Nicky Steylen and Vicky Kuek.

Section 1
Renal Structure and Function

1: *Anatomy of the Urinary System*

THE KIDNEYS

The kidneys are paired bean-shaped organs which lie behind the peritoneum on either side of the 12th thoracic to third lumbar vertebrae (Fig. 1.1). Each is about 10 to 12 cm in length, although they appear about 1 cm longer in abdominal X-rays because of the magnifying effect of the rays diverging through the patient to the film (see Fig. 2.2). The diaphragm is above and behind their upper poles so that kidneys move downward on inspiration. The right kidney is below the liver and, therefore, about 1 to 2 cm lower than the left. It is also 0.5 to 1 cm shorter.

The concave medial aspect of each kidney has a longitudinal slit, the renal hilum, through which pass the renal vessels and nerves, and the renal pelvis — the funnel-shaped upper end of the ureter (Fig. 1.2). There is also a variable amount of sinus fat around the pelvis. Because of the bulk of the vertebral bodies and paravertebral muscles the renal pelvis is directed anteromedially to the kidney (see Fig. 2.5).

In cut section the substance of each kidney can be seen to comprise an outer cortex and an inner medulla (Fig. 1.2).

The renal cortex

The cortex contains scattered dark specks, each about 0.2 mm in diameter. These are the renal corpuscles (or glomeruli).

The renal medulla

The medulla has a striated appearance because the blood vessels which it contains run to and from the pelvis. The medulla is divided into the renal pyramids; each with its base abutting the cortex and its apex forming a nipple-like renal papilla which projects into a cup-shaped cavity, or *calyx*, in the renal pelvis.

Between the pyramids the cortex extends towards the renal hilum as the renal columns of Bertin. The renal vessels and nerves pass from the hilum to the corticomedullary junction in these columns.

The renal pelvis has 7 to 13 minor calyces, each around one papilla. These converge into two or three major calyces and finally into the main cavity of the pelvis. The renal pelvis then funnels into the upper end of the ureter. The renal papillae

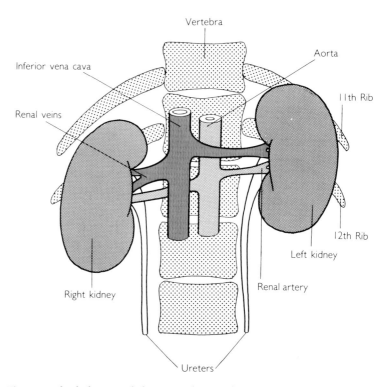

Fig. 1.1 The kidneys and their vascular supply

consist of either simple papillae, each draining one pyramid, or compound papillae each draining several pyramids. The latter arrangement commonly occurs at the renal poles where the tips of the pyramids tend to be crowded. The relevance of this to focal renal scarring in reflux nephropathy will be discussed in Chapter 21.

The junction of the minor and major calyces can also vary, leading to bifid systems, or in extreme cases a total duplex system with two ureters entering the bladder on that side (Chapter 31).

The kidneys are surrounded by perinephric fat which is enclosed behind and in front of the kidney by a sheath of condensed connective tissue known as the renal fascia. The fat and fascia make up the renal capsule.

The nephron

The functional and anatomical excretory unit of the kidney is the nephron (Fig. 1.3). There are 1 to 1.2 million nephrons in each kidney and each consists of two main parts: the renal corpuscle and the renal tubule. Within the corpuscle an ultrafiltrate of plasma is formed which then passes along the renal tubule

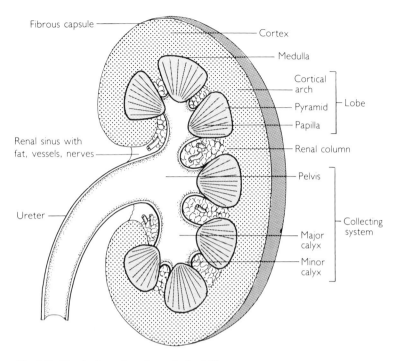

Fig. 1.2 Vertical section through the kidney

toward the pelvis. During this course the tubule modifies the composition of the filtrate by resorption or secretion to form the final product — urine.

The renal corpuscle   Renal corpuscles are about 0.2 mm in diameter and are distributed throughout the cortex. Each consists of an outer, Bowman's, capsule, which encloses a tuft of capillaries called the glomerulus (Fig. 1.4).

The glomerulus   The glomerulus is an anastomosing plexus of capillaries fed by an afferent arteriole and drained by a slightly smaller efferent arteriole. These arterioles enter and leave the glomerulus side by side at the vascular pole which is usually opposite the point where the capsule is attached to the proximal tubule. The capsule is formed by invagination of the blind upper end of the tubule such that the inner layer of epithelial cells covering the capillary tuft, and the outer parietal layer are separated from the glomerulus by a space filled with filtrate from the capillaries. The outer layer is then continuous with the cells of the connecting segment of the proximal tubule. Commonly the term glomerulus is used to refer to the entire renal corpuscle, not only the tuft.

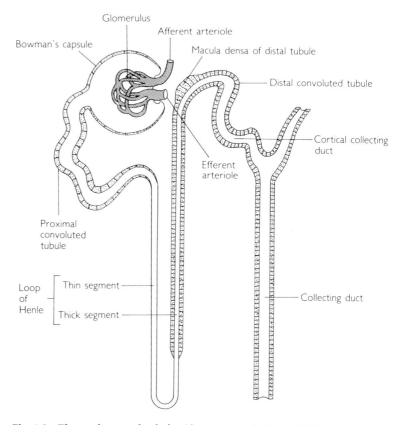

Fig. 1.3 The nephron and tubules (diagrammatic). Note: (1) The glomerulus — filtration of plasma. (2) Proximal tubule — resorption of sodium, chloride, potassium, water, glucose, amino acids, phosphate. (3) Loop of Henle — concentration of renal interstitial fluid. (4) Distal tubule and cortical collecting duct — resorption of sodium, chloride, water acidification, excretion of potassium. (5) Collecting duct — concentration of urine by water resorption. (6) Macula densa — monitoring tubular chloride, part of juxtaglomerular apparatus

There are three main types of cell in the glomerulus (Figs 1.5 & 1.6).
- *The mesangium and its mesangial cells* make up the stalk of the tuft continuous with vascular smooth muscle and connective tissue cells at the vascular pole. The mesangial cells are within a matrix forming a connective tissue-like support for the fragile capillaries. There are several types of cells in the mesangium, including contractile cells and cells with phagocytic properties.
- *The endothelial cells* of the glomerular capillaries run on the outer aspect of the mesangial stalk, and are continuous at each end with the endothelial cells of the arterioles. The cells are flattened such that only a thin layer of cytoplasm covers most of

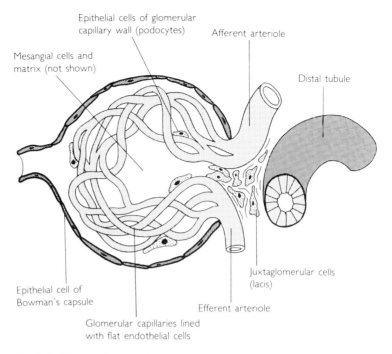

Epithelial cells of glomerular
capillary wall (podocytes)

Afferent arteriole

Mesangial cells and
matrix (not shown)

Distal tubule

Epithelial cell of
Bowman's capsule

Juxtaglomerular cells
(lacis)

Efferent arteriole

Glomerular capillaries lined
with flat endothelial cells

Fig. 1.4 The renal corpuscle

the capillary lumen and most nuclei lie against the mesangial aspect of the loop. The sheet of cytoplasm has numerous fenestrae each about 100 to 200 Å in diameter, bridged only by a thin diaphragm.

• *The epithelial cells* are separated from the endothelial cells by the glomerular basement membrane (GBM). These cells are highly specialised, consisting of stellate cells which stand on the GBM on complex foot processes. These foot processes interdigitate with each other forming zipper-like junctions between adjacent foot processes, with a narrow slit pore between cells.

The glomerular basement membrane

The GBM is about 300 nm thick. It has a central dense lamina and less dense inner and outer zones. The GBM and the epithelial cell membranes have a nett negative charge due to the presence of glycosamines such as heparan sulphate. This appears to be of great importance in the selectivity of macromolecule filtration, particularly regarding negatively charged molecules such as albumin (Chapter 3).

The renal tubule

The glomerular filtrate passes in turn from Bowman's space into the proximal tubule, the loop of Henle and the distal tubule

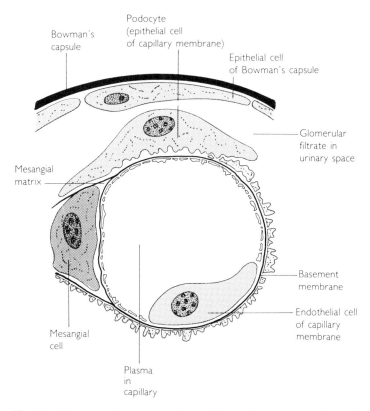

Fig. 1.5 Diagrammatic representation of the cell types of the glomerulus

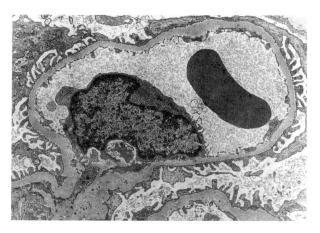

Fig. 1.6 Electron microscopic appearance of one capillary loop in the glomerulus. The lumen of the capillary is indented by an endothelial cell nucleus and a red blood cell is seen as a dark, sausage shape in the lumen. For cell types refer to Fig. 1.5

(Fig. 1.3). The distal tubules join to form collecting tubules. The collecting tubules in turn empty into papillary ducts which open on the papillae.

The proximal tubule

The proximal tubule has a short neck leading into the tortuous proximal convoluted tubule. Here the cells are cuboidal, with many mitochondria, a brush border on the luminal surface and basal nuclei. These cells are extremely active particularly in resorption of sodium chloride, potassium, phosphate, urate, bicarbonate, glucose and aminoacids. Water follows these solutes passively (Chapter 3).

The loop of Henle

The loop of Henle is a segment of tubule that loops down toward the medulla. Superficial cortical nephrons have short loops which do not reach the medulla while about 20% of nephrons, in the juxtamedullary region, have long loops which descend deep into the medulla before making a hairpin turn and returning to the cortex. These long loops have thick segments at either end while the cells of the deeper loop are thin. The loop plays a critical role in the concentration of urine (Chapter 3).

The distal convoluted tubule

The distal convoluted tubule originates between the afferent and efferent arterioles of the same nephron. The cells of the distal tubule are cuboidal, as in the proximal tubule, but they have a less developed brush border, apical nuclei and numerous mitochondria and clefts at their bases.

Functionally the distal convoluted tubule and the cortical section of the collecting ducts have many similarities. This region of the tubule is concerned with the final resorption or secretion of hydrogen ion, sodium chloride, calcium and other solutes as well as secretion of unwanted solutes such as potassium, phosphate and uric acid. The short segment in apposition to the afferent arteriole has narrow cells with crowded nuclei where they form the macula densa of the juxtaglomerular apparatus (see below).

The collecting tubule

The collecting tubule is comprised of cuboidal cells with few organelles. The early cortical segments are functionally similar to distal tubule cells and the remainder plays a passive role in urine concentration as the filtrate descends toward the papillary tip.

The juxtaglomerular apparatus

The juxtaglomerular apparatus (JGA — Fig. 1.7) is found at the vascular pole of the glomerulus where the distal tubule comes back to lie against the afferent arteriole as it enters the glomerulus.

The JGA is comprised of three parts:
• The macula densa — a group of narrow, crowded distal tubule cells sited where the tubule abuts the adjacent afferent arteriole.
• The granular cells of the afferent arteriole — epithelioid cells packed with renin precursor secretory granules.
• The lacis cells — in continuity with, and closely resembling mesangial cells, these cells are also in intimate contact with the granular cells and the macula densa.

The juxtaglomerular apparatus is, therefore, ideally situated to monitor the composition of the distal tubular fluid and to modify the behaviour of the glomerulus by renin secretion into the afferent arteriole (Chapter 4).

The renal vessels   Each kidney normally has one renal artery arising from the abdominal aorta and one vein draining to the inferior vena cava (IVC). Since the aorta lies behind and to the left of the IVC, the right artery is longer than the left and passes behind the IVC,

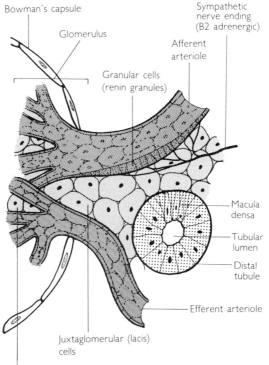

Fig. 1.7 Juxtaglomerular apparatus. Note: (1) Macula densa of distal tubule. (2) Juxtaglomerular (lacis) cells. (3) Granular renin secreting cells of afferent arterioles

while the left renal vein is the longer and passes across the front of the aorta (Fig. 1.1). The left renal vein usually receives the left adrenal and testicular or ovarian vein. Multiple renal arteries are quite common, being found in over 25% of people.

Each renal artery breaks up into anterior and posterior branches which divide to supply one of the five to six segments of each kidney (Fig. 1.8). The interlobar arteries enter the renal substance in the columns of Bertin and pass to the level of the cortico-medullary junction where they divide into arcuate branches. These run in the corticomedullary junction supplying interlobular branches into the renal cortex. The interlobular arteries give rise to the afferent arterioles and sometimes form minor anastomoses with capsular vessels. The renal veins, however, have an extensive system of anastomoses.

The arrangement of the smaller vessels is critical to control of

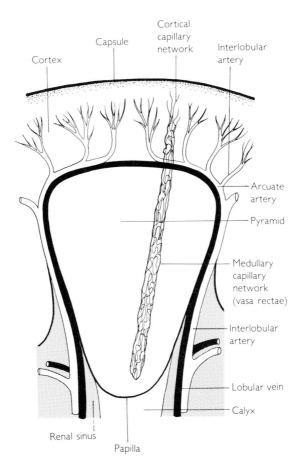

Fig. 1.8 Intrarenal arterial supply of the kidney

glomerular and tubular function. Each afferent arteriole supplies one glomerulus and the blood then emerges in the efferent arteriole which breaks up into a plexus of capillaries which descends and ascends around the loop of Henle. The blood reaching the tubule has, therefore, already passed through glomerular capillaries of the same nephron. Where there are long loops this means that long thin vessels, the vasa rectae, descend into the medulla with the loop and, like the loop, bend sharply to ascend back to the cortex. This arrangement is important to the countercurrent mechanism for urine concentration (Chapter 3).

Renal lymphatics A system of lymphatics surrounds the tubules and drains through the hilum. There are also lymphatics in the subcapsular region and the perirenal fat.

Renal nerves The kidneys are innervated by the autonomic nervous system which forms a rich plexus around the renal vessels. Vasomotor, secretory and pain fibres are included. The pain fibres are conducted to the T10−L1 spinal level. Renal pain, usually felt in the loin, can be provoked by stretching of the renal pelvis or capsule.

THE URETERS, BLADDER AND URETHRA

The ureters pass retroperitoneally to enter the bladder on each side of the posterior aspect of the bladder base, forming the trigone with the internal urethral orifice. The upper ureter is supplied by vessels anastomosing with capsular vessels while the rest of the ureter is supplied from below. With renal arterial or venous obstruction large collaterals can open up around the ureters.

Nerves carry pain from the ureters to spinal segments T11−L2. Pain due to stretching of the ureteric wall can be felt in the loin (T11) or groin (T12, L1). Pain from stretching the ureteral orifice may radiate to the testis or labia (T10−11). Bladder pain can be felt suprapubically and irritation of the internal urethral orifice may cause pain at the tip of the penis.

The urethra in the female is about 4 cm long while in the male it is about 20 cm. This is believed to be the main reason for the much greater incidence of urine infection in the female (Chapter 13).

2: *Assessment of Urinary Anatomy*

The clinical assessment of the kidneys and urinary system will be dealt with in Chapter 7. Here we will outline the investigations that are employed to demonstrate:

1 Macroscopic anatomy — imaging techniques.
2 Microscopic anatomy (histopathology) — renal biopsy.

RENAL IMAGING TECHNIQUES

Over the last decade there have been a plethora of new methods of imaging. Many methods are complementary, some have a varying place depending on constraints of time, experience and equipment, while others have yet to find their role. Each method will be discussed in the context of its place in the evaluation of a patient with suspected renal tract disease.

RADIOLOGICAL RENAL IMAGING

Plain abdominal X-ray

An X-ray of the abdomen including diaphragm and pelvis, an X-ray centred on one or other kidney (zonogram) or tomograms of the kidney are all simple non-invasive methods which can give useful information on renal size and the presence of radiopaque abnormalities such as renal or ureteral stones. Advantages include speed, simplicity, general availability and the avoidance of contrast agents. The disadvantage is poor definition — the kidneys may not be visible, and only radiopaque abnormalities are usually obvious.

The plain abdominal film should be examined for:
* *Renal outline* — shape, position and size — as has been mentioned the kidneys are rarely well seen in plain films, though sometimes a reasonable idea of the renal outlines can be ascertained.
* *Radiopaque abnormalities* — renal stones, calcified papillae, nephrocalcinosis.
* *Air in the renal areas* — with intestinal fistulae and occasionally severe infections with gas producing organisms.
* *Bone abnormalities* — renal osteodystrophy, lytic or blastic metastases, developmental abnormalities associated with urinary

13

disease such as spina bifida associated with neurogenic bladder or widely separated pubic bones associated with ectopia vesicae.

The intravenous pyelogram

The intravenous pyelogram or IVP (appropriately called an intravenous urogram by many since it outlines all urine containing tissue rather than just the renal pelvis) remains the most readily available and cost effective method of renal imaging. An iodine-containing compound which is concentrated by the kidney and excreted in the urine is injected intravenously and radiographs of the renal tract are taken at timed intervals thereafter. A good example of the images which can be obtained is given in Fig. 2.1.

The nephrogram

The renal substance is opacified by dye concentrated in renal tubules. The nephrogram should be observed for position, size and shape of the kidneys. They should measure 11 to 13 cm in bipolar length. It should be noted that this is about 1 cm longer than the renal size as assessed at autopsy or by ultrasound. This is due to the divergence of the rays as they pass from the emitting anode through the patient to the film (Fig. 2.2). The renal length is roughly that of the first three to four lumbar vertebral bodies.

The right kidney is usually lower by 1−2 cm and 0.5−1 cm shorter than the left. The renal outline should be smooth. Tomograms in this phase may reveal intrarenal lucent areas if cysts are present.

The pyelogram

The density of contrast medium in the renal pelvis can be enhanced by applying a constricting band around the patient's abdomen, compressing and hence partially obstructing the ureters.

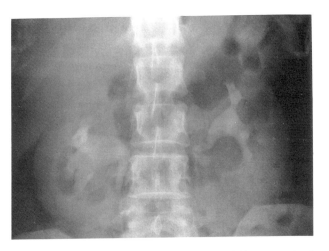

Fig. 2.1 Normal intravenous pyelogram (IVP) film at 5 min showing the kidney substance (nephrogram) and the pelvis (pyelogram)

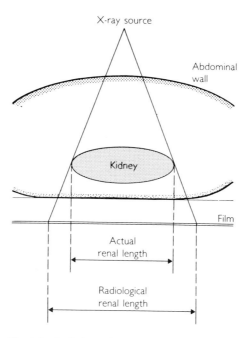

Fig. 2.2 Radiological renal size. In an IVP the kidney length is magnified by about 1 cm because of the divergence of the X-ray beams from the source to the film

This can be quite uncomfortable so the patient should be warned if this is to be part of the routine. During this phase the renal pelvis should be examined to determine:

- *size* — increased in obstruction or hydronephrosis.
- *papillary and calyceal abnormalities* — deformities are seen in many diseases such as reflux nephropathy, renal papillary necrosis, renal tuberculosis or when the pelvis is disturbed by adjacent renal cysts or tumours.
- *space lesions* — radiolucent calculi of uric acid or cystine, pedunculated tumours, loose papillae in renal papillary necrosis, blood clots.

The pyelograms and nephrograms usually form simultaneously in both kidneys and should be well developed by the 5 to 10 min films. Delay in the rate of development in one kidney may indicate unilateral obstruction or renal artery stenosis. In both the nephrogram may become visible later and remain denser in the affected kidney. Pelvic dilatation in delayed films or failure of contrast to clear from the pelvis can be a furth r indication of obstruction.

Films of the ureters and bladder

Information on stones, tumours, anatomical abnormalities and obstruction in the ureters or the bladder can be obtained as these structures fill with excreted contrast medium over the subsequent 30 to 90 min. In the absence of obstruction the ureters are rarely visible in their entire length in the one film.

Post-voiding films

These can demonstrate the volume of residual urine in the bladder, and sometimes will allow demonstration of vesicoureteral reflux particularly if they are delayed until the renal pelvis has cleared of contrast medium.

Variations in IVP technique and results

The results of the IVP will vary with different methods and patients.
- *Patient preparation* — patients are usually deprived of fluid for 12 hours before the IVP to enhance concentration of contrast medium, and given a laxative to reduce faecal and gas shadows obscuring the renal outline. Dehydration should be avoided in elderly patients, in diabetics and in patients suspected of having multiple myeloma since there is evidence that this can exacerbate nephrotoxicity due to the injected contrast agent (see below).
- *Radiocontrast agent* — the volume and nature of radiocontrast agent affects the radiopacity of the urine excreted and hence the quality of the pictures obtained. Usually sodium diatrizoate (50–100 ml of 50–60%) is given after a small test dose for allergy. Recently low osmolarity contrast agents have been introduced, with reported lower risks of toxic side-effects, but greater expense. They are currently recommended for patients with a variety of risk factors such as cardiac or renal disease and diabetes.
- *Radiological technique* — technical factors such as focusing, X-ray intensity, the use of coned or tomogram films, abdominal compression and even the quality of the equipment can greatly affect the information obtained. The referring physician is wise always to view the films, not only to confirm the diagnosis, but also to gain an appreciation of the quality of the examination and hence the likelihood of misinterpretation.
- *Renal function* — good dye concentration is required for optimal results. Since renal failure is accompanied by a loss of concentrating ability in the kidneys (Chapter 6) very poor or even useless films maybe result. In patients with an elevated plasma creatinine, larger (and potentially more hazardous) volumes of contrast media may be required. Once the plasma creatinine exceeds about 0.3 mmol/litre it is rare to obtain useful pictures, even with large doses of contrast medium.

Hazards in performing an IVP

Many are common to all techniques involving the injection of iodinated radiocontrast media, such as in enhanced computerized tomography (CT) scanning, arteriography and digital subtraction studies (see below). Important hazards include:

- *Allergic reactions to iodine* — ranging from transient urticaria to fatal bronchospasm or hypotension. Patients must be asked about allergy to iodine or contrast agents. In those with previous minor reactions some protection can be obtained by premedication with steroids and antihistamines. Adrenaline and antihistamines should be readily available before iodine containing compounds are injected. A small test dose of contrast medium must be given before the main injection.
- *Nephrotoxicity* — acute renal failure following injection of contrast agent can occur (Chapter 34). Predisposing factors include:
  - (a) old age,
  - (b) diabetes,
  - (c) multiple myeloma,
  - (d) volume depletion, and
  - (e) already impaired renal function.

The risk is reduced but not eliminated by prior hydration rather than dehydration in such patients.
- *Cardiac failure* — the injection of radiocontrast agents, all of which are hypertonic, is followed by osmotic volume expansion. In patients with poor renal or cardiac function this can lead to acute fluid overload with pulmonary oedema.
- *Cardiac arrythmia* — can occur with rapid intravenous injection of dye.
- *Fetal irradiation* — abdominal irradiation should be avoided in pregnant women and those in the postovulatory period (who could be pregnant).

Percutaneous antegrade urography

With fluoroscopic or ultrasound guidance a fine needle can be introduced through the skin into the renal pelvis, particularly if it is abnormally dilated. Using this as a guide a larger bore needle or catheter can then be used for the injection of a contrast agent. This is particularly useful in the investigation of ureteral obstruction since it will show the site and cause of obstruction and, if a catheter is left *in situ*, will relieve the obstruction. This is therefore the procedure of choice when the obstruction has caused renal failure (Fig. 2.3).

Retrograde pyelography

Through a cystoscope a catheter can be placed in the ureter and contrast medium injected back toward the kidney (Fig. 2.4). Disadvantages include the need for anaesthesia and the coordination of the urologist, theatre and radiology services to allow films to be taken before the catheters fall out. This procedure is therefore gradually being replaced by other techniques but it is still used

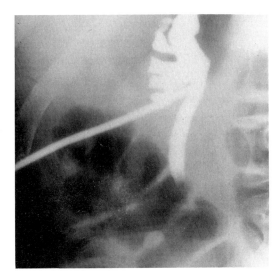

Fig. 2.3 Antegrade pyelogram. The ureter is obstructed by a radiolucent uric acid stone

occasionally when they are not available or when they yield dubious information. The procedure will sometimes dislodge or bypass an obstruction and can also be used for the selective collection of bacteriological, cytological or biochemical samples from each kidney.

Renal angiography

There are now a variety of methods for demonstrating renal arterial anatomy.

Conventional arteriography

This first involves aortography with a catheter usually introduced via the femoral artery (see Fig. 12.1). The renal arteries are then selectively catheterised and even branch vessels can be entered. These techniques have lead to development of a range of percutaneous interventional techniques including dilatation of arterial stenoses and the injection of materials to cause obstruction of vessels in cases of renal arterial bleeding.

Digital subtraction angiography (DSA)

This less invasive technique can be performed as an outpatient procedure. Computerised equipment is used to subtract the image before injection of dye from that obtained when dye is passing through the renal vessels (see Fig. 12.2).

Subsequent images can also be used to give most of the information usually obtained from the IVP. It is likely that with further development this technique will largely replace conventional radiocontrast studies.

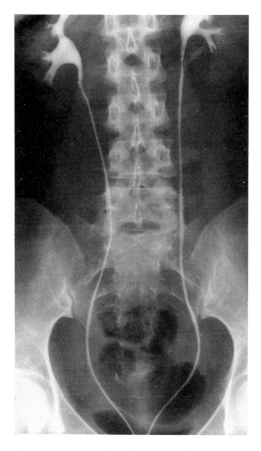

Fig. 2.4 Retrograde pyelogram. Catheters are passed up from the bladder and contrast injected into the renal pelvis

Renal venography

Using catheters, inserted usually via the femoral veins, contrast medium is injected into the renal veins to diagnose renal vein thrombosis. Simultaneous injection of adrenaline into the renal arteries is often used to decrease the blood flow in the veins, enhancing the retrograde filling by dye. Samples of blood from the renal veins can be assayed for renin content (Chapter 12).

Cystography and urethrography

Cystography is used to demonstrate bladder abnormalities with voiding films to demonstrate bladder outlet obstruction or vesico-ureteric reflux. Retrograde urethrography can be used to demonstrate urethral stricture.

Computerised tomography (CT scanning)

The role of CT scanning has increased rapidly in the investigation of renal disease, despite the relatively high cost. Multiple radiographic images are reconstructed by computer to produce cross-sectional images across the renal areas (Fig. 2.5). Common uses include the evaluation of abnormal renal masses, demonstration of the causes and level of ureteral obstruction, and visualisation of the adrenal, perirenal, retroperitoneal and pelvic areas where neoplastic and inflammatory masses and collections otherwise can be very difficult to define. The CT scan should be modified according to the indication. Multiple 'cuts' can be taken through the area of interest, and films can be taken to follow the sequence of contrast passage through a lesion. Uric acid calculi invisible on IVP invariably appear radiopaque on CT scan.

Disadvantages include the cost, limitations on availability of the procedure, and the large volumes of radiocontrast used in contrast-enhanced studies.

RENAL ULTRASOUND

This technique is quickly becoming the first imaging technique in a wide range of renal conditions. A major advantage is the minimal risk or inconvenience to the patient, since the technique is non-invasive and does not involve radiation or the use of contrast agents. The results are independent of renal function. Unfortunately the results are very dependent on operator experience and equipment quality. Moreover, even in the best case the definition is very poor when compared with radiography (Fig. 2.6). With colour Doppler techniques the flow of blood in the renal vessels may be demonstrated, allowing diagnosis of

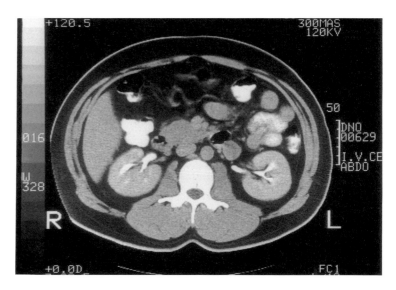

Fig. 2.5 Abdominal computerised tomogram (CT). Note both kidneys with the renal pelvis highlighted by the radiocontrast agent

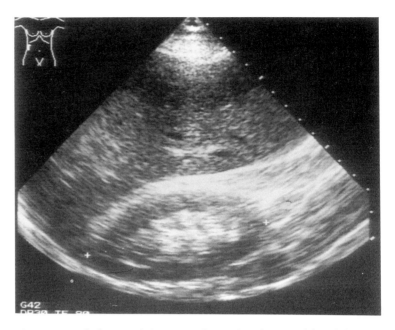

Fig. 2.6 Renal ultrasound showing right renal outline, renal length (+ to +). Renal pelvic fat appears white

renal artery stenosis or venous thrombosis in some cases.

Particular indications for renal ultrasonography include:

● *Acute and chronic renal failure* — since radiocontrast agents are poorly concentrated.

● *Renal cysts and tumours* — to distinguish fluid from solid contents.

● *Guidance for percutaneous procedures* — such as percutaneous renal biopsy, cyst puncture, antegrade pyelography and nephrostomy.

OTHER TECHNIQUES

Radionuclear imaging

In these studies a substance which is excreted by the kidneys is radiolabelled and injected intravenously. The pattern of radioactivity over the kidneys is then followed to give an assessment of renal blood flow, function and anatomy. The radiation doses are far lower than in radiography. Common studies include:

● *Technetium DTPA scans.* Diethylaminetriamine penta-acetic acid (DTPA) is filtered by the glomeruli and passes to the pelvis and ureters within 5 to 10 min. The rate of accumulation and excretion can be followed in the isotope renogram. This gives no indication of renal shape but will indicate poor renal perfusion or obstruction. This is most used in the early assessment of renal transplants when confirmation of renal blood flow is important. It can also be used in screening for unilateral renal artery stenosis.

• *Technetium DMSA scans.* Dimercaptosuccinic acid (DMSA) is not filtered but is selectively removed from the blood by tubular cells to which it binds strongly. Maximal renal parenchymal concentration takes several hours, and the resulting picture resembles a radiographic nephrogram (Fig. 2.7). Renal cysts, tumours and scars can be seen. In renal infarction or infection the parenchymal abnormality can be visualised before renal scarring is apparent in the IVP. It is therefore valuable as an early screening test for renal scarring, particularly since the discomfort and radiation dose is low. Technetium glucoheptonate (GHA) is also used in this way.

• *Radionuclear renal function studies.* Though not used for imaging, the excretion rates of chromium labelled ethylenediamine-tetra-acetic acid (EDTA) and iodinated hippuran can be used to measure accurately GFR and effective renal plasma flow (ERPF) respectively (Chapter 5).

Magnetic resonance imaging

A definite role in nephrology for this expensive technique has not yet been established though the ability to give some information on the chemical content of tissues is likely to prove very useful in the future (see Fig. 29.5).

RENAL BIOPSY

Some of the most common serious diseases of the kidney cause no diagnostic macroscopic morphological abnormality and can be diagnosed only by microscopic examination of renal tissue. The technique requires considerable expertise to be performed safely, and the subsequent tissue processing and examination is a specialised branch of histopathology. It is recommended that renal biopsy be performed only by nephrologists trained and expert in the technique, and with access to appropriate specialised pathological services, including light and electron microscopy as well as immunostaining by immunofluorescent, immunoperoxidase or other techniques.

Indications

The indications for renal biopsy are diverse but may be summarised as the presence of significant glomerular bleeding and/or proteinuria or the presence of renal failure not explained by the clinical picture or by renal imaging techniques.

Method

Renal biopsy is carried out under radiological (fluoroscopic or in difficult cases by CT) or ultrasound control. With the patient

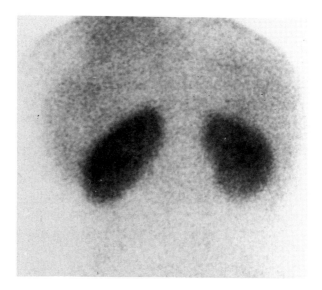

Fig. 2.7 Technetium DMSA nuclear scan of the kidneys

prone on the couch a fine needle is introduced into the renal angle to determine exact renal depth and position, the former by close attention to the 'swing' of the needle with respiration. A biopsy needle is then used to obtain a sample of the renal cortex from the lower and outer border of the kidney. The procedure requires considerable patient cooperation, particularly since the breath must be held in deep inspiration as the biopsy is being taken to prevent tearing of the kidney. The procedure is nearly always performed with only local infiltrative anaesthesia but in rare uncooperative patients and some children general anaesthesia may be required.

After the biopsy the patient should rest prone in bed for at least 6 hours and stay in bed for 24 hours, with frequent observation of pulse and blood pressure. The urine should be checked for macroscopic haematuria before discharge.

Precautions and contraindications

Before renal biopsy the patient is checked for bleeding disorders (skin bleeding time, prothrombin time, partial thromboplastin time and platelet count). The presence of two functioning kidneys should be proven, or at least the presence of two kidneys by ultrasound if renal function is poor. Blood pressure must be controlled before and after the procedure.

The only absolute contraindication is the presence of a significant uncontrolled bleeding disorder. Relative contraindications, each of which must be balanced against the likelihood of obtaining information helpful to the patient, include the presence of only one functioning kidney, severe renal failure where loss of a kidney would precipitate end-stage renal failure, and the presence of small shrunken kidneys where the risk of bleeding is high and the likelihood of obtaining sufficient unscarred tissue to make a diagnosis low. In some of these cases open renal biopsy or CT guided biopsy may reduce the risk.

Complications

Significant complications occur in less than 1% of patients.

• *Renal bleeding* is by far the most common. This may cause haematuria and occasionally clot colic or urine retention. Perirenal bleeding can cause loin pain, and sometimes a perirenal haematoma with a palpable loin mass. Very rarely severe bleeding can lead to shock or can be persistent. Patients should remain in bed and be adequately transfused. If bleeding continues angiography should be performed. The bleeding point, usually a traumatic arteriovenous anastomosis, can be identified and treated by ablation of the feeding segmental artery by injection of material through the arteriography catheter. With modern procedures it is exceedingly rare for a kidney to be removed for postbiopsy bleeding.

• *Intrarenal arteriovenous fistula* occasionally occurs after renal biopsy. Most commonly these are small and discovered coincidentally when arteriograms are performed soon after the biopsy. Occasionally they are large and cause a continuous renal bruit with associated hypertension or even haemorrhage. In these cases they should be ablated.

• *Biopsy of the wrong organ,* including liver, spleen or bowel,

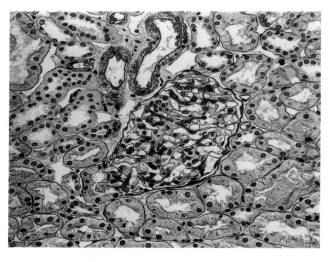

Fig. 2.8 Normal renal biopsy: light microscopy

occurs occasionally and with surprisingly little consequence other than that the renal biopsy may need to be repeated and the patient watched more closely.

Tissue processing and examination

The tissue obtained by renal biopsy is about 1–2 cm long and 1.5 mm thick. Although the usual aim is to obtain only cortex, not uncommonly medulla, in which there are no glomeruli, is also present. A dissecting microscope is used at the bedside to identify the cortex. A large segment of cortex is fixed for light microscopy, with smaller portions frozen or fixed for immunostaining and electron microscopy. This is necessary because no single fixative is ideal for all three procedures. As a consequence immunostaining or electron microscopy tissue is sometimes inadequate.

Light microscopy is performed using a variety of different stains on consecutive sections, each 1 to 2 μm thick. Each stain is chosen to highlight nuclei, cytoplasm, basement membrane, collagen, fibrin or protein deposits and commonly combinations are used on the same section. Haematoxyphil–eosin (H & E), periodic acid–Schiff (PAS) and various silver and trichrome stains are only a few of the many important stains used. In some cases special techniques, e.g. Congo red to identify amyloid (Chapter 27), are also employed. In each section detailed observations can be made of the glomeruli, vessels, tubules and the interstitium (Fig. 2.8).

Electron microscopy (EM) allows detailed observations of renal ultrastructure and is particularly useful in defining glomerular disease (Fig. 1.6).

Immunofluorescent studies involve staining the glomeruli with fluorescein-labelled antibodies to various human proteins such as IgG, IgA, IgG, fibrinogen and complement components (C3, C4, C1q). This allows inferences to be drawn about immunopathology and a useful subclassification of the basic morphological abnormalities seen in light and EM studies.

Further developments include the use of monoclonal antibodies, other stains including chemical stains as in immunoperoxidase immunostaining and the combination of immunostaining with EM. Most of these are in their infancy but can be expected to produce advances not only to help classify diseases into the current diagnostic groups but also to provide new diagnostic subgroups and insights into pathogenesis.

3: Excretory Functions of the Kidney: the Formation of Urine

The major functions of the kidneys (Table 3.1) are:
- Excretory functions, i.e. the formation of urine.
- Metabolic functions, particularly the synthesis or degradation of hormones (Chapter 4).

The production of urine from the blood perfusing the kidney occurs in two steps, each performed in an anatomically discrete segment of the nephron:
- Filtration of plasma in the glomerulus.
- Selective resorption or excretion in the tubules.

The magnitude of the changes occurring are summarised in Tables 3.2 & 3.3.

Table 3.1 Functions of the kidneys

Production of urine
Elimination of wastes:
  metabolic products
  ingested toxins such as drugs
Control of water balance:
  maintenance of total body water
  maintenance of plasma osmolarity
Control of electrolyte balance:
  sodium, chloride
  calcium, phosphate
  potassium
  acid–base
  magnesium and others

Metabolic
Synthesis of hormones and similar molecules:
  renin
  vitamin D
  erythropoietin
  autocoids – prostanoids, kallikrein
Degradation of polypeptide hormones:
  insulin
  parathormone
  prolactin, growth hormone, vasopressin
  glucagon, gastrointestinal hormones
Other metabolic functions:
  gluconeogenesis

Table 3.2 Volume changes in urine production

	Volumes	
	Per minute	Per day
Cardiac output	5 litre	7200 litre
Renal blood flow	1.2 litre	1728 litre
Renal plasma flow	0.66 litre	950 litre
Glomerular filtration rate (GFR)	0.125 litre (125 ml/min)	180 litre
Urine volume	1 ml	1.5 litre

Table 3.3 Formation of urine from glomerular filtrate: changes in the concentrations and amounts of solutes

Solute	Plasma	Glomerular filtrate*	Urine
Protein g/litre	60–80	0.01–0.03	<0.2
Sodium mmol/litre mmol/day	135–145	135–145 24 000–26 000	5–>160 5–300
Potassium mmol/litre mmol/day	3.5–5.5	3.5–5.5 630–990	10–80 5–>200
pH	7.36–7.42	7.36–7.42	4.5–8.5
Osmolarity mosmol/litre	280–300	280–300	30–1400
Urea mmol/litre mmol/day	2.5–8.3	2.5–8.3	100–2100
Creatinine mmol/litre mmol/day	0.05–1.2	0.05–1.2	7–24

* The glomerular filtrate is an ultrafiltrate of plasma and thus has the same composition except for the higher protein concentration in plasma

First, systemic arterial blood is filtered in the glomerulus. Protein and cells are separated from plasma, and about 180 litre of glomerular filtrate passes into the renal tubules per day. Each minute at rest about 25% of the cardiac output, i.e. 1200 ml of blood, passes through the kidneys, and of this about 125 ml/min (2 ml/s) becomes glomerular filtrate.

In the tubules, this large amount of glomerular filtrate is reduced from 125 ml/min (2 ml/s) to result in a urine volume of about

1 ml/min (about 1.5 litre/day), i.e. to less than 1% of the original volume. This is mainly due to active resorption of sodium with consequent passive resorption of water and chloride by the tubular cells. By selective resorption and secretion by the tubule the filtrate is gradually changed to urine, which contains very high concentrations of waste substances such as urea and creatinine. Energy is consumed by the tubular cells in the processes of resorption and secretion, hence the tubular cells are more susceptible to hypoxia, ischaemia and metabolic poisons than the glomeruli. Most of the kidneys' oxygen consumption is used for the resorption of sodium.

GLOMERULAR FILTRATION

The glomerular filtration rate (GFR) is an important measure of renal excretory function. About 125 ml of filtrate is formed every minute (2 ml/s), with the filtrate passing through the filtration barrier imposed by:
• The endothelium.
• The basement membrane.
• The epithelium of the glomerular capillary wall.

The GFR is not fixed. The GFR of individual glomeruli — the single nephron GFR (SNGFR) — and the overall GFR can increase by 25% or more in response to various stimuli including high protein diets and pregnancy. Moreover some glomeruli, particularly the larger juxtamedullary glomeruli, have a higher SNGFR than others.

Glomerular filtration membrane permeability

Early studies suggested that the filtration membrane acted as a semipermeable membrane with pores about 50 to 60 Å in diameter. This means that molecules of molecular weight (MW) over 60 000 Da should not enter the filtrate. This roughly accords with the observation that albumin (MW 66 500) and haemoglobin (MW 68 000) are poorly filtered, while vitamin B_{12} (MW 1360), urea (MW 60) and creatinine (MW 113) are freely filtered. Since electron microscopy failed to demonstrate 'pores' of the appropriate size it was concluded that this molecular sieving function depended on the mesh-like fibrillar construction of the basement membrane matrix.

Recently a more dynamic and complex system has been shown to exist. First, an important contribution of the negative charge of the basement membrane (see Chapter 1) has been shown, resulting in poorer permeability to negatively charged molecules such as albumin. The maintenance of this charge barrier is important in preventing heavy albuminuria, since the MW of albumin is so close to the estimated pore size. In addition the 'permselectivity' of the capillary membrane varies with different pressure and flow conditions, suggesting that the permeability coefficient can alter with hydrodynamic changes.

Control of the glomerular filtration rate

The driving force for glomerular filtration is the glomerular capillary pressure (Pg). This is opposed by the colloid osmotic pressure (COP) of the glomerular capillary blood, and the hydrostatic pressure in Bowman's space (Pbs). The GFR depends also on the permeability coefficient of the filtration membrane (Kf). Thus:

$$GFR = Kf\,[Pg - (Pbs + COP)].$$

The Pg varies with changes in systemic blood pressure, and with constriction of the afferent or efferent arterioles.

Since Pg falls as plasma passes along the capillary, and the COP rises as water is filtered leaving a higher protein concentration, it is likely that in the normal state a 'filtration equilibrium' is reached in the glomerular capillaries such that in their latter portions no effective filtration occurs. A consequence of this is that GFR increases with increased plasma flow, since there is a greater length of capillary involved in filtration. Sustained increases in plasma flow, as occur in diabetes (Chapter 26) and pregnancy (Chapter 33) will thus lead to sustained increases in SNGFR (Table 3.4).

Of great interest recently has been the observation that the mesangium contains cells which can contract and in doing so decrease the surface area and thus the ultrafiltration coefficient (K) by decreasing the filtering surface area. There is considerable evidence that SNGFR can be altered by a variety of factors which act via alterations in mesangial contractility.

Angiotensin is a particularly powerful stimulant of mesangial contraction, and the renin–angiotensin system, centred in the juxtaglomerular apparatus (Chapter 1), seems to be in an ideal situation for monitoring and controlling glomerular function,

Table 3.4 Factors which elevate individual nephron glomerular filtration rate

Residual nephrons in renal failure
Diabetes mellitus
Pregnancy
Damaged glomerular wall:
  glomerulonephritis
  diabetes
  other glomerular disease
High protein diet
Acromegaly (high growth hormone)

both by its effect of increasing GFR by causing efferent arteriolar vasoconstriction and decreasing GFR by mesangial contraction. The relative importance of these has yet to be determined though the first seems best demonstrated clinically where the administration of angiotensin-converting enzyme inhibitors to patients with poor renal blood flow can cause a sudden fall in GFR (Chapter 10). Antidiuretic hormone (ADH), noradrenaline, parathormone and various prostanoids (PGE1, PGE2, PGI2) also cause mesangial contraction.

Understanding the factors modulating SNGFR may prove important in the treatment of progressive renal failure, since one hypothesis is that glomerular damage slowly occurs when SNGFR is persistently elevated as in the remnant glomeruli after loss of renal tissue. This so-called 'hyperfiltration' theory will be discussed in Chapter 6.

Renal blood flow

In isolated perfused kidneys, renal blood flow and GFR change little as renal arterial pressure changes over the range 80–160 mmHg. This 'autoregulation' occurs in the kidneys themselves, and is believed to be a result of changes in intrarenal vascular tone. One theory is that the smooth muscle cells of the precapillary vessels spontaneously contract in response to increased pressure. In addition, other complex neural and hormonal mechanisms exist to maintain renal blood flow and GFR in states of low renal artery pressure. In this situation some agents which interfere with these mechanisms may produce acute renal failure, as with administration of angiotensin-converting enzyme inhibitors or non-steroidal anti-inflammatory drugs which block prostaglandin production (Chapter 10).

RESORPTION AND SECRETION BY THE RENAL TUBULES

The renal tubules convert glomerular filtrate, a protein-free ultrafiltrate of plasma, into urine. Urine is formed in far smaller volumes and has a very different chemical constitution (Tables 3.2 & 3.3). The process involves controlled resorption and secretion of a wide variety of important plasma components:
1 Water.
2 Sodium and chloride.
3 Potassium.
4 Glucose.
5 Calcium and phosphate.
6 Urea.
7 Amino acids.
8 Polypeptides and proteins.

Many of these tubular functions are interrelated, particularly with tubular handling of sodium and water. The tubular cells contain a variety of 'pumps' or active transport mechanisms capable of moving molecules against a concentration gradient. The most important of these is the $Na-K-ATPase$ mechanism which couples sodium resorption and potassium excretion with ATP consumption. This is responsible for the majority of renal oxygen consumption.

Excretion of water

Under normal circumstances over 99% of filtered water is resorbed (Table 3.2).
● Normal body fluid content and plasma osmolarity (280 to 300 mosmol/litre) are maintained despite wide variations in fluid intake and load of osmotically active wastes.
● The urine volume is around 1.5 litre/day, but can vary from 400 ml to over 20 litre/day in situations of extreme water deprivation or load.
● The load of osmotically active products is about 600 mosmol/day. This can increase to over 1200 mosmol/day in states of severe catabolism, as in patients with extensive burns. The concentration of solutes in the urine can be adjusted by the kidneys such that the urine osmolarity can vary from about 30 to 1400 mosmol/litre.
● With maximum urine concentration 400 ml of urine are required to excrete the basal osmotic load of 600 mosmol/day. This is the minimal urine output compatible with maintaining adequate excretion of waste products.

Water resorption

Most water is resorbed in an iso-osmotic fashion with sodium and chloride, i.e. as sodium chloride is resorbed water follows. Since 99% of sodium filtered is actively resorbed (see later in this chapter) this results in the movement of most of the water back into the circulation.

In addition further water is resorbed in the process of urine concentration, which occurs in the distal tubule and collecting duct.

Urine concentration

The urine concentrating mechanism results in the resorption of water in excess of nitrogenous and other solutes, so that in urine the concentration of urea is about 60 times that in plasma. In states of maximal urine concentration urine osmolarity can quickly be raised to about 1200 mosmol/litre. If the situation persists for several days, urine osmolarity can reach 1400 mosmol/litre.

The mechanism is based on the production of a hypertonic interstitium in the medulla through which the collecting tubules pass. The collecting tubules can be rendered selectively permeable to water by the action of antidiuretic hormone (ADH — otherwise known as pitressin or vasopressin — Chapter 4), secreted by the posterior pituitary. In the presence of antidiuretic hormone (ADH), water flows along the concentration gradient from the tubule lumen to the papillary and medullary interstitium leaving the tubular contents hyperosmolar. The water is then carried away into the renal veins by the extensively fenestrated vasa recta and renal venules.

The steps are as follows:

1 The establishment of a hypertonic (i.e. high salt and urea concentration) deep medullary interstitium.

2 Passive resorption of water but not solutes in the distal tubule and collecting duct, with water moving along the osmotic gradient from the lumen to the hypertonic interstitium.

3 The removal of the water from the papillary and deep medullary interstitium by the loops of the vasa recta.

Establishment of the hypertonic medulla. The medulla is rendered hypertonic by the countercurrent multiplier system involving the loop of Henle.

The mechanism of a countercurrent multiplier system is outlined in Fig. 3.1. In this system a very high concentration can be reached at the tip of a hairpin loop, even though the 'pump' at any point in the system can only maintain a small concentration gradient.

The ascending thick portion of the loop actively resorbs sodium and chloride (and to a lesser extent urea) from the tubular lumen to the interstitium which becomes hypertonic. The descending thin segment of the loop is freely permeable to solutes and water and equilibrates with this space. The result is that the tubular and interstitial fluid become progressively more concentrated as the tip of the loop is reached (Fig. 3.2).

In effect there is recirculation of sodium chloride and urea in the deep medulla. They are pumped out of the ascending tubule into the interstitium, then diffuse back into the lumen in the more proximal descending tubule, whereupon they are delivered again to the ascending limb. In states of prolonged antidiuresis the concentration in the medullary interstitium gradually builds up to about 1400 mosmol/litre. On the other hand in prolonged diuresis the medullary hypertonicity can be reduced, with a consequent reduction in acute urinary concentrating capacity.

Urine concentration in the collecting duct. In the presence of ADH the walls of the collecting duct (and the very end of the

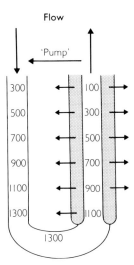

Fig. 3.1 Principle of a countercurrent loop multiplier. In this system a large overall change in concentration at the tip of the loop can be generated by a pump which is only capable of achieving a much smaller gradient between the ascending and descending limbs of the loop. In this diagram a concentration of 1300 units is achieved by a pump capable of a 200 unit gradient

distal tubule) are rendered permeable to water but not sodium chloride. As the duct passes through the hypertonic medulla, water is removed along the osmotic gradient from the lumen to the interstitium, resulting in concentration of the solutes in the lumen, i.e. the production of small volumes of urine with a high concentration of urea and creatinine.

The sodium and chloride content of the urine depends on the extent of their resorption in the proximal and distal tubule (see later in this chapter). In most cases where ADH secretion is high there is also a stimulus to sodium chloride retention, so the urinary sodium and chloride concentrations are low.

Removal of water from the interstitium by the vasa recta. The hairpin loop structure of the vasa recta, and their free permeability to water and solutes, facilitates the removal of the water which has diffused from the collecting ducts. The loop structure minimises the loss of sodium chloride and urea from the medulla, maintaining medullary tonicity which would be lost if the blood flowed in one direction only.

Urine dilution

The minimal osmolarity of urine is 30 mosmol/litre, far less than the normal lower limit of plasma osmolarity (280 mosmol/

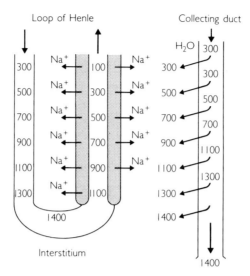

Fig. 3.2 Countercurrent mechanism in the kidney. In the kidney the loop of Henle acts as a countercurrent multiplier system, capable of generating a deep medullary (tip of the papilla) concentration of about 1400 mmol/litre under conditions of severe dehydration. Sodium chloride is pumped by the thick ascending limb into the interstitium, which it renders hypertonic, and then diffuses into the permeable thin descending limb. In the late distal and collecting tubule ADH renders the walls permeable to water but not solutes. Accordingly water diffuses by osmosis into the interstitium, leaving the tubular fluid progressively more concentrated

litre). Dilution is firstly achieved by sodium chloride and urea resorption in the ascending thick limb of the loop of Henle, which results in hypotonic luminal fluid (150–200 mosmol/litre) at the beginning of the distal tubule (Fig. 3.2). In maximal diuresis there is still some resorption of water from the terminal collecting tubule into the inner medullary interstitium. This dilutes the inner medulla, from its maximum of 1400 mosmol/litre to around 600 mosmol/litre, reducing the concentrating capacity. Active resorption of sodium and urea in excess of water also continues in the collecting duct, further lowering urine osmolarity to the minimum of 50 mosmol/litre.

Sodium and chloride excretion

Sodium and chloride excretion are considered together, not only because they constitute the major intravascular electrolytes and hence must move in similar directions to preserve electroneutrality, but also because their transport is usually linked.
• There is a wide variation in dietary sodium intake, from below 70 to over 350 mmol/day in different persons and populations.
• With a normal plasma sodium concentration of 135–145

mmol/litre over 25 000 mmol are filtered per day and of this over 99% must be resorbed if a steady state is to be achieved.

A fine balance is required since sodium retention can result in hypertension and oedema, while sodium depletion can lead to hypotension or shock.

The mechanisms for tubular sodium (chloride) resorption can be followed down the nephron.

Proximal tubule. In the proximal tubule over two-thirds of filtered sodium is resorbed mainly by the Na−K−ATPase system. This creates an electrochemical gradient favouring resorption of anions, particularly chloride. Water is resorbed along with these molecules by osmotic diffusion since the cells of the proximal tubule are highly permeable to water. Thus this mechanism is also responsible for over two-thirds of water resorption.

Glomerulotubular balance describes the linking of tubular resorption to the glomerular filtration. Since the peritubular capillary bed lies downstream and 'in series' with the glomerulus, alterations in pressure and flow in glomerular capillaries will have direct effects on the peritubular capillaries. Accordingly increased flow in the glomerular capillaries with increased GFR may be balanced by enhanced tubular resorption due to increased flow in peritubular capillaries. Similarly if there is a high filtration fraction at the glomerulus, blood in the peritubular capillaries will be more concentrated, resulting in a compensatory increase in tubular resorption.

Loop of Henle. In the thin segment no active transport occurs. In the thick ascending limb sodium and chloride are resorbed from the tubular lumen by an active process against a concentration gradient and not accompanied by water, resulting in resorption of a further 5−10% of filtered sodium chloride.

Distal convoluted tubule and collecting duct. At the commencement of the distal tubule is the juxtaglomerular apparatus with the specialised segment of the tubule — the macula densa. Here intraluminal sodium chloride concentration and resorption are monitored to provide feedback control of both GFR and tubular sodium resorption via the renin−angiotensin system. In the distal and early collecting tubules further sodium chloride resorption occurs, resulting in the removal of a further 10% of filtered sodium.

Only about 2% of filtered sodium reaches the cortical collecting duct. The majority of adrenocorticosteroid-modified sodium chloride resorption occurs in the cortical collecting duct and the more distal segments of the distal convoluted tubule. Mineralo-corticoids produce sodium retention and an increase in potassium excretion. The remainder of the collecting duct plays little role in sodium resorption, but continues to be active in water resorption under ADH control.

Control mechanisms in sodium chloride excretion

Hormones and autocoids. These are discussed in Chapter 4. Mineralocorticoids such as aldosterone and glucocorticoids promote sodium resorption, while many prostanoids, atrial natriuretic peptide, kallikrein−kinins and dopamine promote natriuresis.

Diuretics are drugs which increase excretion of both sodium and water. Their mechanisms of action vary.
- *Osmotic diuretics* (e.g. mannitol). These are osmotically active molecules which are filtered at the glomerulus but not resorbed in the tubules, where they act to retain fluid in the tubular lumen. In renal failure the high urea content of glomerular filtrate contributes to polyuria.
- *Loop diuretics.* These very powerful diuretics (e.g. frusemide, ethacrynic acid and bumetanide) inhibit sodium chloride resorption in the ascending limb of the loop of Henle.
- *Thiazides.* These inhibit tubular sodium resorption and increase potassium excretion in the distal tubule.
- *Aldosterone antagonists.* Spironolactone competitively antagonises mineralocorticoid effects on the collecting duct. A similar effect can be obtained by blocking the renin−angiotensin system with converting-enzyme inhibitors (captopril, enalapril). Unlike the other diuretics they may produce hyperkalaemia.
- *Carbonic anhydrase inhibitors and mercurial diuretics.* These inhibit sodium transport in proximal tubules, leading to sodium and potassium loss. Their effects are weak.

Potassium excretion

Potassium is a predominantly intracellular cation. Precise control is required for optimal operation of many cell functions including membrane excitability.
- Of the total body potassium (about 3500 mmol) only about 2% is found in the extracellular fluid.
- Plasma potassium concentrations are maintained in the range 3.5−5.5 mmol/litre.
- Dietary potassium intake varies widely, usually between 50 and 120 mmol/day.
- Renal excretion can easily be increased to cope with increased load, but cannot be decreased below 10−20 mmol/day. In addition obligate sweat and faecal losses are 15−20 mmol/day. Faecal

losses increase with diarrhoea and when renal excretion is inadequate.

• Urinary potassium excretion reflects diet and is about 50–100 mmol/day. Since plasma potassium concentration is 3.5–4.5 mmol/litre, and filtrate volume around 180 litre/day, this is about 10–20% of the filtered load.

Renal handling of potassium involves virtual total resorption in the proximal tubule and loop of Henle followed by controlled secretion in the distal tubule and collecting duct. In practical terms, therefore, potassium excretion is entirely a tubular function. The tubular mechanism for potassium excretion has a massive capacity for increase, particularly if the load is increased gradually.

Accordingly hyperkalaemia is rarely a problem in chronic renal failure until most tubules are destroyed, usually with a GFR of less than 15–20 ml/min, or the disease particularly involves renal tubules. In acute renal failure hyperkalaemia is common, both because the patient is often catabolic and acidotic, and the tubules non-functioning (Chapter 10).

The steps involved in excreting potassium are:

• *Glomerular filtration* results in delivery to the proximal tubule of fluid with a potassium concentration of 3.5–5.5 mmol/litre (about 700 mmol/day).

• *Total resorption in the proximal tubule, loop and early distal tubule.* The proximal tubule resorbs 60–70% of filtered potassium and further absorption occurs in the ascending thick limb of the loop of Henle and early distal tubule. By the end of the loop all but 5–15% of filtered potassium has been resorbed, and virtually all of the remainder is resorbed by the mid-distal tubule.

• *Secretion by the distal convoluted tubule and collecting duct.* Potassium secretion occurs in the cortical collecting duct, and perhaps to a lesser extent in the final (connecting) segment of the distal tubule. In these portions of the tubule, potassium (and hydrogen ions) can be secreted against significant concentration gradients into the tubular lumen while sodium and chloride are transported in the opposite direction.

A major factor in potassium secretion appears to be the electronegativity of the tubular lumen consequent on sodium resorption. Poor sodium delivery to the distal tubule will limit potassium secretion, while increased sodium delivery as with diuretic therapy or saline infusion will enhance potassium excretion.

Control of renal potassium excretion

The major mechanisms for regulating potassium excretion act on the tubular secretion of potassium in the distal tubule and cortical collecting duct. These modulating factors include:

- Mineralocorticoid effects.
- Distal tubular flow rate and sodium delivery.
- Acid—base balance.

Mineralocorticoid effects. Hyperkalaemia is a potent direct stimulus to the adrenal cortex to secrete aldosterone. Aldosterone causes a rise in potassium excretion and a fall in sodium excretion. The main effect is on distal and collecting tubules. Protracted mineralocorticoid treatment maintains kaliuresis, although sodium retention is only temporary due to the 'escape' phenomenon variously attributed to volume expansion with enhanced depression of proximal tubular sodium excretion or to the presence of natriuretic factor(s). Glucocorticoids have a more rapid and less prolonged kaliuretic effect which reflects increased tubular flow.

Distal tubular flow rate. A high rate of fluid and sodium delivery to the distal tubule encourages potassium excretion. Volume loading with sodium chloride and administration of diuretics are therefore likely to promote potassium excretion. Saline loading with frusemide administration is therefore a method of encouraging potassium excretion in hyperkalaemia.

Acid—base balance. Acute acidosis depresses, while acute alkalosis stimulates urinary potassium excretion. A simplistic explanation is that in the distal tubule and cortical collecting duct hydrogen ions and potassium ions compete for excretion in exchange for sodium resorption into cells.

Regulation of normal plasma potassium concentration

There are two major regulatory mechanisms for maintaining plasma potassium concentration.
- Intracellular—extracellular balance. With about 98% of potassium inside cells, and the constant equilibrium, driven by Na—K—ATPase, between intracellular and extracellular potassium, it is not surprising that this is the major mechanism for acute plasma potassium control.
- Renal potassium excretion maintains normal body potassium balance and corrects abnormal plasma concentrations more slowly than the above mechanism.

In addition to intra—extracellular balance, and renal potassium excretion it is likely that increased faecal losses due to increased colonic secretion of potassium help to prevent hyperkalaemia in severe chronic renal failure.

Intracellular—extracellular potassium balance. Nett movement of potassium into cells can be rapidly promoted by several factors, notably insulin, increased plasma pH and β_2-adrenergic stimulation. All of these have clinical relevance.

• *Insulin* promotes potassium uptake into cells independently of its effect on plasma glucose. This is the basis of insulin–glucose treatment of hyperkalaemia (Chapter 14).

• *Plasma pH*. Acidosis is often associated with hyperkalaemia, and correction of the acidosis will usually result in a fall in plasma potassium. The effect is most marked when a metabolic acidosis with a low plasma bicarbonate concentration is present. A rise in plasma pH by 0.1 units may cause a fall of plasma potassium by over 0.5 mmol/litre. The repair of acidosis by bicarbonate administration is a potent acute method of dealing with hyperkalaemia, particularly in metabolic acidosis.

• *Beta-adrenergic hormones*. Beta$_2$-adrenergic stimulation with adrenaline (or more specifically salbutamol) stimulates potassium uptake. This can be blocked by β_2-blocking drugs such as propranolol. Accordingly β_2-blocking drugs may potentiate hyperkalaemia, and salbutamol administration can be associated with hypokalaemia, as in asthma. Recently, salbutamol administration has been proposed as a therapy for acute hyperkalaemia.

• *Other factors*. Both mineralocorticoids and glucocorticoids promote potassium excretion by sweat glands and colonic epithelia. Hypertonicity is associated with a rise in plasma potassium concentration, as has been demonstrated with mannitol infusion.

Acid and base excretion

Plasma pH is maintained in the normal range of 7.35 to 7.45 by combined renal and pulmonary mechanisms. These will compensate for any disturbance leading toward a change in plasma pH, and usually prevent overt acidaemia (pH < 7.35) or alkalaemia (pH > 7.45). The terms acidosis and alkalosis may also be used in patients whose plasma pH is still in the normal range, but who have metabolic or respiratory acidosis or alkalosis with renal and/or pulmonary compensation returning the pH toward the normal range. We do not intend to discuss acid–base physiology in depth. Rather we will outline the renal mechanisms for excretion of acid and alkali.

• Urinary pH is normally about 6, but can be varied in the range 4.5 to 10.

• The products of normal metabolism include about 70 mmol/day of acids whose bases such as phosphate, sulphate and urate are non-volatile, i.e. cannot be further metabolised to carbon dioxide and excreted by the lungs.

• In addition about 15 000 mmol/day of volatile acids such as pyruvate, lactate and ketoacids are also produced. These are usually metabolised through bicarbonate to carbon dioxide, but in states of overproduction, as in diabetic ketoacidosis or lactic acidosis,

they may be inadequately metabolised and cause metabolic acidosis.
• In states of metabolic alkalosis, such as with ingestion of sodium bicarbonate, or prolonged vomiting with loss of hydro-chloric acid from the stomach, renal excretion of the excess alkali may be required.

Renal excretion of acid

Since bicarbonate is freely filtered, and the basal rate of non-volatile acid production is 70 mmol/day, to maintain normal pH in the presence of a normal metabolic load the tubules must:
• Resorb virtually all filtered bicarbonate (25 mmol/litre).
• Excrete 70 mmol/day of hydrogen ion.
   In so doing the urinary pH cannot be reduced below about pH 4.5, since the tubules cannot sustain a plasma to urine pH gap of more than about 3 units. In practice this means the tubules must secrete buffers into the urine so that added hydrogen ions do not inordinately reduce pH. The major urinary buffers are ammonium and phosphate (Table 3.5).

Bicarbonate resorption. 75% of the bicarbonate is resorbed in the proximal tubule mainly by passive resorption along with sodium and water. Further bicarbonate resorption occurs as a consequence of active hydrogen ion excretion into the tubular lumen. The overall equation is:

$$H^+ + HCO_3^{2-} \xleftrightarrow{pK\ 6.1} H_2CO_3^- \xleftrightarrow{carbonic\ anhydrase} CO_2 + H_2O.$$

The reaction is facilitated by carbonic anhydrase which is found in the tubular brush border and speeds the conversion of $H_2CO_3^-$ to $CO_2 + H_2O$.

Table 3.5 Buffers of urinary acid. In alkalosis, bicarbonate is not all resorbed, and up to 140 mmol/day may be excreted in prolonged severe alkalosis

Ammonium (30−50 mmol/day)
$H^+ + NH_3 \rightarrow NH_4^+$ (pK 9.4)
Can rise to 700 mmol/day in chronic acidosis

Phosphate (20−30 mmol/day)
$H + HPO_4^{2-} \rightarrow H_2PO_4^-$ (pK 6.8)
Can increase with acidosis

Other titrable acids
Creatinine − 10−24 mmol/day (pK 4.97)
Uric acid − 1−4 mmol/day (pK 5.75)

Bicarbonate − normally all resorbed
$H^+ + HCO_3^{2-} \rightarrow H_2O + CO_2$ (pK 6.1)

Ammonium excretion. 30–50 mmol/day of hydrogen ion excretion is accounted for by ammonium secretion. In the proximal tubule ammonia (NH_3) is produced by deamination of glutamine:

$$glutamine \xrightarrow{glutaminase} glutamate + NH_3.$$

Ammonia is converted to ammonium (NH_4^+) in the tubular lumen:

$$NH_3 + H^+ \longrightarrow NH_4^+ \text{ (pK 9.4)}.$$

The excretion of NH_4^+ can be increased by chronic acidosis to over 700 mmol/day by increased ammonia synthesis in the proximal tubular cells.

Phosphate buffering. About 20–30 mmol/day of urinary hydrogen ion is buffered with inorganic phosphate.

Most plasma inorganic phosphate (0.7–1.4 mmol/litre) is filtered and then resorbed, resulting in a urinary phosphate excretion of 10–50 mmol/day, varying considerably with dietary phosphate intake. In chronic acidosis the renal excretion of phosphate is increased due to a decrease in tubular phosphate excretion. The mechanism is poorly understood. Phosphate is the major titrable acid in normal urine.

In plasma at pH 7.4 the equilibrium:

$$HPO_4^{2-} + H^+ \longleftrightarrow H_2PO_4^- \text{ (pK 6.8)}$$

is such that the ratio $HPO_4^{2-} : H_2PO_4$ is about $4:1$. With acidosis the proportion of H_2PO_4 increases.

Other buffering acids. Urate (pK 5.75), up to 3.6 mmol/day, and creatinine (pK 4.97), 7–24 mmol/day, are two minor urinary buffers for hydrogen ion. In diabetic acidosis β-hydroxybutyrate (pK 4.7) and acetoacetate (pK 3.6) contribute to the urinary titrable acids, the total of which may rise to over 100 mmol/day.

Renal excretion of alkali

Alkalinisation of the urine is achieved by excretion of bicarbonate, with elevation of urine pH to levels as high as 10.

Excretion of an alkaline load is particularly rapid when the load is combined with extracellular fluid expansion. Addition of sodium bicarbonate to the body results in extracellular volume expansion, increased tubular flow, reduced proximal tubular bicarbonate resorption due to suppression of proximal acidification by alkalaemia, reduced excretion of ammonium and titrable acid and overwhelming of distal tubular hydrogen ion excretion. The result is bicarbonate in the urine and extremely rapid repair of the alkalosis. Indeed it is difficult to maintain an alkalosis in this way, even when as much as 24 mmol/day/kg (140 g for a 70 kg human) of bicarbonate is ingested for weeks.

When extracellular volume contraction, chloride deficiency or potassium deficiency are present the situation is significantly modified. Since all three commonly coexist with excessive gastrointestinal or renal losses of bicarbonate this is important clinically. The volume of distribution of chloride is roughly equal to extracellular volume, hence volume depletion is equivalent to chloride depletion. There is thus a requirement for chloride and potassium repletion in treatment of metabolic alkalosis with volume contraction.

Calcium excretion

The renal role in calcium and phosphate metabolism is critical, so much so that bone disease is one of the more troublesome aspects of chronic renal failure. The endocrine role of the kidney in bone metabolism, through activation of vitamin D, is discussed in Chapter 4. Although renal excretion of calcium plays a major role in total body calcium balance, its role in the regulation of plasma calcium concentration is minor when compared with factors regulating blood–bone calcium balance.
- 99.5% of total body calcium is in bone and teeth, and 0.5% in soft tissues. The extracellular fluid contains only about 0.1% of body calcium.
- In plasma the normal concentration of calcium is 2.1–2.6 mmol/litre. About half of this is bound to plasma proteins, particularly albumin, and not filtered at the glomerulus.
- Daily urinary excretion of calcium is about 5 mmol/day (3.7–6.2 mmol/day). Since 180 litre of glomerular filtrate are formed, and ultrafilterable (ionised) plasma calcium is around 1.3 mmol/litre it follows that less than 2% of filtered calcium is excreted in the urine, indicating considerable tubular resorption of calcium.

Calcium resorption occurs:
1 75–90% in the proximal tubule and ascending loop of Henle, in proportion to sodium resorption;
2 10–25% in the distal tubule and proximal collecting duct by mechanisms capable of regulation according to physiological requirements.

Factors influencing calcium excretion

- *Plasma calcium concentration.* Hypercalcaemia leads to inhibition of both calcium and magnesium resorption.
- *Parathormone* decreases GFR and increases resorption of calcium by a cyclic AMP (cAMP) mediated effect on distal nephron segments.

- *Plasma phosphate.* Renal calcium excretion varies inversely with phosphate load.
- *Tubular sodium and fluid flow rates.* Increased tubular sodium flow increases calcium excretion along with sodium excretion by reducing tubular resorption of calcium.
- *Acid-base balance.* Acidosis enhances renal calcium excretion.
- *Vitamin D.* Vitamin D dependent calcium binding protein is found in the distal tubule where active calcium resorption takes place. It has been suggested that vitamin D may have a calciuric effect.
- *Diuretics.* The loop diuretics, e.g. frusemide and ethacrynic acid, cause a marked increase in fractional excretion of calcium. They are thus useful in treatment of hypercalciuria. On the other hand thiazide diuretics eventually cause a fall in urinary calcium excretion. This is thought to be a result of a fall in ECF and body sodium as well as an enhancing effect on distal calcium resorption by an unknown mechanism. Thiazides, therefore, may cause elevation of plasma calcium and have been used in the treatment of calcium nephrolithiasis, particularly in the presence of hypercalciuria (Chapter 25).

Phosphate excretion

Phosphate exists in plasma as organic and inorganic moeities.
- The plasma inorganic phosphate concentration is $0.7-1.4$ mmol/litre.
- Urinary phosphate excretion is $10-50$ mmol/day, varying with dietary intake.
- $80-95\%$ of filtered phosphate is resorbed in the proximal tubule by an active mechanism using the energy of the $Na-K-ATPase$ system.
- Further phosphate resorption occurs in the distal tubule, particularly in the early straight segment.

Control mechanisms

Both proximal and distal tubular resorption is influenced by many factors including dietary phosphate, parathormone and acidosis.

Adaptation to phosphate requirement. Tubular phosphate resorption increases in response to reduction in dietary intake and increased body phosphate requirements, as occur in growth, pregnancy and lactation. The effect is largely due to changes in the brush border of the proximal tubule. The mechanism is unknown.

Parathormone (PTH) decreases renal phosphate resorption and causes major increases in renal phosphate excretion. The main effect is on the proximal tubule where surface binding of PTH results in activation of adenyl cyclase, production of cAMP and consequent activation of membrane bound protein kinase which stimulates phosphorylation of tubular brush border phosphate transport protein.

Acidosis. Chronic metabolic acidosis produces a significant decrease in phosphate resorption by unexplained mechanisms. This provides more phosphate for the buffering of urinary hydrogen ion excretion.

Renal handling of proteins

The normal glomerular filtration barrier excludes the larger plasma proteins, such as fibrinogen (MW 340 000), albumin (MW 66 500) and the globulins (MW 150 000 to 900 000), from the glomerular filtrate. On the other hand smaller polypeptides, including virtually all circulating peptide hormones, immunoglobulin fragments such as light chains (Bence-Jones proteins), many small enzymes such as lysozymes and ribonuclease, and membrane antigens (β_2-microglobulin), are filtered at the glomerulus and extensively resorbed and metabolised by the tubular cells. Since resorption appears to be 'saturable' proteinuria can result from excessive filtration of protein, or diminished tubular resorption. The total concentration of protein in normal glomerular filtrate is a matter of controversy, though all agree it is low.

Albumin

Micropuncture studies suggest rat glomerular filtrate contains something less than 10 to 30 mg/litre of albumin (MW 66 500). In man, with 180 litre/day of glomerular filtrate, a filtrate albumin concentration of only 1 mg/litre, would result in filtrate albumin losses of 180 mg/day. This is more than the normal upper limit for albumin excretion in the urine (40–60 mg/day). If the glomerular filtrate had 30 mg/litre, which is the upper limit of the range reported in rats, the tubules would be obliged to resorb over 5 g/day to prevent significant proteinuria.

It seems likely that a considerable amount of tubular resorption of albumin occurs to reduce the daily urine output of albumin in man to less than 40–60 mg/day. In states of impaired glomerular permselectivity seemingly minor increases in filtrate albumin can therefore quickly swamp tubular resorption. Urinary albumin excretion is accordingly a very sensitive test for glomerular diseases affecting permselectivity.

Renal amino acid handling

Amino acids are filtered but it would be metabolically wasteful if they were freely excreted. There are therefore active mechanisms for resorption of amino acids in the proximal tubule. Several distinct mechanisms are each responsible for resorption of a group of structurally related amino acids. For example the basic amino acids lysine, ornithine, arginine and cystine appear to be resorbed by, and compete for, the same mechanism.

A wide variety of inherited and acquired tubular transport defects can lead to selective or non-selective amino acidurias (Chapter 28).

Renal glucose handling

Glucose (MW 180) is freely filtered but normally does not appear in urine. An active D-glucose resorptive mechanism, linked to the $Na-K-ATPase$ pump, is present in the proximal tubule. This can be saturated when glomerular filtration of glucose exceeds the tubular capacity for resorption. This critical point is known as the tubular maximum resorptive capacity for glucose (TM_{gluc}), and can be measured as described in Chapter 5.

4: *Hormones, Metabolism and the Kidney*

A wide variety of systemically and locally acting hormones are produced by the kidney, and the functions of the kidney are affected by hormones produced elsewhere. In addition, the tubular cells are the site of degradation of most polypeptide hormones, and are an important site of gluconeogenesis (Table 4.1).

HORMONES PRODUCED BY THE KIDNEY

Renin and the renin–angiotensin system

The secretion of renin by the juxtaglomerular apparatus (JGA) is an important regulatory mechanism for systemic blood pressure via effects on sodium excretion (aldosterone) and vasoconstriction (angiotensin II) as well as intrarenal and glomerular blood pressure and flow. The system is outlined in Fig. 4.1.

The juxtaglomerular apparatus

The juxtaglomerular apparatus is situated at the vascular pole of the glomerulus (Fig. 1.7), and is comprised of:
1 The macula densa cells of the distal tubule.
2 The juxtaglomerular (or lacis) cells.
3 The granulated cells of the efferent arteriole.

Renin

Renin is an acid protease secreted by the specialised granular cells of the wall of the afferent arteriole in the JGA.

Stimulation of renin secretion. Release of renin from the JGA is thought to be stimulated in two main ways:
• Beta-adrenergic stimulation.
• Distal tubular sodium or chloride concentration.

Reduction in blood pressure or volume stimulates baroreceptors in the aortic arch or volume receptors in the great veins and atria. This leads to β-adrenergic signals stimulating renin release through sympathetic nerve endings in the JGA. Beta-adrenergic blocking drugs (e.g. propranolol, metoprolol, atenolol) interfere with this mechanism.

Decrease in sodium or chloride resorption in the distal tubule, as occurs with reduced perfusion or in states of sodium depletion, is monitored by the cells of the macula densa and leads to renin release.

46

Table 4.1 Hormones, autocoids and the kidney

Hormones and autocoids produced in the kidney
Renin
Erythropoietin
Vitamin D (1,25-dihydroxycholecalciferol)
Prostanoids
Kallikrein–kinin
Dopamine

Hormones with major effects on tubular functions
Antidiuretic hormone (ADH)
Angiotensin II
Mineralocorticoids and glucocorticoids
Atrial natriuretic peptide
Parathormone

Hormones catabolised in the kidney
Insulin and glucagon
Parathormone
Prolactin
Growth hormone
Gastrin and other gastrointestinal hormones

Action of renin. Renin acts on the globulin, angiotensinogen (renin substrate), to cleave off the inactive decapeptide, angiotensin I. Angiotensin I is then converted to the active octapeptide, angiotensin II by angiotensin-converting enzyme (ACE).

Angiotensin-converting enzyme

Angiotensin-converting enzyme is widely distributed in vascular endothelium, and is in high concentration in the lungs. It converts angiotensin I to angiotensin II, and also cleaves bradykinin, hence it is also known as kininase II. ACE inhibitors (e.g. captopril, enalapril) are used in a variety of situations including the treatment of hypertension (Chapter 12).

Angiotensin II

Effects of angiotensin II include:
• Vasoconstriction, affecting vascular resistance and hence blood pressure.
• Stimulation of aldosterone secretion.
• Regulating intrarenal blood flow and GFR.
• Stimulation of thirst.
• Feedback inhibition of renin release.

Angiotensin II and hyperkalaemia are the major stimuli to aldosterone secretion by the adrenal cortex. Aldosterone promotes sodium retention and potassium secretion by the kidney (see later in this chapter).

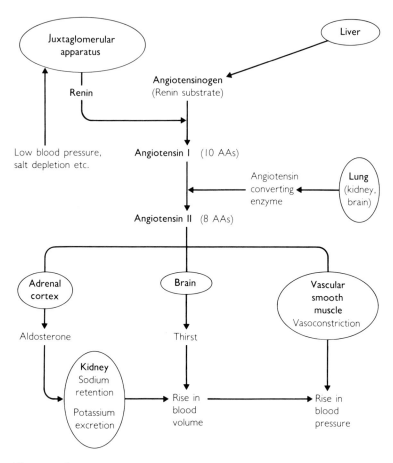

Fig. 4.1 The renin–angiotensin system

Angiotensin II is a potent vasoconstrictor, and also has complex effects on intrarenal vasculature. It participates in regulation of renal blood flow, GFR, urine flow rate, sodium excretion and urine osmolarity. These effects are due to both angiotensin II delivered via the renal arteries and from angiotensin II generated in the kidney by intrarenal ACE. The effects on GFR are discussed in Chapter 3.

The stimulation of thirst may be a direct effect on the brain and has been suggested as yet another method by which angiotensin II works to preserve blood pressure and volume.

Erythropoietin

Erythropoietin is a glycoprotein (MW 34 000 Da) produced in the renal cortex whose main effect is to increase marrow red cell production thus increasing red cell count and haematocrit. The stimulus appears to be cellular hypoxia, most commonly initiated by anaemia or by inadequate haemoglobin oxygenation as in cyanotic pulmonary or cardiac disease.

The anaemia of chronic renal failure (Chapters 6 & 11) is characterised by inappropriately low erythropoietin levels for the severity of anaemia. Increased erythropoietin levels and poly-cythaemia have been reported in occasional patients with cystic disease of the kidney, renal transplants and renal artery stenosis.

Erythropoietin-like activity in the blood with polycythaemia has also been documented in a variety of tumours including about 2% of renal cell carcinomas, also Wilm's tumours, cerebellar haemangioblastoma, hepatoma, uterine fibroma and dermoid cysts of the ovary.

Recently recombinant human erythropoietin has become available and has proven effective in raising haemoglobin in anaemic dialysis patients in a dose-dependent fashion. Side effects include hypertension, thrombosis and convulsions. Assays for circulating erythropoietin levels are not generally available.

Vitamin D (1,25 dihydroxy-cholecalciferol)

The most active form of vitamin D is 1,25-dihydroxycholecalci-ferol (1,25-DHCC), a hormone produced in the kidney by the addition of a hydroxyl group to the liver-produced precursor, 25-hydroxycholecalciferol (25-HCC) (Fig. 4.2). 1,25-DHCC is about 100 times as active as 25-HCC. Production of 1,25-DHCC by the kidney is stimulated by parathormone and hypophosphataemia. The exact site of synthesis is unknown, although the 1-hydroxylase enzyme is found in proximal tubule cells.

Effects of vitamin D

The major effects are to:
• Increase gastrointestinal calcium absorption.
• Promote normal bone calcification.

Vitamin D is necessary for the normal formation of bone matrix and maturation of the growth plate, even in the presence of normal plasma calcium and phosphate levels. 1,25-DHCC de-ficiency is a major contributing factor in uraemic renal bone disease (Chapters 6 & 11).

There are other circulating vitamin D metabolites, including 25-hydroxy D_3 and 24,25-dihydroxy D_3, which have differing effects from 1,25-DHCC. 25-hydroxy D_3 appears to be important in normal muscle physiology, restoring muscle strength in vitamin D deficiency.

1,25-DHCC is available as an orally active preparation (calci-triol) widely used in the prevention and treatment of renal bone disease (Chapter 11). Other vitamin D preparations are slower in onset of action and therefore more difficult to titrate against

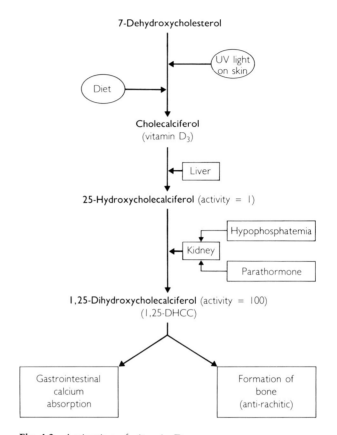

7-Dehydroxycholesterol

UV light on skin

Diet

Cholecalciferol
(vitamin D_3)

Liver

25-Hydroxycholecalciferol (activity = 1)

Hypophosphatemia

Kidney

Parathormone

1,25-Dihydroxycholecalciferol (activity = 100)
(1,25-DHCC)

Gastrointestinal
calcium
absorption

Formation of
bone
(anti-rachitic)

Fig. 4.2 Activation of vitamin D

patient response. Measurement of plasma vitamin D is not widely used in the management of renal bone disease.

Prostanoids

Prostanoids are a group of cell messengers important in renal function. They are derived from oxidation of arachidonic acid and other polyunsaturated fatty acids and have great diversity of structure and biological effects (Fig. 4.3). Different cells appear to be highly specific in their prostanoid production. It is likely that renal prostanoids are produced in the kidney mainly to regulate local processes. They are not strictly hormones, since they act in the organ in which they are produced. The term 'autocoids' has been introduced to describe such locally acting agents. The kidney has the enzymes to produce all known primary prostanoids, and appears to be able to adapt production according to circumstances.

Actions of prostanoids

Prostanoids may be divided into those with vasodilator, diuretic and antithrombotic effects, and those with opposing actions. The major renal effects of prostanoids are listed below.

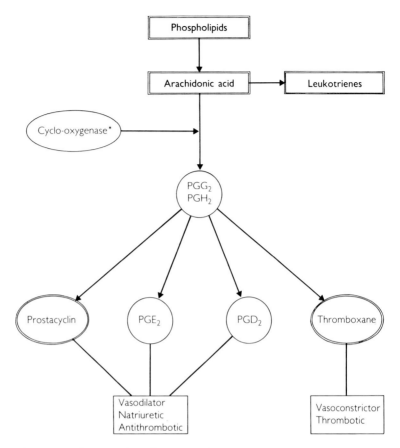

Fig. 4.3 Production of renal prostanoids. * Cyclo-oxygenase is blocked by non-steroidal anti-inflammatory drugs (NSAIDs)

Regulation of intrarenal blood flow. The kidney contains vasodilator (PGE2, PGI2, PGD2) and vasoconstrictor (thromboxane) prostanoids. When renal perfusion is compromised the vasodilator prostanoids help to maintain renal blood flow, perhaps in response to the high angiotensin II levels. Accordingly in such circumstances (hypotension, sodium depletion, liver failure) non-steroidal anti-inflammatory drugs (NSAIDs) can precipitate acute renal failure by inhibiting cyclo-oxygenase and thus vasodilator prostanoid production (Chapters 10 & 34).

Effects on sodium excretion. Natriuretic prostanoids such as PGE2 act both directly on tubular cells and by enhancing renal perfusion. NSAIDs decrease the effects of thiazide diuretics and can precipitate cardiac failure in patients with heart disease.

Effects on water excretion. PGE2 inhibits the tubular effect of ADH (Chapter 3) while the NSAID indomethacin has been shown to potentiate the antidiuresis.

Interactions with the renin–angiotensin system. Prostanoids stimulate release of renin from the granular cells of the juxta-glomerular apparatus (Chapter 1), in response to reduced chloride resorption in the macula densa. Furthermore local prostaglandins (particularly prostacyclin and PGE2) decrease the vasoconstrictor effects of angiotensin II within the vascular pole of the glomerulus.

Other effects. The prostanoids are critical messengers in a renal regulation network involving stimulation of renal prostanoids by bradykinin, angiotensin II, vasopressin, noradrenaline, sympathetic nerve stimulation, ischaemia and decreased renal perfusion; and prostanoid modulation of the effects of many of these stimuli on the kidneys.

Kallikrein–kinin (bradykinin)

Kallikrein and bradykinin are vasodilator autocoids found particularly in the renal cortex (Fig. 4.4). The enzyme kininase II, which converts the vasodilator bradykinin to inactive fragments also converts angiotensin I to the active vasoconstrictor angiotensin II (Fig. 4.1) and is thus also called angiotensin-converting enzyme (ACE).

Effects of kallikrein–kinin

These include modification of:
• *renal blood flow.* Renal kinins decrease renal vascular resistance, particularly in low sodium states;
• *renal electrolyte and water excretion.* Endogenous kinins augment renal sodium and water excretion. This could be a direct tubular, a haemodynamic effect or both;
• *interrelationships with other hormones and autocoids.* Kinins activate prostaglandin synthesis and appear to have a role in complex interrelationships with other regulatory substances.

HORMONES ACTING ON THE KIDNEY

Antidiuretic hormone (vasopressin)

In humans antidiuretic hormone (ADH) is a nonapeptide (MW 1084 Da) — argininine vasopressin (AVP). It is produced by cells of the supraoptic nucleus of the hypothalamus and released from the posterior pituitary.

Effects of ADH

The major effects are:
• increasing collecting tubule water permeability leading to urine concentration (Fig. 3.2);

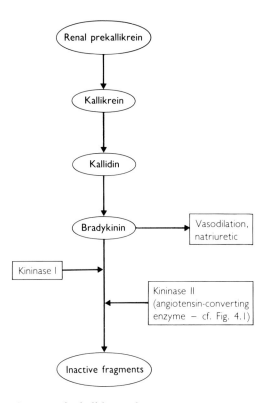

Fig. 4.4 The kallikrein−kinin system

- vasoconstriction, leading to a rise in arterial blood pressure.

Stimuli to secretion of ADH

ADH secretion is stimulated by several factors which are listed below.
- *Decreased effective blood volume.* Pressure sensors in the cardiac atria, aortic arch and carotid sinuses respond to changes in blood pressure and effective blood volume. The response curves are exponential, therefore volume stimuli will override osmolar stimuli. By this mechanism decreased effective blood volume results in ADH release in a wide range of conditions, including sodium depletion, cirrhosis and cardiac failure, and may contribute to hypo-osmolarity and hyponatraemia, since the volume stimulus is overriding the osmotic response (Chapter 14).
- *Increased plasma osmolarity.* Sensitive osmoreceptors exist in the hypothalamus, and the response is linear, from a threshold of 280 mosmol/litre. The nature of the osmotic stimulus is critical. Sodium chloride is a powerful stimulant, while urea, glucose and ethanol are very poor stimulants.
- *Other.* Many other stimuli, including nausea, hypoglycaemia,

high ambient temperature, anxiety and stress are associated with release of ADH.

Synthetic analogues of ADH

Synthetic ADH (8-arginine vasopressin — AVP) is available for parenteral or intranasal use in ADH deficiency. Desamino-D-arginine vasopressin (DDAVP) is a synthetic analogue which has increased antidiuretic but decreased vasoconstrictor effects compared with AVP, suggesting that the antidiuretic and vasoconstrictor properties reside in different aspects of the molecule.

Mineralocorticoids and glucocorticoids

Aldosterone is a steroid hormone produced by the adrenal cortex mainly in response to one of three stimuli:
- angiotensin II, stimulated by the renin–angiotensin system;
- hyperkalaemia;
- adrenocorticotrophic hormone (ACTH).

The main effect of aldosterone is to reduce excretion of sodium and consequently to promote excretion of potassium. The site of action in the kidney is the late distal tubule and the early collecting duct.

Aldosterone excess can occur as a primary phenomenon (Conn's syndrome) or, far more commonly, secondarily to an increase in plasma renin, as in oedematous states, renal artery stenosis and malignant hypertension.

Glucocorticoids at high concentration have mineralocorticoid effects, and also promote potassium excretion by increasing tubular flow rates.

Atrial natriuretic peptide

Atrial natriuretic peptide (ANP) is a 28 amino acid peptide released from granules in the cardiac atria in response to stretch. ANP has both renal (diuretic and natriuretic) and haemodynamic (hypotensive) effects. It also has important hormonal actions, e.g. suppression of renin and aldosterone.

Dopamine

Dopamine is released by renal nerves, probably secondary to stimulation of vascular baroreceptors. It causes renal vasodilation and natriuresis. This results mainly from stimulation of the kallikrein–kinin system (see above). Dopamine is used as an infusion to maintain urine output in incipient acute renal failure (Chapter 10).

PEPTIDE HORMONE CATABOLISM

The kidney removes many peptide hormones from the circulation, either by glomerular filtration with subsequent tubular resorption and degradation, or by removal of the hormone from the peritubular circulation by binding to receptors in the basolateral tubular cell membrane. It is by this latter effect that some peptide hormones such as PTH, calcitonin and vasopressin reach their receptors and exert their effects on tubular function.

Insulin

About 25% of insulin (MW 6000) is extracted from the circulation by the kidney; mainly by glomerular filtration but also by peritubular extraction. Proinsulin (MW 9000) and the inactive C-peptide split from proinsulin during formation of the insulin are also renally excreted. In advanced renal failure the basal plasma levels of insulin, proinsulin and C-peptide are all elevated. In diabetics insulin requirements often fall in end-stage renal failure. On the other hand peripheral resistance to insulin action in uraemia may cause carbohydrate intolerance.

Parathormone

About 30% of overall metabolism of PTH occurs in the kidney. Glomerular filtration removes intact hormone (MW 9500) and both carboxyl and amino-terminal fragments, while only the intact hormone and amino-terminal are removed by specific binding in the peritubular circulation. Elevated plasma PTH and particularly C-terminal PTH concentrations in uraemia are partially due to failure of renal metabolism (Chapters 6 & 11).

Prolactin

Most prolactin (MW 23 000) catabolism is via renal (glomerular filtration) mechanisms. Elevated prolactin levels are found in over 60% of dialysis patients, suggesting pituitary feedback is also deranged. This is probably responsible for gynaecomastia and galactorrhea, and contributes to infertility and impotence in chronic renal failure.

Growth hormone

The kidney removes 40–70% of growth hormone (MW 21 500) from the circulation, mainly by glomerular filtration. Elevated growth hormone levels may be found in uraemia, but feedback and control mechanisms are complex, and the contribution of the decreased metabolism to the growth aberrations in renal failure requires clarification.

Vasopressin

The kidneys remove 30–50% of this renally active hormone by both glomerular filtration (MW 1084) and peritubular removal.

Glucagon

This hypoglycaemic hormone (MW 3500) is about 30% renally excreted.

Gastrointestinal hormones

Gastrin, vasoactive intestinal polypeptide (VIP) and gastric inhibitory polypeptide are all partially renally degraded, and elevated

levels are often found in uraemia. The contribution of immunologically reactive but functionless metabolites to elevated levels,
and their clinical significance is unclear. Uraemic patients have a
high incidence of peptic ulceration. This is multifactorial but
elevated gastrin levels may contribute.

5: *Assessment of Renal Function*

Renal function tests are usually assessments of glomerular function, or measurements of various tubular functions. The latter are dependent on normal glomerular filtration rate, i.e. they are not valid tests of tubular function in chronic renal failure.

ASSESSMENT OF GLOMERULAR FUNCTION

The usual tests of glomerular function address two separate aspects:
1 Glomerular membrane permeability.
2 Glomerular filtration rate.

Tests of glomerular membrane permeability

Damage to the glomerular filtration membrane usually leads to increased permeability, reflected clinically by the appearance of proteinuria and/or haematuria. The investigation of patients with proteinuria and haematuria will be discussed in detail in Chapter 7.

Proteinuria

Normally there is less than 150 mg of protein in a 24-hour collection of urine. Only about 10 mg of this is albumin; the rest being low molecular weight proteins such as β_2-microglobulin (MW 11 800 Da) and Tamm–Horsfall glycoprotein which is secreted by the tubules. With glomerular injury the absolute amount and proportion of albumin in the urine increases (Chapters 7 & 8).

Glomerular haematuria

In many glomerular diseases large numbers of red blood cells are found in the urine. In such cases renal biopsy occasionally demonstrates actual ruptures in the glomerular basement membrane, or electron microscopy demonstrates red cells transgressing the basement membrane or free in the capsular space. In most cases, however, the exact mechanism by which glomerular haematuria occurs is not readily apparent, though passage of the cells through the filtration membrane is assumed. Haematuria can occur with minimal or no proteinuria. Urinary red cells in glomerular disease are varied in shape and may be associated with red cell casts (Chapter 8, Fig. 8.2).

Assessment of glomerular filtration rate

Measurement of the GFR gives the best index of overall renal excretory function, and with allowance for hypertrophy and increases in single nephron GFR (SNGFR) also gives an indication of the number of functioning nephrons.

The concept of renal clearance

Renal physiologists have found the concept of 'clearance' very helpful in estimating various aspects of renal function. The calculations depend on determining the amount of a substance appearing in the urine in a certain time (usually per minute or per second), then calculating the volume of blood that contains that amount of the substance. Though useful, the concept is confusing because only in cases where the kidney completely removes all of a substance from the blood in one passage through the kidney does the term 'clearance' really mean the volume of blood actually 'cleared' of the substance in the time. This only occurs with low concentrations of substances which are both filtered and very actively secreted by the tubules, as with para-amino hippurate which is used to determine renal blood flow.

To measure GFR the substance measured should be filtered at the glomerulus and neither resorbed or excreted by the tubules. In a steady state, if the plasma concentration of the substance is P, the amount filtered at the glomerulus per minute will be $P \times GFR$. This should equal the amount appearing in the urine per minute, which can be calculated from the urine concentration (U) multiplied by the urine volume per minute (V), i.e. $U \times V$.
Hence:

$$P \times GFR = U \times V$$

i.e.: $GFR = UV/P$.

The clearance of the polysaccharide, inulin, is the most accurate measure of GFR, however, this is impractical clinically since an inulin clearance study requires an intravenous infusion to maintain a constant plasma inulin concentration, and the measurement of inulin concentration is technically demanding.

Creatinine clearance

Creatinine is mainly an endogenously generated nitrogenous substance formed from creatinine in muscle. The normal adult excretes 7 to 24 mmol/day, with the larger amounts in muscular persons. Daily excretion equals production and overall balance, with a constant plasma level, is maintained unless renal function is changing rapidly. Creatinine is readily filtered and is not resorbed by the tubules, although a small amount of tubular secretion occurs. This potential for overestimation of GFR is cancelled out in practice by the fact that the techniques for measurement of plasma creatinine overestimate the concentration by about the same proportion.

GFR can therefore be reasonably deduced in practice from the creatinine clearance. A blood sample for plasma creatinine concentration (PCr) and a timed urine collection (usually 24 hours) for urine flow rate (V) and urine creatinine concentration (UCr) are required. Then:

Creatinine clearance = $UCr \times V/PCr$.

This is usually about 125 ml/min in males and 110 ml/min in females (1.5 to 2.5 ml/s). Due to tubular excretion of creatinine this overestimates renal function when GFR is very low.

The main disadvantage in practice is the unreliability of unsupervised timed urine collections, and the inconvenience to the patient of having to collect the urine.

EDTA clearance and radioisotopic methods

EDTA is handled by the kidney like inulin. Radioactive ^{51}Chromium-labelled EDTA can be used to assess GFR. A bolus injection of EDTA is given and serial blood samples taken over the following 4 hours. Advantages include greater accuracy than creatinine clearance, particularly when GFR is low, and the elimination of the need for a timed urine collection. The method is time-consuming for the patient and more expensive than creatinine clearance and is therefore not often used outside specialist nephrology centres.

Other radionuclide-labelled substances which are renally cleared, such as DTPA, can be injected and the excretion in each kidney followed by surface scanning (Chapter 2). This can provide an assessment of the relative contribution of each kidney to the overall GFR, which may be important in severe unilateral renal disease. This has replaced previous methods requiring bilateral ureteral catheters.

Plasma creatinine concentration

Measurement of the plasma creatinine concentration (PCr) is the simplest way to assess renal function. The normal plasma concentration is 0.05 to 0.11 mmol/litre (0.6 to 1.2 mg/100 ml). Since $CCr = UCr \times V/PCr$ (see above), and $UCr \times V$ is the generation rate of creatinine which should be relatively constant in any individual under constant conditions, it follows that in a given patient CCr is inversely proportional to the plasma creatinine, i.e.:

Creatinine clearance (CCr) is proportional to $1/PCr$.

Repeated measurement of the PCr is the best way of frequently assessing renal function in a given individual, but is a poor screening method for renal damage because it does not rise above the laboratory normal level until the GFR is below about 60% of normal (Fig. 5.1).

Plasma urea concentration

Urea is the major urinary nitrogenous waste, and therefore the plasma urea concentration (or the blood urea nitrogen — BUN) has long been used as a test of renal function. However:
- Most of the urinary urea is derived from dietary protein, therefore the plasma urea fluctuates with diet.
- Tissue breakdown (catabolism) also leads to a rise in plasma and urinary urea.
- Urea back-diffuses from the tubules into the blood, particularly with low tubular flow rates.

For these reasons urea measurements do not give a good indication of renal function or GFR, since situations exist when the plasma urea is inappropriately high or low when compared with the plasma creatinine or GFR (Table 5.1).

Measurement of renal blood flow

Para-aminohippuric acid excretion

At low concentrations para-aminohippuric acid PAH is filtered by the glomerulus and actively secreted by the tubules so that very little reaches the renal veins. The clearance of PAH therefore equals the effective renal plasma flow (RPF), i.e.:

$$RPF = U_{PAH} \times V/P_{PAH}$$

where U_{PAH} and P_{PAH} are the urine and plasma concentrations of PAH and V is the urine flow rate. The renal blood flow (RBF) can then be calculated from RPF and the haematocrit (normally 45%). Hence:

Table 5.1 Causes of a high plasma urea/creatinine ratio which is normally about 80:1 (urea 8:creatinine 0.11 mmol/litre)

Increased urea production due to catabolism
Infection
Trauma
Corticosteroid therapy
Tetracycline therapy

Increased gastrointestinal protein load
High protein diet
Upper gastrointestinal bleeding

Increased tubular resorption of urea
Dehydration
Salt depletion
Prerenal renal failure (Chapter 10)

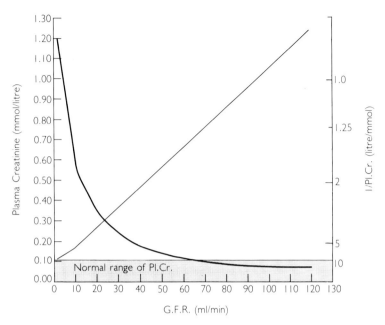

Fig. 5.1 Relationship between the plasma creatinine concentration and glomerular filtration rate (GFR). The plasma creatinine (darker line) rises almost reciprocally with falling GFR, and does not reliably exceed the normal upper limit until the GFR is below about 50−60% of normal. As the GFR falls the reciprocal of plasma creatinine increasingly overestimates GFR because of tubular and gastrointestinal secretion of creatinine

$$RBF = RPF \div (1 - \text{haematocrit})$$
$$= 660 \div (1 - 0.45)$$
$$= 1200 \text{ ml/min.}$$

Other methods

Hippuran renogram. I^{131}-hippuran is handled by the kidney like PAH. By injecting this substance and monitoring the appearance of radioactivity over the kidneys an assessment can be made of individual kidney blood flow.

Other radiological and isotope imaging. Slow accumulation of radiocontrast or isotope labels in imaging techniques (Chapter 2) can be the result of poor blood flow. Renal angiography can demonstrate vascular stenosis as well as poor flow through intra-renal vessels (Fig. 12.1).

TESTS OF TUBULAR FUNCTION

These tests are only valid indicators of tubular function when GFR is near normal; in other instances they only measure the overall ability of the kidneys to perform a certain task.

Assessment of water excretion mechanisms

Detailed investigation of renal mechanisms for urine concentration is uncommonly performed, but many simple tests are useful.

Urine specific gravity

The specific gravity (SG) of urine varies between 1.003 and 1.035. In chronic renal failure a fixed SG of 1.010 is common due to loss of the concentrating mechanism.

Urine osmolarity

Urine osmolarity can be measured to determine concentrating ability (for simplicity we will use the term osmolarity, even when the technique actually measures the osmolality; the units for the former are mosmol/litre and the latter mosmol/kg). The plasma osmolarity (normal 280 to 300 mosmol/litre) should always be measured at the same time. Although urine osmolarity can reach 1400 mosmol/litre, this only occurs after severe and prolonged stimulation.

Urine concentrating tests

Clinically useful stimuli for urine concentration are fluid deprivation and ADH injection.

Water deprivation test. This test should be performed with great care, since severe dehydration can occur in patients with a concentrating defect. Up to 24 hours of water deprivation, to a maximum of 4% loss of body weight, should result in a urinary osmolarity of above 900 mosmol/litre or SG >1.025. As a screening test urine passed after overnight fluid deprivation should have an osmolarity exceeding 600 mosmol/litre or SG >1.015.

Exogenous ADH test. Pitressin tannate in oil subcutaneously (remember to shake the oily suspension well) should provoke a urine osmolality of over 750 mosmol/litre in the next 8 hours, or over 900 mosmol/litre if the test is preceded by water deprivation.
  In interpreting the results of these tests it must be remembered that prolonged polyuria can blunt the response to ADH because of medullary hypotonicity (Chapter 3).

Plasma osmolarity

Plasma osmolarity can be measured directly (actually osmolality is measured — normal 280 to 300 mosmol/litre) or extrapolated from plasma sodium, potassium, glucose and urea concentrations where these are expressed in mmol/litre:

Calculated osmolarity = 2(Na + K) + glucose + urea.

For example in a normal individual:

= 2(140 + 4) + 5 + 6
= 299 mosmol/litre.

This usually slightly overestimates osmolarity.

Free water clearance This estimates the urinary 'clearance' of water. It is calculated by:

$$\text{Free water clearance} = V \times \left(1 - \frac{\text{urine osmolarity}}{\text{plasma osmolarity}}\right).$$

It is positive when water is being excreted in excess of solutes, i.e. when urine is being diluted.

Water load test This test measures the ability to excrete a sudden large water load. A 70 kg person with a GFR of 120 ml/min should be able to excrete over 1050 ml (75%) of a 1400 ml water load in 4 hours. This is more dependent on adequate GFR than on tubular function.

Assessment of sodium excretion
Urinary sodium excretion and concentration

Normally 70 to 300 mmol/24 h; 20 to 100 mmol/litre of urine. Urinary sodium excretion can be measured in 24-hour samples, and interpreted on the basis of oral sodium intake, with, if necessary, deliberate loading or depletion. In normal individuals urinary sodium output reflects dietary sodium content. In some renal diseases affecting the tubules 'salt wasting' can occur with inappropriately high urinary sodium losses in the face of clinical salt depletion (Table 5.2). A similar situation occurs in mineralocorticoid deficiency (Addison's syndrome) and can be provoked by diuretic drugs.

Random samples of urine can show very low sodium concentrations, often below 10 mmol/litre, in situations of poor renal

Table 5.2 Urinary sodium excretion

High
High salt diet
Mineralocorticoid deficiency
Diuretic therapy
Salt-wasting renal diseases:
  renal papillary necrosis
  recovering tubular necrosis
  recovering or partial obstruction
  renal cystic disease
  reflux nephropathy

Low
Low salt diet
Poor renal perfusion:
  dehydration
  shock
  cardiac failure
  hepatorenal syndrome

perfusion such as in dehydration, shock, and severe liver or cardiac failure (Chapter 11). Urinary sodium estimations are not reliable if the patient has been given diuretic drugs.

Plasma sodium concentration

Normally 135–145 mmol/litre. Plasma sodium concentration bears little relationship to total body sodium content. It is a better reflection of the state of the water-handling mechanisms of the kidney (Chapter 14).

Plasma renin concentration

High peripheral plasma renin concentrations indicate activity of the renin–angiotensin system as in salt depletion and mineralocorticoid deficiency. The effect of many drugs on plasma renin concentrations, such as β-adrenergic blocking drugs which profoundly depress levels, must always be considered (Chapter 12).

Assessment of potassium excretion
Plasma potassium concentration

Normally 3.5–5.5 mmol/litre. Even though it represents only a small portion of total body potassium the measurement of plasma potassium is important because of the profound effect of hypokalaemia and hyperkalaemia on neuromuscular and cardiac excitability. Because of the tenuous relationship between plasma and total body potassium it is important to monitor closely plasma potassium during repletion or depletion.

Urinary potassium excretion

Normally 40–90 mmol/24 hours. The finding of a urinary potassium concentration greater than 10 mmol/litre in the face of hypokalaemia suggests renal potassium loss, e.g. in diuretic therapy, renal tubular acidosis and adrenocortical insufficiency. Urinary potassium conservation, i.e. less than 10 mmol/litre suggests extrarenal loss, particularly gastrointestinal (Chapter 13).

Assessment of renal acid–base regulation

Renal disorders resulting in acid–base disturbance are covered in Chapter 13. In all acid–base disturbances several investigations are required to determine the cause, as not all measure renal mechanisms. The tests of renal mechanisms include:

Urine pH. Urine pH can be readily measured by dipstix and usually varies between 4 and 8. A pH meter is more accurate and is essential in tests of urinary acidification.

Urinary acidification test. The capacity of the tubules to acidify the urine is measured by the ammonium chloride urine acidification test. An oral load of 0.1 g/kg of ammonium chloride should reduce urine pH to less than 5.3, provided plasma pH falls and the urine is not infected.

Tests of acid–base status. Further assessment may require measurement of plasma pH, plasma P_{CO_2} and bicarbonate, urine pH, urine bicarbonate and urine titratable acid estimation.

Renal glucose handling

Since glucose should be fully resorbed by the proximal tubule, and the mechanism can be saturated, measurement of the maximum tubular resorptive capacity is a useful test of tubular function. This can be saturated. The critical point is when glomerular filtration of glucose exceeds the tubular capacity for resorption, and is known as the tubular maximum resorptive capacity for glucose (TMgluc).

TMgluc can be calculated from the GFR and the plasma glucose concentration at which glycosuria appears, i.e. the renal threshold. Since the amount filtered is the GFR multiplied by the plasma glucose concentration, and the amount in the urine is the urine concentration multiplied by the urine volume then:

TMgluc = (GFR × plasma glucose concentration)
        − urine volume × urine glucose concentration).

The normal TMgluc is about 15–20 mmol/min.

6: *The Failing Kidney: Pathophysiology of Renal Failure*

Several reasons for the kidneys' limited response to damage are:
• The nephron is an anatomical functional unit. Any cause of death of either the glomerulus or tubule will result in death of the whole nephron.
• New nephrons are not formed after birth.
• As nephrons are lost through disease the remaining nephrons must compensate for the reduced nephron numbers. This is achieved by complex haemodynamic and metabolic mechanisms, and by hypertrophy of residual nephrons.
• With further nephron loss the capacity of the remaining nephrons to preserve homeostasis will eventually be lost. Since the ability to compensate for different function varies, some functional derangements will become obvious before others. Many of the functional inadequacies are not obvious to the patient or clinician. In fact, renal failure is largely an asymptomatic disease until a very late stage. Most patients with a GFR above about 25% of normal (i.e. above about 30 ml/min) are asymptomatic. Even in patients with a GFR as low as 10–20 ml/min symptoms may only be mild. It is unusual for patients whose GFR is less than 10 ml/min to remain symptomless, but as the symptoms are often vague and non-specific (malaise, fatigue) it is not uncommon for patients to first present with end-stage chronic renal failure, these symptoms having been ignored or attributed to depression or anaemia.
• The primary renal disease will impose its own special pathophysiology, resulting in an overlap of abnormalities. These usually precede the derangements purely due to nephron loss. There may also be a bias in the dysfunction because of attack on a specific portion of the nephron, e.g. glomerulus or tubule. Broadly, glomerular disease is more likely to give problems with fluid retention, oedema and hypertension than tubular disease where polyuria, salt and water depletion, and acidosis are more likely.

NEPHRON RESPONSE TO RENAL DAMAGE

Glomerular hyperfiltration and hypertrophy

Reduction in glomerular numbers by unilateral nephrectomy in the adult usually results in a fall in GFR by only about 25%. The mechanisms by which the residual glomeruli act to preserve total GFR have been well studied in animals but less so in humans. It has been shown that after uninephrectomy the remnant kidney increases its GFR by 40–60%, with a rise in mean single nephron GFR (SNGFR). Most of this response is evident in a few days and virtually all has occurred by 2 weeks.

This response in residual glomeruli has been termed *hyperfiltration* by Brenner and his colleagues. The increase in SNGFR is accompanied by increases in blood flow, *hyperperfusion*, attributable to dilatation of both afferent and efferent arterioles. The dilatation of the efferent arteriole is less than that of the afferent vessel, hence the pressure as well as the flow in the glomerular capillaries is increased. Both these alterations tend to increase SNGFR. Commonly with renal damage there is also systemic hypertension, further increasing afferent pressure, aggravating the hyperfiltration.

The residual glomeruli also increase in size. In animals this occurs within weeks. The rate in humans is unknown, but the residual glomeruli in patients with reduced renal function are larger than normal. Subsequently the residual glomeruli are progressively destroyed by a sclerosing process which effects segments of glomeruli, focal and segmental glomerulosclerosis (FGS – Fig. 6.1). It has, therefore, been postulated that this glomerulosclerosis is a deleterious side effect of the mechanisms related to hyperfiltration (see below).

Tubular hyperfunction and hypertrophy

With nephron loss and increase in SNGFR the tubular functions of secretion and resorption must also increase if solute homeostasis is to be maintained. Major alterations in function and structure have been demonstrated.

Within hours of uninephrectomy normal glomerulotubular balance is re-established. Salt and water resorption, nett acid secretion and all other tubular functions are sufficient to cope with the load which has, on average, doubled for each tubule. This is brought about primarily by the complex osmotic, circulatory and hormonal mechanisms believed to match tubular function to SNGFR (glomerulotubular balance, Chapter 3) as well as subsequent hypertrophy.

The tubules increase in both diameter and length. This process is mainly completed in 2 weeks in experimental animals and probably also in humans although some suggest that continuing hypertrophy may continue for months in young kidneys. Since tubules make up the bulk of renal mass it is this increase in tubular size that is largely responsible for the contralateral renal hypertrophy characteristic of juvenile onset unilateral disease in humans.

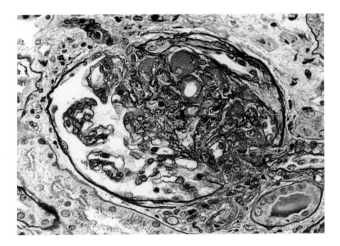

Fig. 6.1 Secondary focal glomerulosclerosis (FGS) occurring in a patient with reflux nephropathy

FACTORS STIMULATING RENAL HYPERTROPHY AND HYPERFILTRATION

Though there is still much to be learnt about hypertrophy and hyperfiltration some stimuli and mechanisms are becoming clear.

Hyperfiltration does not only occur in the situation of reduced renal mass. Some known stimuli include loss of renal tissue, high protein feeding, pregnancy and diabetes (Table 3.4).

The situation relating to high protein feeding has been the subject of most interest. A similar but less pronounced effect can be achieved by intravenous infusion of amino acids, and the effect is blunted by severe liver disease. The message to the glomerular vessels in response to the protein load seems to involve the renin–angiotensin system since the effect is ameliorated by angiotensin-converting enzyme inhibitors. It is assumed that similar mechanisms pertain in the residual nephron situation. The response has its limitations, however, since no increase in GFR is seen after protein feeding of patients with severe renal failure. The picture is sufficiently cohesive to suggest that this mechanism is involved in the genesis of glomerulosclerosis in chronic renal failure.

THE INTACT NEPHRON HYPOTHESIS

This most useful theory states that since the nephrons are functional and anatomical units, each undamaged nephron in a diseased kidney should behave in a physiologically integrated and appropriate manner. In effect each nephron acts in a normal fashion given its biochemical milieu.

A relevant clinical example occurs with intravenous pyelography in renal failure. The concentrating defect in the residual nephrons, perfused as they are with plasma with a high urea concentration, is largely due to an osmotic diuresis. The contrast agent injected into the bloodstream is thus not sufficiently concentrated by the tubules to be seen as a nephrogram or pyelogram. However, if the plasma urea level is artificially lowered by dialysis immediately prior to the injection of dye sometimes a nephrogram can be seen. A similar effect occurs in severe unilateral renal disease where a very small kidney with little function can often be seen to excrete dye because the opposite kidney is holding the plasma urea in the normal range.

PROGRESSION OF RENAL FAILURE

In many patients with renal damage a progressive decline in GFR occurs even after the insult which produced the original damage has gone. This is usually accompanied by proteinuria, hypertension, and focal and segmental glomerulosclerosis (FGS).

It seems likely that this progression is related to the hyperperfusion and hyperfiltration mentioned above. It has been suggested that this can be ameliorated by low protein feeding, control of hypertension, and control of hyperphosphataemia. Much is still to be learnt about the mechanisms, and other techniques, such as the use of angiotensin-converting enzyme inhibitors to lower the intraglomerular capillary pressure, in slowing of the progression of chronic renal failure.

COURSE OF PROGRESSION OF RENAL FAILURE

In most patients with renal disease the GFR falls in a fairly steady fashion, presuming a complication such as accelerated hypertension (Chapter 12) does not occur.

This can be accurately followed by radionuclear EDTA clearance (Chapter 5) but this is inconvenient and the alternative, i.e. creatinine clearance, is so dependent on accurate urine collection that it may have limited accuracy in outpatients.

Since the creatinine clearance is proportional to 1/plasma creatinine (Chapter 5) it follows that if the creatinine clearance is falling in a linear fashion then the plot of 1/plasma creatinine will be a straight line whose slope gives a good indication of the rate of decrease of creatinine clearance (Fig. 5.1). In many patients plotting the reciprocal of their plasma creatinine against time gives a fairly straight line, allowing estimates to be made of the likely prognosis and highlighting any significant change in course.

Whenever using plasma creatinine or creatinine clearance to estimate GFR in patients with renal failure it must be remembered that the worse the renal function the more the creatinine clearance overestimates GFR, because of an increasing proportion of creatinine cleared by tubular and gastrointestinal secretion.

CONSEQUENCES OF RENAL FAILURE

These are:
1 Failure of excretory functions,
  (a) reduction in GFR, and
  (b) disturbances in tubular resorption and secretion.
2 Failure of hormonal functions,
  (a) reduction of erythropoietin,
  (b) reduction of active vitamin D,
  (c) disturbance in renin secretion, and
  (d) others.
The clinical consequences will be covered in detail in Chapter 11.

Failure of excretory functions
Glomerular filtration

As GFR falls there is accumulation in the blood of products whose excretion normally depends on glomerular filtration. Plasma urea and creatinine concentrations first rise above the laboratory upper limits of normal when GFR is about 60% of normal (Fig. 5.1) — they are insensitive indices of mild to moderate renal damage. Subsequently since their plasma concentrations are roughly inversely proportional to their clearance (clearance — UV/P — as discussed above) they rise in an exponential manner with falling GFR. Other measurable products whose excretion depends on renal function, such as phosphate and urate also accumulate in the blood.

As will be discussed later in this chapter these molecules do not account for many of the clinical abnormalities seen in patients with renal failure. A great many can be attributed to fluid, electrolyte, acid–base or hormonal derangements but some very characteristic signs and symptoms are generally attributed to accumulation of unknown, normally renally excreted, 'uremic toxins' (see the last section in this chapter).

Water excretion

Inability to concentrate the urine is an important indicator of renal dysfunction since it is responsible for the very common early symptom of nocturia when the diurnal rhythm of urine excretion is lost. Later polyuria and thirst may occur. It is mainly due to an osmotic diuresis occurring in surviving nephrons. The body continues to produce around 600 mosmol/day of osmotically active substances which are now being filtered by fewer glomeruli, hence the osmotic burden on each tubule is increased. The effect is similar to that which occurs if an osmotic diuretic (such as urea or mannitol) is administered to a normal person. Each nephron thus produces a larger amount of urine which is less concentrated.

There is usually little effect on overall water balance, only on the minimal amount of urine which must be excreted to deal with the osmotic load. Briefly, if normally 500 ml is required to excrete 600 mosmol/day at the maximal urine concentration of 1200 mosmol/litre, if the urine is isotonic with plasma (300 mosmol/litre), 2000 ml will be required; an increase of 1500 ml. The situation becomes critical when water intake is reduced or increased water losses occur, particularly if there is also greater catabolism producing a greater load of osmotically active waste products. Patients with renal functional impairment are therefore prone to dehydration with intercurrent illnesses. Dehydration leads to a further fall in GFR, increasing uraemia, with consequent anorexia and nausea and further decrease in fluid intake. Hypernatraemia is uncommon because there is often concomitant sodium loss.

Inability to dilute the urine is a late manifestation of renal failure. In near end stage failure the urine passed has a fixed specific gravity (SG) of 1.010, and osmolarity similar to that of plasma — 300 mosmol/litre. This is still fairly dilute urine since in health the urine osmolarity can be varied between about 50 mosmol/litre (SG 1.001) and 1300 mosmol/litre (SG 1.040).

More importantly there is a limitation in the rate with which the kidneys can excrete a water load. This is attributable to the reduction in GFR rather than a diluting defect. A simplified explanation can be given by the following calculation. A 70 kg person with a GFR of 120 ml/min should be able to excrete over 1050 ml (75%) of a 1400 ml water load in 4 hours (see Water load test, Chapter 5). This represents a water excretion rate of over 4 ml/min, which may exceed the total GFR of a patient with renal failure and a water load can thus precipitate dilutional hyponatraemia (Chapter 14).

Sodium excretion

As the number of glomeruli decreases and SNGFR increases, sodium resorption in each tubule adjusts (as does the accompanying water and chloride) such that body salt and water balance is maintained. This adjustment of tubular resorption is accomplished by a variety of mechanisms including glomerulotubular balance and probably activation of hormonal mechanisms such as atrial and other natriuretic factors (Chapter 4).

The ability to adjust to fluctuations in sodium intake gradually fails. At a GFR of about 10 ml/min minimal urinary sodium excretion may be raised from the normal of less than 10 mmol/litre to about 30 mmol/litre. An intercurrent illness with decreased sodium intake, or non-renal losses due to vomiting, diarrhoea or fever with sweating can lead to negative salt and water balance; this saline depletion further reduces GFR and acute-on-chronic renal failure occurs.

In most patients gradual salt and water retention occurs. This is a major factor in the genesis of hypertension in renal failure. In over 90% of dialysis-dependent patients hypertension can be controlled by salt and water restriction. Oedema and signs of cardiac failure may be seen in severely overloaded patients.

In others salt and water depletion dominates the clinical picture. This occurs particularly in diseases primarily attacking renal tubules, such as analgesic nephropathy (Chapter 22), cystic kidney diseases (Chapter 29) and chronic tubulointerstitial nephritis (Chapter 20). These 'salt-losing' diseases (Table 5.2) are particularly important because salt supplementation may be required. Skin pigmentation may accompany chronic salt depletion (as in Addison's disease).

Potassium excretion

The kidneys have an enormous functional reserve for potassium excretion, particularly if the load is gradually increased (Chapter 3). Accordingly serious hyperkalaemia rarely occurs unless the GFR is less than 5–10 ml/min or there is another reason for hyperkalaemia, such as excessive load, as is often the case in acute renal failure (Chapter 11), or specific interference with kaliuresis as in so-called hyporeninaemic hypoaldosteronism (see Diabetic nephropathy, Chapter 26), or severe acidosis with volume contraction (Chapter 14).

In severe renal failure (acute renal failure and end-stage chronic disease), hyperkalaemia becomes a serious problem not only because it is common but also because it can prove so rapidly fatal (Chapter 14).

Acid–Base balance

Metabolic acidosis with depressed plasma bicarbonate is characteristic of renal failure. It is usually only mild, even in quite advanced renal failure, but in end-stage failure it can dominate the clinical picture with typical Kussmaul 'air hunger' respiration. The major mechanisms producing acidosis are:

• *Decreased GFR*, hence decreased excretion of the important titratable acids such as phosphate, creatinine, and urate.

• *Inadequate ammonia production* by the proximal tubule.
• *Lowered threshold for bicarbonate excretion* also exists so bicarbonate administered to reduce acidosis may spill into the urine in the manner that it does in proximal (type 1) renal tubular acidosis (Chapter 28).

The patients usually have a urine pH less than 5.0 in the presence of acidosis but less acid is being excreted with the dilute buffers present. Acidosis is more prominent in diseases affecting renal tubules such as analgesic nephropathy, cystic disease and interstitial nephritis and can be markedly exaggerated by saline depletion or increased acid load, as is often the case with intercurrent infection or trauma.

In chronic acidosis much of the buffering of hydrogen ion occurs in the bones and chronic acidosis is thought to contribute to skeletal calcium loss in renal bone disease.

| *Calcium and phosphate excretion* | The disturbances of calcium-phosphate metabolism in renal failure are complex, relating to both the excretory and vitamin D activating (i.e. hormonal) roles of the kidney. The major direct effect of failure of renal excretory mechanisms is reduction in the excretion of phosphate. As GFR falls below about 30% of normal, hyperphosphataemia begins to be seen. It has been argued that prior to this there are increasing waves of postprandial hyperphosphataemia, resulting in rises in parathormone secretion, gradually causing parathyroid hyperplasia. The complex relationships between urinary and plasma calcium and phosphate, vitamin D, parathormone and the bones in renal failure will be discussed later in this chapter. |

| *Glucose, amino acid and phosphate resorption* | The proximal tubular functions of resorption of glucose, amino acids and phosphate are usually sufficient to cope with the increased SNGFR and greater tubular delivery. Glucose occasionally spills into the urine (renal glycosuria) in predominantly tubular disorders. |

| *Uric acid* | Uric acid excretion is usually well maintained until GFR is less than about 20 ml/min. Hyperuricaemia is common in severe renal failure although clinical gout is perhaps less common than one might suppose. It is easily confused clinically with acute calcium phosphate arthropathy, otherwise known as pseudogout. |

| *Drugs* | Care must be taken when using renally excreted drugs such as digoxin and aminoglycosides in patients with renal disease. Like other renally excreted substances they can accumulate and produce drug toxicity in renal failure (Chapter 34). |

Failure of hormonal functions

Erythropoietin

Erythropoietin deficiency is the main cause of the anaemia seen in chronic renal failure. Uraemic patients have lower plasma erythropoietin levels than non-uraemic patients with the same degree of anaemia, and anephric patients have even lower levels, presumably with some being produced by the liver.

In some patients, notably some of those with adult polycystic kidney disease (Chapter 29), haemoglobin levels are high despite severe renal failure, presumably because of continued erythropoietin production. Two situations in which the haemoglobin rises without any improvement in renal function are in uraemic acquired-polycystic kidney disease (Chapter 35) and in hepatitis when regenerating liver seems to form erythropoietin.

In end-stage renal failure haemoglobin concentrations are usually between 5 and 10 g/100 ml. This anaemia is refractory to haematinic vitamins or iron therapy and can be made worse by repeated transfusion which seems to further depress the drive to erythropoietin production. Fortunately the symptoms of the anaemia are not as severe as one might expect. Patients with haemoglobin levels as low as 5–6 g/100 ml are often able to continue normal activity. This is attributed to the shifting to the right of the oxygen-dissociation curve by a rise in intracellular 2,3-DPG and acidosis, the former a result of phosphate retention. This results in increased availability of oxygen to the tissues (and, incidentally, lowers the drive for erythropoietin production). The anaemia can be reversed by administration of erythropoietin.

Vitamin D activation, renal failure and renal bone disease

Renal bone disease is one of the most important aspects of morbidity in chronic renal failure, particularly in children and dialysis patients.

The major aspects of pathogenesis of renal bone disease are the failure of two important renal functions:

1 Failure of 1-hydroxylation of 25,OH-cholecalciferol to produce the active hormone 1,25(OH)$_2$-cholecalciferol (Chapter 4).

2 Failure of phosphate excretion with consequent secondary hyperparathyroidism.

Failure of 1,25-dihydroxy-cholecalciferol production. 1,25(OH)$_2$-Cholecalciferol (1,25(OH)$_2$D3) is 100 times more potent than its precursor and is produced by the mitochondria of proximal tubule cells. Its main actions are:

• To enhance gut absorption of calcium.

• To facilitate normal mineralisation of bone.

It also prevents the proximal myopathy of vitamin D deficiency.

Failure to produce this renal hormone leads to a fall in plasma calcium concentration and abnormal ineffective bone mineralisation.

Phosphate retention and secondary hyperparathyroidism. As GFR falls, transient, then permanent elevation of plasma phosphate (P) concentration occurs due to the fall in P excretion. The high plasma P causes a fall in plasma Ca because a dynamic equilibrium exists. This is aggravated by the hypocalcaemia secondary to 1,25(OH)$_2$D3 deficiency. The fall in plasma Ca acts to stimulate the parathyroid glands to secrete parathormone (PTH). The effects of hyperparathyroidism may be potentiated by reduction in renal metabolism of PTH (Chapter 4).

The main effects of PTH are to promote:
• Resorption of bone by stimulating osteoclasts. This raises plasma Ca but depletes bone Ca.
• Renal phosphate excretion. This effect is blocked by severe renal failure.

In addition to demineralisation of bone other important effects of secondary hyperparathyroidism are as follows.
• Promotion of extra-osseus calcification because of the high plasma Ca × P product. Calcification occurs in arterial walls, conjunctivae, and skin as well as other soft tissues.
• Fibrosis of the bone marrow aggravating anaemia.

With prolonged severe secondary hyperparathyroidism the parathyroid glands hypertrophy and eventually become so large that they cannot decrease PTH production in response to a normal or even elevated plasma Ca: so-called tertiary or autonomous hyperparathyroidism.

In summary, renal bone disease is a mixture of two processes:
1 Vitamin D deficiency; rickets in children, osteomalacia in adults.
2 Hyperparathyroidism.

Renin, blood pressure and renal failure

The renin–angiotensin system is only one of many factors in blood pressure control. As renal failure progresses salt and water retention contributes increasingly to raised blood pressure. Other vasoactive renal products or hormones including bradykinins and prostaglandins are also deranged.

Inappropriately high renin levels for the ambient blood pressure and hydration status are found in many patients with renal disease, and about 5% of patients with end-stage renal failure continue to produce abnormally large amounts of renin from their otherwise seemingly functionless kidneys. Overall about 80% of patients commencing dialysis are hypertensive, and in over 90% of these the hypertension can be controlled by reducing body salt and water content. It has therefore been concluded that salt and water retention is the main cause of hypertension in dialysis dependent patients.

THE URAEMIC SYNDROME

The uraemic syndrome is a consequence of severe failure of both the excretory and endocrine functions of the kidney. The manifestations can therefore be regarded as being due to:
- accumulation of 'uraemic toxins', and/or
- derangements in fluids, electrolytes and hormones.

Uraemic toxins

Although it has long been assumed that the many manifestations of uraemia that cannot be readily attributed to fluid, electrolyte or endocrine disturbances (Table 6.1) are due to accumulation of toxic products of metabolism, probably nitrogenous in nature, these toxins have not been convincingly identified.

Urea represents over 90% of urinary nitrogenous products. It was an early favourite for the 'uraemic toxin' and lent its name to the clinical syndrome, 'uraemia'. However studies in which patients were dialysed against high concentrations of urea showed that a very high blood urea produced only mild lethargy, anorexia and malaise.

Creatinine and uric acid are the next most common nitrogenous urinary products but also do not produce the uraemic syndrome.

Table 6.1 Uraemic manifestations attributed mainly to uraemic toxins

General
Lethargy, malaise, nausea

Cardiovascular
Pericarditis

Pulmonary
Pleurisy

Gastrointestinal
Uraemic colitis

Nervous system
Depression
Tremor
Flap
Myoclonus
Convulsions
Peripheral neuropathy

Haematological
Platelet dysfunction
Immune deficiency

Middle molecules are substances of molecular weight 300 to 2000 Da, i.e. larger than urea (MW 60) and creatinine (MW 113) yet well within the upper limit for glomerular filtration (MW 60 000), and smaller than most polypeptide hormones. Their presence in uraemic serum has been postulated as the basis for uraemic symptoms, again without any proof.

Other substances which have been blamed for various uraemic abnormalities include polyamines (spermine, putrescene), guanidines, phenols, inositol and products of nucleic acid breakdown, but none of these has been convincingly demonstrated to be the uraemic toxin.

The 'trade-off' hypothesis

It has been postulated that all or most of the manifestations of uraemia could be the result of compensatory responses to the abnormalities in body fluids and hormones, i.e. one disease has been 'traded' for another. The best example of this is bone disease due to secondary hyperparathyroidism, which compensates for failure of the vitamin D activating and phosphate excreting roles of the kidney. One theory blames PTH for other uraemic abnormalities, since anorexia, psychological disturbances, gastrointestinal illness and many other symptoms can occur in primary hyperparathyroidism where the plasma levels of PTH are often much lower than those found in uraemia.

Section 2
Clinical Nephrology:
the Approach to
Presenting Problems

7: Clinical Approach to Patients with Renal Disease

HISTORY AND EXAMINATION

The symptoms of many renal diseases are so vague or trivial that they may be neglected until a complication or progression to renal failure occurs. Increased attention to detection of hypertension in the community and routine testing of urine for protein and blood is gradually leading to earlier detection of renal abnormalities in patients who have not complained of renal symptoms. As a result the 'presenting complaint' is commonly asymptomatic hypertension, proteinuria or haematuria. Even in these cases however, careful history taking and examination can often give some clue as to the likely underlying diagnosis and hence appropriate investigation.

Common presenting complaints

These are listed in Table 7.1. Since many renal diseases are chronic and the symptoms vague, the patient should be quizzed in detail about both current and past history of these symptoms.

Insurance, pre-employment and military service examinations have often been performed. Patients should be asked about past screening for hypertension and proteinuria, since this often helps in indicating the chronicity or otherwise of their renal disease.

Age and sex

These are important in differential diagnosis, since most renal diseases have a tendency to present at certain ages and may have a striking difference in incidences between sexes (Table 7.2).

In childhood the symptoms of renal disease, particularly urine infection, may be obscure. Persistent enuresis, unexplained fevers and abdominal pain may indicate a history of urine infections suggesting developmental anatomical abnormalities, the commonest of which is vesicoureteric reflux (Chapter 21). Failure to thrive is apparent in many young children with severe renal disease.

Adolescence and early adulthood is a time when females are particularly prone to develop urine infection, which may only be recalled as episodes of 'bladder' or 'kidney chills'. Prescription of

81

Table 7.1 Common symptoms of renal disease

	Chapter
Pain Renal pain, ureteric colic	7
Disturbances of micturition Dysuria, oliguria, incontinence, strangury, nocturia, nocturnal enuresis, frequency, polyuria	7
Urine abnormalities Haematuria*, smelly urine, frothy urine, proteinuria*	7–9
Oedema Mild with periorbital oedema, severe and generalised	7 and 9
Uraemic syndrome Fatigue, itch, bone pain, malaise, Anorexia	10 and 11
*Urinary tract infection**	13
*Hypertension** Occasionally accelerated with severe headache or visual disturbance	12
*Electrolyte or acid-base disturbances**	14

* Often these are asymptomatic, but detected at routine or other medical examinations.

the oral contraceptive pill should have stimulated the doctor to screen for hypertension, proteinuria and haematuria, and sometimes 'the pill' can precipitate hypertension.

The elderly patient is at risk since renal functional reserve is less, disease of other systems with secondary renal involvement is common and old age brings special problems such as neoplasia, prostatic disease in the male and pelvic floor weakness in the female. Disturbances of micturition such as poor stream, frequency, nocturia and urge or stress incontinence are frequent, and symptoms suggesting neoplasm and cardiac failure must be assessed.

Pregnancy

Tests for urine infection, proteinuria, hypertension and even renal function are routine in most obstetric practices. Even though abnormalities may not be followed by disease the patient is often aware of the result. Urine infection is often precipitated by preg-

Table 7.2 Age/sex bias in renal disease

	Chapter
Female preponderance	
Reflux nephropathy	21
Analgesic nephropathy	22
Systemic lupus erythematosus	17
Pregnancy-related disorders	33
Male preponderance	
Alport's syndrome	31
Fabry's disease	31
Childhood preponderance	
Minimal change glomerulonephritis	15
Poststreptococcal glomerulonephritis	15
Haemolytic uraemic syndrome	32
Gross anatomical abnormalities	31
Gross tubular biochemical abnormalities	28
Geriatric preponderance	
Drug-related renal disease	34
Prostatic obstruction (male)	23
Pelvic floor weakness (female)	
Iatrogenic disease	

nancy, and hypertension, proteinuria or pre-eclampsia commonly occur in patients with renal disease. A past history of such trouble can be a valuable indicator of chronicity of disease, particularly if it occurred in second or subsequent pregnancies (Chapter 33).

A full drug and toxin history

Drug side effects are particularly likely either as a cause or consequence of renal disease (Chapter 34). Information from the local doctor is often useful. Environmental toxins (lead, hydrocarbons) should not be neglected in this search for toxic chemicals.

The family history

A familial predisposition can be found with many diseases, the former much more likely in patients with a defined genetic defect (Table 7.3).

Examination of patients with renal disease

Renal failure causes important abnormalities in every system of the body (Chapter 11, Fig. 11.1). Moreover, renal disease often occurs as a complication of disease primarily of another system (e.g. diabetic nephropathy) or of a multisystem disease (e.g. SLE, scleroderma). Accordingly a complete examination of all body systems is required in patients with renal disease. On the other hand there are particular aspects which are crucially important in patients with renal disease and worth highlighting.

Table 7.3 Renal diseases with familial predisposition

	Chapter
Strong predisposition	
Adult polycystic kidney disease (autosomal dominant)	29
Alport's syndrome (autosomal dominant — penetrant in males)	31
Fabry's syndrome (X-linked recessive)	31
Inherited tubular biochemical disorders (all autosomal recessive), e.g. cystinosis, oxalosis, cystinuria	28 / 25
Medullary cystic disease (variable inheritance)	29
Weaker predisposition	
Vesicoureteral reflux	21
Diabetic nephropathy (type I diabetes)	26
Renal stone disease	25
Urate nephropathy	24
Tuberculosis	31
Essential hypertension	12
Occasional familial incidence	
IgA glomerulonephritis	15

General appearance

In uraemia pallor with yellow-tinged (sallow) skin is characteristic, but can be missed in poor light. Acidotic hyperventilation (Kussmaul respiration) may be seen in severe uraemia.

Blood pressure

The blood pressure must always be measured, both lying and standing. Postural hypotension is one of the few physical findings in salt depletion, a feature of salt losing renal lesions (Table 5.2). Hypertension occurs in many renal diseases and can accelerate renal functional decline.

Skin and conjunctivae

These may show pallor indicating anaemia. Skin rashes occur in many systemic diseases with renal involvement, while bruising and scratch marks are common in uraemia.

Cardiovascular and respiratory systems

These should be checked for evidence of fluid overload or depletion. Fluid depletion may cause postural hypotension, tachycardia, a low jugular venous pressure (JVP) and poor tissue turgor. With fluid overload the JVP is elevated, and there may be basal crepitations in the lungs and peripheral oedema. Oedema may also be seen with the nephrotic syndrome and acute glomerulonephritis (Chapter 9). Occasionally pericarditis or pleurisy may be found in uraemia or connective tissue disease.

The kidneys

The kidneys are examined for tenderness, size, shape and the presence of vascular bruits. Each kidney is examined with one hand in the flank and one hand in the front, palpating the anterior abdomen upward from the iliac fossa and noting whether a renal mass can be detected on inspiration. It is usual in thin people to be able to feel the lower pole of the right (depressed by the liver) kidney but not the left. Enlarged kidneys are usually resonant to anterior percussion (though with massive kidneys occasionally the bowel will be displaced anteromedially, this often occurs with polycystic kidney disease) and move longitudinally up and down with respiration. Renal masses must be distinguished from liver and spleen.

The more common causes of grossly enlarged kidneys are given in Table 7.4. Mild enlargement is found in many renal diseases, including acute pyelonephritis, acute glomerulonephritis, compensatory enlargement, infiltration and hydronephrosis.

The bladder and genitalia

These should be examined, the first for urine retention with bladder distention, the second for congenital and acquired abnormalities of the urethra and genitalia (often associated with urinary tract abnormalities). A prostatic examination should be carried out in adult males.

The nervous system

There may be uremic tremor or flap, and peripheral neuropathy can occur with uraemia or systemic diseases (e.g. diabetes, arteritis, amyloidosis).

The fundi

Fundal examination may reveal haemorrhages and exudates in accelerated hypertension (Fig. 12.4) and in a variety of systemic diseases including diabetes, vasculitis and subacute bacterial endocarditis. In accelerated hypertension there may also be papilloedema.

Urinalysis and urine microscopy

Urinalysis is part of physical examination. The presence of protein, blood or glucose should be recorded. Microscopic examination of

Table 7.4 Causes of gross renal enlargement. The diagnosis should be obvious with renal ultrasound in all these conditions

Polycystic kidneys
Gross hydronephrosis
Renal tumour — primary or secondary
Massive staghorn calculus

a freshly voided urine specimen provides invaluable information about the underlying renal lesion (Chapter 8).

HAEMATURIA

Blood in the urine is one of the most important symptoms or signs of renal disease. The appearance of the urine depends on the site and severity of bleeding, and the pH of the urine.

Macroscopic haematuria is present if the blood is visible to the naked eye as discoloured urine. Blood in the urine is usually seen as red if the urine is alkaline, but in acid urine denaturation of the haemoglobin leads to brown urine, commonly described as weak tea (without milk) or 'Coca-Cola'. There are a variety of other causes of red or brown urine which may be distinguished by history, urine testing or urine microscopy (Table 7.5). In macroscopic haematuria the urine contains over 1 million RBC/ ml. Common causes of macroscopic haematuria are listed in Table 7.6.

Table 7.5 Causes of dark urine

	Colour	Hemastix	Microscopy
Endogenous pigments			
Haematuria (see Table 7.6)	Red or brown	++++ Granular	Red cells
Haemoglobinuria in haemolysis	Red or brown	++++ Diffuse	—
Myoglobinuria in muscle damage	Brown	++++ Diffuse	—
Bile in jaundice	Brown	— (Bile+)	—
Porphyrins in porphyria	Brown	—	—
Alkaptonuria after standing	Brown/black	—	—
Melanin in melanoma	Brown/black	—	—
Exogenous pigments			
Foods			
Beetroot	Red	—	—
Food dyes	Red	—	—
Drugs			
PAS	Red/brown	—	—
Phenolphthalein	Red/brown	—	—
Pyridium	Red	—	—

Table 7.6 Causes of macroscopic haematuria

Non-glomerular bleeding
Tumours — renal, bladder
Trauma
Stones — renal, ureteral, bladder
Urine infection
Renal infarction
Renal papillary necrosis

Glomerular bleeding
Primary glomerulonephritis (GN), particularly proliferative GN such as:
  IgA disease
  Poststreptococcal
  Mesangiocapillary GN

Secondary glomerulonephritis
  Goodpasture's syndrome
  Vasculitis
    polyarteritis
    Wegener's granulomatosis
    Henoch–Schönlein purpura
  Systemic lupus erythematosus
  Subacute bacterial endocarditis

Familial glomerular disease
  Alport's syndrome

Microangiopathic disease
  Haemolytic uraemic syndrome
  Thrombotic thrombocytopenia

Exertional haematuria

Microscopic haematuria is present when urine on testing is found to contain blood which is not apparent to the naked eye.

Blood clots indicate non-glomerular bleeding, and can be associated with renal or ureteral colic if the blood comes from the upper tract, or bladder outlet obstruction with clot retention with upper or lower tract bleeding. Stones, trauma, tumours and cysts are common causes of clot haematuria.

Initial or terminal haematuria, i.e. with blood being seen only at the beginning or end of the urine stream usually indicates bladder or urethral bleeding, whereas blood of renal or ureteral origin is usually mixed throughout the stream.

Painless haematuria is suggestive of tumour or glomerular bleeding, while pain is usually present with calculi, bleeding into cysts or severe urine infection.

Cloudy urine may be noted by some patients. Since amorphous phosphate debris or other crystals forming in concentrated urine can give a cloudy appearance, particularly in the initial urine of the morning, cloudiness which persists or appears later in the day is of greater significance.

Investigation of haematuria

Investigation should first confirm haematuria is present, then determine the cause.

Urine test strips

Urinary dipstix for detection of haematuria (e.g. Hemastix) are now widely available. These are sensitive to both haemoglobin and red blood cells in the urine.

False positive tests can occur with myoglobinuria and the presence of large amounts of ascorbic acid ('megavitamin therapy' with vitamin C) can reduce the sensitivity. Used in accord with the manufacturers instructions these tests are very sensitive. A trace or more of blood will be detected at around 5000–10 000 RBC/ml (phase contrast microscopy — see Chapter 8). A slightly different pattern, granular rather than diffuse, is found in haematuria when compared with haemoglobinuria or myoglobinuria.

Urine microscopy

The microscopic examination of a fresh midstream urine specimen (Chapter 8), preferably with phase contrast, is an essential part of the investigation of a patient with haematuria.

Using a counting chamber the concentration of red cells can be accurately determined. The upper limit of normal for red cells in the urine with light microscopy (not phase contrast) is about 1000 RBC/ml, however with phase contrast microscopy a great many cells not visible with light microscopy are detected, accordingly the upper limit of normal rises to around 8000 RBC/ml. If a counting chamber is not available more than about 2 cells per high power field on a plain glass slide with a cover slip usually indicates significant haematuria. This is neither a sensitive nor accurate way to assess the severity of haematuria.

Distinction of glomerular from non-glomerular haematuria

The next step is to distinguish where the blood is coming from. Evidence that bleeding is from the glomeruli is provided by the following.
- *Red cell casts* in the microurine (Fig. 8.4).
- *A polymorphic pattern of urinary red cells.* In most patients with glomerular haematuria the red cells in the urine appear in many different shapes on phase contrast microscopy. In non-glomerular bleeding only one to three populations of red cell shapes are found (Fig. 8.2). This distinction requires some skill on the part of the observer. Systems by which the distribution

of red cell sizes are plotted by Coulter counter are now being introduced.

• *Heavy proteinuria.* Though glomerular bleeding can occur with minimal proteinuria, significant proteinuria suggests glomerular bleeding. This is apparent if we consider that in glomerular bleeding protein leakage may exceed red cell leakage, while in other forms of urinary tract bleeding there will usually be loss of whole blood into the urine. If we assume a blood red blood cell count of 5×10^{12}/litre, a haematocrit of 45% and a plasma protein concentration of 80 g/litre, then 1 ml of blood contains 5×10^9 RBCs and 55% of 80 mg, i.e. 44 mg of protein. The effect of 1 ml of whole blood in a daily urine volume of 1 litre will be to raise the RBC count to 5 million RBC/ml, i.e. to apparent macroscopic haematuria, yet only elevate the urinary protein excretion by 44 mg/day, well within normal limits. Bleeding with whole blood will therefore not result in significant protein-uria until quite gross macroscopic haematuria is evident.

Further investigation   The cause of haematuria should always be determined. An IVP is usually the next step. With glomerular bleeding the final investi-gation is usually renal biopsy (Chapter 2), while in non-glomerular bleeding, cystoscopy, renal cytology and sometimes other forms of imaging are required.

PROTEINURIA

Patients almost never complain of proteinuria, since the only direct symptom is of urine frothing in the toilet bowl due to the action of protein in lowering surface tension. Since this is also seen with other detergents such as bile or toilet-cleanser it seldom in itself causes a patient to complain, though it is a useful part of the history since if it has been noticed it may help determine the date of onset of proteinuria. In severe proteinuria, usually greater than 3.5 g/24 hours, inadequate hepatic protein synthesis leads to hypoproteinaemia, and the patients will present with gross oedema and the nephrotic syndrome (Chapter 9). On the other hand testing of the urine for protein has now become part of normal physical examination, hence along with hypertension and microscopic haematuria this has become a common present-ing abnormality for asymptomatic patients with renal disease.

Mechanisms of proteinuria   There are four main mechanisms.

• *Excessive smaller proteins in the blood.* These can be filtered by the glomerulus if they are below MW about 60–70000, e.g. immunoglobulin light chains, haemoglobin and myoglobin.

- *Abnormally permeable glomerular filtration membrane*, due to perturbations of glomerular haemodynamics or glomerular disease. This is the usual cause of significant proteinuria.
- *Inadequate tubular resorption of normally filtered proteins*, i.e. those of MW < 60 000, i.e. polypeptides such as β_2 microglobulin, and polypeptide hormones (Chapter 4).
- *Secretion of Tamm−Horsfall protein* (urinary glycoprotein) by renal tubular cells.

Tests for proteinuria   The various tests employed to detect proteinuria and to determine the type of protein present are discussed in Chapter 8. Usually proteinuria is first detected by urinary reagent strips (dipstick testing) which are sensitive for albumin but much less so for Bence-Jones proteins. The severity is then assessed by quantification of total protein or albumin in a 24-hour collection of urine. In a few instances, such as childhood nephrotic syndrome (Chapter 9), Bence-Jones proteinuria and suspected tubular proteinuria, further tests to determine the nature of the proteins present may be employed.

Causes of proteinuria   Some of the many causes are listed in Table 7.7.

Haemodynamic causes   *Postural proteinuria*. This condition, otherwise known as orthostatic proteinuria, is very common in the young, being present in about 30% of children but only 5% of young adults. Characteristically mild proteinuria can be found when the patient has been upright for some time, as is usually the case when medical screening is carried out at school or for military service. However, if the urine is tested before the patient gets out of bed in the morning it is negative for protein. It is said that this proteinuria results from hepatic pressure on the inferior vena cava (IVC) in the upright or lordotic position causing a rise in renal vein pressure. There is little proof for this hypothesis.

Febrile, cardiac failure and other forms. Transient proteinuria occurs during acute illnesses of many kinds. Whether this is the result of haemodynamic changes in the glomerulus or due to actual transient structural damage is unknown. With exertion proteinuria is common, probably originating from similar mechanisms to postural proteinuria. With extreme exercise macroscopic glomerular haematuria can occur.

In fever it is quite possible that transient minor glomerular disease could occur since many infections can cause glomerulonephritis. In these cases the usual management is to monitor renal function until the proteinuria subsides. If renal function

Table 7.7 Causes of proteinuria

Abnormal protein load
Bence-Jones proteinuria
Myoglobinuria
Haemoglobinuria

Glomerular protein leak
due to increased glomerular permeability to proteins

Haemodynamic
  febrile proteinuria
  orthostatic proteinuria
  renal artery stenosis
  malignant hypertension
  cardiac failure

Glomerulonephritis — all forms

Other glomerular diseases
  diabetic glomerulopathy
  amyloidosis

Tubular proteinuria
due to failed tubular resorption especially of low MW polypeptides
Acute tubular necrosis
Tubulointerstitial disease
Analgesic nephropathy
Heavy metal poisoning
Fanconi's syndrome
Reflux nephropathy
Transplant rejection
Medullary cystic disease

Tamm—Horsfall proteinuria
due to excessive secretion of uromucoid
Chronic tubulointerstitial nephritis

Chronic renal failure
in which all the above mechanisms may play a role

deteriorates, haematuria occurs, or proteinuria persists, further investigation including renal biopsy is usually indicated. Persistent proteinuria does not occur in the absence of disease, though the disease may prove to be so insignificant that no other abnormalities will result.

Glomerular diseases With many cases of glomerular proteinuria there is also haematuria. There are some diseases, however, where proteinuria can be found either alone, or grossly out of proportion to associated haematuria (Table 9.3). Renal functional impairment and hypertension are two other markers that glomerular disease is present (Chapter 9).

Tubular proteinuria

In diseases which primarily attack the renal tubules, the tubular capacity to resorb filtered proteins, both albumin and low MW proteins, may be exceeded. Urinary protein electrophoresis will show an abnormally high concentration of low MW (5000–35 000 Da) proteins. Other tubular abnormalities such as a concentrating defect, renal glycosuria, renal tubular acidosis, renal amino aciduria and renal phosphaturia may be also found (Chapter 28).

Tamm–Horsfall proteinuria

In a variety of diseases affecting the tubules, such as obstructive and reflux nephropathies (Chapters 21 & 23) excessive amounts of this glycoprotein are found in the urine.

Chronic renal failure

Proteinuria, usually 1–2 g/day, is found in most patients with chronic renal failure. It is due to a combination of:
• failure of tubular resorption after the compensatory increase in SNGFR has resulted in greater albumin delivery to the tubule;
• haemodynamic changes associated with compensatory elevation of SNGFR (Chapter 6);
• structural glomerular abnormalities culminating in FGS (Chapter 6).

OEDEMA

There are many causes of generalised oedema (Table 7.8). In all forms of generalised oedema there must be an associated disturbance of renal physiology to result in salt and water retention, since there is always weight gain with increasing oedema and weight loss with improvement.

Table 7.8 Causes of generalised oedema

Cardiac failure

Liver failure

Renal oedema
Renal failure
Nephrotic syndrome
Mixed abnormalities (e.g. acute glomerulonephritis, pre-eclampsia)

Generalised capillary vasodilatation
Drugs — minoxidil, diazoxide
Liver failure, renal failure, pre-eclampsia
Sepsis

Oedema of uncertain aetiology
Idiopathic recurrent oedema (cyclical)
Diuretic dependent oedema

Mechanisms of oedema in renal disease

There are several ways in which renal disease can lead to salt and water retention.

• Renal failure can cause inadequate salt and water excretion (Chapter 6).

• Heavy proteinuria can lead to hypoalbuminaemia (Chapter 9) and consequent loss of intravascular fluid to the interstitium. Compensatory mechanisms, including the renin–angiotensin via aldosterone, and antidiuretic hormone (ADH) will then cause salt and water retention.

• Intrarenal mechanisms. Salt and water retention may occur secondary to intrarenal perturbations, particularly in glomerular disease. Decreased glomerular blood flow, decreased GFR, hypoalbuminaemia and increase in intratubular oncotic pressure can all, either directly or via intrarenal hormonal mechanisms, lead to decreased salt and water excretion.

• Congestive cardiac failure often complicates the picture, since hypertensive left ventricular failure and coronary artery disease often occur in patients with renal disease. In uraemia it is likely that generalised capillary vasodilation also plays a contributory role.

Clinical features of oedema due to renal disease

Renal oedema, whether due to renal failure or nephrotic syndrome, is usually generalised and pitting in nature, since the fluid can move freely in the interstitial space. The distribution of oedema depends on gravitational and other hydrostatic factors. For instance, in the nephrotic syndrome (Chapter 9) oedema is usually generalised but most marked in the lower extremities and as ascites, while in the nephritic syndrome (Chapter 9) there is characteristically periorbital and facial oedema. In diseases such as acute glomerulonephritis and chronic renal failure where hypertensive left ventricular failure is common, pulmonary interstitial oedema with pleural effusion may occur.

The first clinical step is to determine whether the oedema is primarily renal or not. Almost invariably there will be associated proteinuria. Cardiac and hepatic oedema are the commonest differential diagnoses and can usually be excluded on clinical grounds. In chronic renal failure the situation is of volume overload, and left ventricular dysfunction due to hypertension, anaemia, or accelerated coronary disease is often associated. In some cases of severe chronic renal failure the cardiac status cannot be reliably ascertained until the fluid overload is resolved by vigorous diuretic therapy or dialysis. Even then the anaemia of chronic renal failure can make minor cardiac dysfunction appear worse clinically.

Ward testing of the urine for protein and blood is essential in all patients with generalised oedema. The presence of significant proteinuria strongly suggests renal oedema, as does the presence of blood in the urine. It should be noted, however, that proteinuria can occur in other causes of oedema, e.g. cardiac failure, and rarely there may no proteinuria in patients with nephritis.

PAIN

Renal pain and ureteric colic

Renal pain is a feature of several diseases (Table 7.9). The main stimuli of the sympathetic pain fibres in the renal nerves appear to be distention of the renal pelvis or of the fibrous renal capsule. Renal pain can be poorly localised, but is usually felt in the loin, (i.e. in the angle between the last rib and sacrospinalis muscle), the flank or in the anterior hypochondrium.

Renal pain is common in acute pyelonephritis, pelviureteric obstruction and renal infarction. Capsular distention by renal tumour, acute glomerulonephritis and renal cysts (particularly if bleeding or infection is present) can also cause renal pain.

The term renal colic is often used to describe the pain of ureteric obstruction — which more properly should therefore be called ureteric colic.

Ureteric colic. Obstruction of the ureter by stone, papilla or clot usually causes pain in the loin radiating around the flank to the groin. If the ureteric orifice is the site of obstruction the pain may radiate to the testicle or vulva. Characteristically the pain is extremely severe, of sudden onset, and constant despite the term 'colic' (Chapter 25).

Table 7.9 Causes of renal pain

Urinary obstruction
Stone
Papilla
Blood clot
Tumour
Pelviureteric junction dyssynergia

Rapid renal swelling
Acute pyelonephritis
Bleeding into a renal cyst
Infection of a renal cyst
Renal tumour (primary or secondary)

Renal infarction
Renal arterial embolus
Acute renal arterial thrombosis
Acute renal vein thrombosis
Arteritis

When pain disappears in cases of urinary obstruction this does not necessarily mean the obstruction has resolved. In cases of complete and permanent obstruction the pain can resolve in only a few days, when the kidney ceases function. If this is unrecognised permanent renal damage can result, leading to a non-functioning kidney. In cases of gradual urinary obstruction (e.g. intra-ureteral tumour, bladder neck obstruction, retroperitoneal tumour or fibrosis) renal pain is often absent or minimal.

In patients with loin pain particular attention should be paid to coincidental haematuria (e.g. ureteral obstruction, renal cyst bleeding or infarction), and to dysuria or frequency (acute pyelonephritis). Low back and loin pain is frequently found in patients without renal disease, and is usually musculoskeletal.

Investigation of renal and ureteric pain

This should include urine microscopy and culture, renal function testing, and an intravenous pyelogram (IVP). The IVP is likely to show an abnormality in most cases of renal or ureteric pain. In an emergency situation, or when the IVP fails to visualise the kidney, renal ultrasound is very useful.

Bladder pain

Suprapubic pain can be a symptom of acute bladder distention or severe bladder wall inflammation.

Prostatic pain

In acute bacterial prostatis, pain may be felt in the perineum or rectum, often made worse by defecation.

VOIDING DISTURBANCES

Nocturia and polyuria are quite common in patients with renal disease but rarely cause patients to consult their doctor. Common disturbances of micturition include changes in the following.

Pattern of micturition

Nocturia is an important early symptom of renal insufficiency, reflecting the early concentrating defect. It is quite non-specific, being also found in insomnia, cardiac failure and bladder neck obstruction, but it is usually well remembered by patients and therefore may be useful to assess the chronicity of disease.

Urinary frequency can result in frequent small volumes being passed, as in cystitis, or in large volumes with polyuria. The distinction is important.

Nocturnal enuresis in children is usually not associated with significant renal or bladder disease, though it may be a marker of these.

Incontinence is important both medically and socially.

Volume of urine

Polyuria, with passage of large quantities of urine, can be difficult to distinguish from simple frequency, but is usually accompanied by excessive thirst.

Oliguria, is defined as the passage of less than 400 ml of urine per day. This is the minimal volume in which a person with normal renal function can excrete the normal daily osmotic load (Chapter 3).

Anuria or the passage of no urine, usually implies complete urinary obstruction or occasionally a fulminant intrarenal cause for acute renal failure (Chapter 10).

Ease of urination

Hesitancy, poor stream and postvoiding dribbling all suggest bladder outlet obstruction as in prostatomegaly.

Dysuria, pain or burning with or after voiding, is a symptom of urethral or bladder base irritation. By far the commonest cause is urine infection (Chapter 13).

8: *Examination of the Urine*

Examination of the urine is an intrinsic part of the routine examination of all patients with suspected renal disease; indeed dipstick testing for blood, protein and glucose is essential in the evaluation of all patients. Normal findings are summarised in Table 8.1.

COLLECTION OF URINE SPECIMEN

The urine specimen can be collected in several ways.

Fresh voided urine

A freshly collected random sample of urine is suitable for inspection and biochemical testing, but not for microscopy or culture.

Midstream urine collection

A properly collected midstream specimen of urine (MSU) is preferred for urine microscopy and culture. The morning urine is preferred because it is concentrated and any organisms have incubated overnight. The MSU is best collected from a full bladder, since this allows passage of at least 200 ml of urine, flushing the urethra of contaminant organisms which are normally found in the outer urethra, before collection of the urine specimen. It is important that the urine flow is continuous, with the collection container moved in and out of the stream, collecting at least 20 ml.

Table 8.1 Properties of normal urine

Colour	Pale yellow to amber	
Specific gravity (SG)	1.01–1.04	
pH	5–8	
Protein, glucose, blood	Negative	

Microscopy	Light	Phase contrast
Red cells	<1000/ml	<8000/ml*
White cells	<2000/ml	<2000/ml
Casts	Hyaline only	Hyaline only

* Centrifuged urine (<13 000/ml in uncentrifuged urine)

97

In women the labia are held apart with two fingers, after insertion of a tampon, and thorough washing of the vulva with clean tap water with no soap or detergent. It is best if the woman watches the urine to see that it passes directly from the urethra into the container. In males the foreskin should be retracted and the glans washed with clean water. In children, pregnant women, the obese, the elderly and those with poor understanding, supervision by a nurse may be helpful.

Ideally the urine is examined and cultured immediately. The urine can be stored for up to a few hours in a refrigerator at 4°C, but during this time a certain amount of damage to cells and casts can occur, particularly in hypotonic and alkaline urine. For culture the urine can be stored at 4°C for up to 24 hours and still give useful results.

Catheter specimen of urine

A catheter specimen of urine (CSU) should be used only in patients with indwelling catheters, those in whom a catheter is to be passed anyway, and occasionally in infirm or uncooperative patients. The disadvantages include:
- Discomfort.
- Cost.
- Risk of introducing infection/contaminants.

Instillation of 40 ml of 0.4% neomycin into the bladder before the catheter is removed decreases the risk of infection. In women the use of a short wide bore catheter with an end-orifice (Fig. 8.1), discarding the first 200 ml, reduces the risk of introducing contamination and provides a specimen almost as good as that obtained by suprapubic aspiration (SPA).

Suprapubic aspiration

Urine obtained by SPA is particularly useful for culture. In infants this is the most reliable method of obtaining a clean specimen.

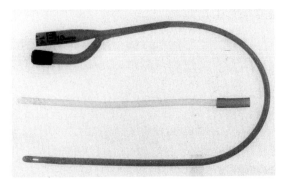

Fig. 8.1 Open ended small bore catheter (centre) compared with the conventional, larger, side holed, Foley catheter

Red cell contamination reduces the usefulness in urine microscopy.

The technique is simple and safe. The bladder should be very full. After cleaning and infiltration of the skin just above the pubic bone, a needle (lumbar puncture needle in adults, smaller needle in infants) is quickly inserted through the anterior abdominal wall into the bladder. Urine is then aspirated by syringe; usually the first 5—10 ml is discarded to eliminate skin contaminants, and then urine is taken for microscopy and culture. This urine should be sterile — any growth at all indicates urine infection (Chapter 13).

Full evaluation of the urine includes:
- Inspection.
- Chemical tests.
- Urine microscopy.
- Urine culture.

URINE INSPECTION

A freshly voided sample of urine should be inspected for colour, turbidity and odour (Table 8.2).

Table 8.2 Inspection of the urine

Colour (see also Table 7.5)
Brown urine
   bilirubin (conjugated in obstructive jaundice)
   blood and haemoglobin (in alkaline urine)
   myoglobin (in myolysis)
   porphyria (after urine has been standing)
   melanin (multiple melanoma)
   homogentisic acid (alkaptonuria)

Red urine
   blood and haemoglobin (in acid urine)
   pyridium (urinary tract analgesic)
   beetroot (beeturia)
   phenylalanine (in laxatives)
   some food dyes

Turbidity
Cloudy urine
   phosphate crystals
   urate crystals
   cells — white, red, bladder, vaginal

Odour
Ammonia
Ketones
Urine infection

Colour　　　　　　Usually fresh urine is pale to dark yellow or amber. While red-brown urine may be due to blood, there are a range of other causes (Table 7.5).

Turbidity　　　　　Cloudiness may be due to cells (haematuria, pyuria) or crystals (phosphate, urate). Crystalluria may occur in normal subjects in the concentrated urine passed in the morning. This can be cleared by adding acetic acid to the specimen.

Odour　　　　　　Heavily infected urine may have an unpleasant odour. An ammoniacal smell is due to bacterial degradation of urea, and is usual in specimens that have stood for any time. The smell of acetone may be obvious in diabetic ketoacidosis.

TESTS FOR PROTEINURIA

Chemical test strips　Urinary dipsticks (e.g. Albustix) to detect proteinuria are based on a change in the colour of buffered acid tetrabromphenol from yellow to green in the presence of protein — particularly albumin. Albumin is detected in the urine at a concentration of about 300 mg/litre. A semiquantitative scale is given up to about 20 g/litre. Trace amounts are therefore found in mild (about 200 mg/day) proteinuria and ++++ amount (over 20 g/litre) in nephrotic syndrome.

These test strips are much less sensitive to proteins other than albumin; hence such proteins as globulins, β_2-microglobulin, globulin light chains (Bence-Jones protein), and Tamm–Horsfall glycoprotein can be present in quite large amounts and not be detected by these reagent strips. This can be helpful, since they are all detected easily by other means and the discrepancy may suggest tubular proteinuria or myeloma.

Chemical strip tests for protein have, for practical purposes, superceded the older methods of sulphosalicylic acid precipitation or urine boiling. They are far more convenient, more specific for albuminuria, and are conveniently combined on the strip with tests for haematuria, glycosuria, pH, specific gravity and a wide variety of other abnormalities.

Sulphosalicylic acid　Eight drops of 20% sulphosalicylic acid are added to 2 ml of urine. A white precipitate indicates proteinuria. This test detects any form of proteinuria but is less specific than test strips. In particular radiocontrast agents in the urine give a positive test.

Urine boiling　　　Urine is heated in a test-tube after acidification with dilute acetic acid. Bence-Jones proteins will precipitate at 70°C and clear with continued heating. Albumin and other protein will remain as a precipitate. This test is now rarely used outside obstetric practice where it is used to give a semiquantitative index of proteinuria. It has largely been superceded by specific antibody tests for light chains in Bence-Jones proteinuria, though it is still a quick method for detecting their presence.

24-hour urine protein excretion

The most accurate method to determine whether significant proteinuria or albuminuria is present is to analyse a 24-hour collection. Because of inaccuracy of 24-hour collection it is wise to measure the 24-hour creatinine excretion since this should be constant (between 8−24 mmol/day) in a given patient. In some cases, where a 24-hour collection is inconvenient, a shorter timed urine collection can be taken and the protein content adjusted according to either time or the urine creatinine concentration.

More than 200 mg/day of urinary protein or 160 mg/day of urinary albumin is considered abnormal.

Tests for tubular proteinuria

The clearance of a low molecular weight protein, such as β_2-microglobulin (MW 11 600), can be used as an indicator of tubular damage since such proteins are handled by glomerular filtration and tubular resorption (Chapter 3).

Tests for selective proteinuria

In patients with heavy proteinuria the ratio of clearance of a large molecule (e.g. IgG, MW 146 000) to the clearance of a smaller molecule (e.g. transferrin, MW 88 000) can be used to determine the selectivity of glomerular proteinuria. Selective proteinuria (e.g. IgG clearance/transferrin clearance <0.2) is highly indicative of minimal change glomerulonephritis (Chapter 9) in children. This test has little value in adults.

OTHER CHEMICAL TESTS BY REAGENT STRIPS

Urine blood and haemoglobin

Blood or haemoglobin can be detected by reagent strips. Like proteinuria this is a common and important presenting abnormality in urinary tract disease, and has been discussed in Chapter 7. False positive tests occur with haemoglobinuria and myoglobinuria while vitamin C decreases the sensitivity.

Urine concentration

The specific gravity (SG) is measured by reagent strips or clinical hygrometer (Table 8.3). A first morning specimen is usually concentrated (SG > 1.020) while in chronic renal failure, diseases affecting the renal tubules and diabetes insipidus the urine has a SG of only 1.010 due to the concentrating defect (Chapter 3). Glucose and IVP dye increase the SG of urine.

Urine pH

Urinary pH varies throughout the day from about pH 5 to pH 8 (Table 8.4). It is more acid in the early morning (after overnight

Table 8.3 Specific gravity of urine (range 1.005–1.040)

High
Concentrated urine
Glycosuria
Recent IVP dye

Low
Dilute urine
Chronic renal failure
Renal tubular abnormality
Diabetes insipidus

respiratory depression with respiratory acidosis) and often alkaline after meals (alkaline tide). In renal tubular acidosis (Chapter 28) the urine pH cannot be reduced below 5.4 even with an acid load, while with urine infection due to *Proteus* spp. the splitting of urea leads to alkaline urine (Chapter 25). Acid urine predisposes to uric acid and cystine calculi while alkaline urine accelerates formation of triple phosphate stones (Chapter 25).

Other urine dipstick tests

Glucose, bile and phenylketones are other substances which are now readily detected with various dipsticks. Glycosuria can occur in renal tubular disorders due to failure of glucose resorption. With aspirin ingestion the test for phenylketones becomes positive — this can be useful in the diagnosis of analgesic nephropathy (Chapter 22).

URINE MICROSCOPY

Careful microscopy of the urine is an essential part of the evaluation of all patients with suspected urinary tract disease, and is best carried out on a freshly collected MSU.

Table 8.4 pH of urine (normal pH range 5–8)

Acid urine
Acidosis
  metabolic (non-renal)
  respiratory
Phenylketonuria, alkaptonuria
Severe chloride depletion

Alkaline urine
Alkalosis (non-renal)
Renal tubular acidosis
Carbonic anhydrase-inhibiting drugs
Primary aldosteronism
Urine infection with urea-splitting organisms

Centrifugation
To concentrate the urine cells and casts it is usual to centrifuge the urine and examine the freshly suspended sediment. Usually 10 ml of urine is spun at around 2000 rpm for 10 min, 9.5 ml removed and the sediment gently resuspended in the remaining 0.5 ml. Quantitative counting is then possible, since the sediment has been concentrated 20 times. On the other hand if there are large numbers of cells or casts it is better to examine an un-centrifuged sample since centrifugation leads to loss of some cells on the side of the centrifuge tube, and casts can be disrupted by vigorous resuspension.

Wet film microscopy
Urine is usually examined without staining. Phase contrast microscopy is more sensitive than ordinary light microscopy, but is not always available. The urine can be examined as a wet film on an ordinary microscopy slide, in which case quantitation is not possible, though vague assessments such as 'over 10 red cells per high-power field' can be made. A counting chamber (Fuchs–Rosenthal) is preferable, since then the number of cells seen can be expressed in terms of 'cells per ml of urine'.

Urinary red cells
Normal urine contains less than 1000 RBC/ml and 2000 WBC/ml in a MSU collection examined under ordinary light microscopy. Phase contrast microscopy increases the sensitivity considerably, and red cell counts of up to about 8000 RBC/ml can be found in normal individuals (Table 8.1).

Excessive numbers of red cells in the urine can occur in a wide variety of conditions (Table 7.6 lists the causes of macroscopic haematuria). The investigation of haematuria has been discussed in Chapter 7. It is important to distinguish glomerular from non-glomerular bleeding, both because the causes and the diagnostic approach differ. Using phase contrast microscopy, urinary red cells in cases of glomerular bleeding vary in shape and size ('poly-morphic'), while in non-glomerular bleeding only one to three populations of red cells are seen (Fig. 8.2). Red cell casts (see below) only occur with glomerular bleeding.

Urinary white cells
Over 2000 leucocytes/ml in an MSU is abnormal (Fig. 8.3). Leuco-cytes are commonly seen in the urine in urinary tract infection (Chapter 13) and a variety of other conditions (Table 13.4).

Urinary casts
Urinary casts (Fig. 8.4) are formed in the tubules of the kidney, by aggregation of Tamm–Horsfall (Chapter 7) and other urinary proteins with other constituents of tubular fluid such as red cells, leucocytes or tubular cells.
● *Hyaline casts* are found in normal urine. They are glassy trans-parent cylinders which dissolve in alkaline urine.

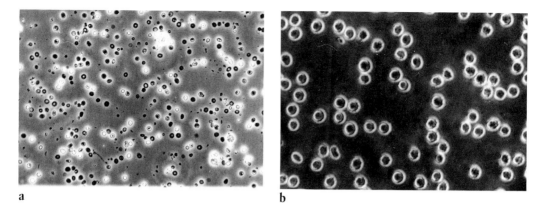

a   b

Fig. 8.2 Red cells seen in urine (phase contrast). (a) Glomerular haematuria. Cells of many shapes and sizes (magnification ×50). (b) Non-glomerular haematuria. Red cells of only one or two populations of size and shape (magnification ×100)

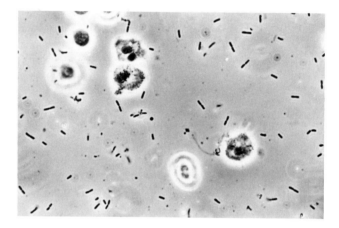

Fig. 8.3 Leucocytes and bacteria in bacterial cystitis (magnification ×200)

- *Red cell casts* occur with glomerular bleeding, and are therefore pathognomonic of glomerulonephritis.
- *White cell casts* composed of leucocytes attached to hyaline casts, occur in pyelonephritis and other causes of renal interstitial inflammation.
- *Epithelial cell casts* contain tubular cells and may be seen in acute tubular necrosis.
- *Granular casts* contain amorphous debris, resultant upon break-down of the cells in white cell or epithelial cell casts.
- *Waxy casts* are thought to be degenerate granular casts.
- *Broad casts* are hyaline casts of larger tubules seen in renal failure.

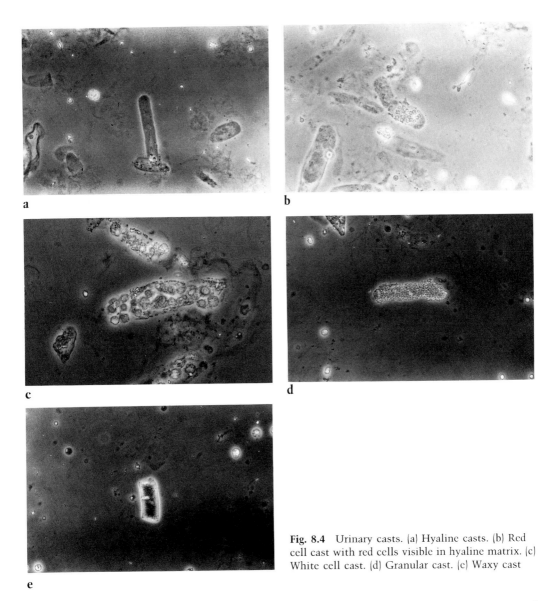

Fig. 8.4 Urinary casts. (a) Hyaline casts. (b) Red cell cast with red cells visible in hyaline matrix. (c) White cell cast. (d) Granular cast. (e) Waxy cast

- *The 'telescoped urine'* of lupus nephritis contains a mixture of virtually all types of casts.

Crystals

Crystals of many types may be seen in the urine (Fig. 8.5). The presence of the hexagonal 'benzene ring' crystals of cystinuria provide an instant diagnosis of cystinuria (Chapter 25).

Fat bodies

Oval fat bodies, which show as Maltese crosses when examined under polarised light (Fig. 8.6), occur in the nephrotic syndrome (Chapter 9), and are associated with the hyperlipidaemia.

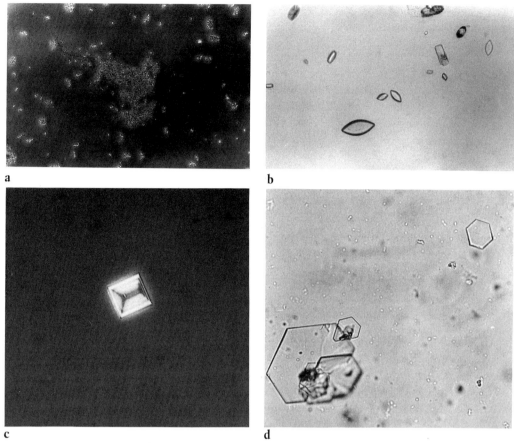

Fig. 8.5 Urinary crystals. (a) Amorphous phosphates. (b) Uric acid — red rhombic prisms. (c) Oxalate 'Envelopes'. (d) Cystine 'Benzene ring' shapes

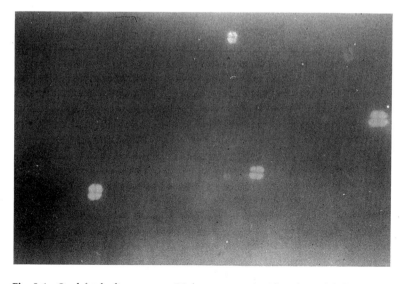

Fig. 8.6 Oval fat bodies seen as 'Maltese crosses' with polarised light

URINE CULTURE

Quantitative urine culture is important in the management of urinary tract infection (Chapter 13). Since the quantitation is performed by counting the number of colonies of organisms growing on an agar plate the results should be expressed as colony forming units per ml (cfu/ml) rather than organisms/ml. The interpretation of MSU culture results is covered in Chapter 13. Although simple dipstick or other tests for bacterial infection are available they are not sufficiently accurate other than for use in screening or in following patients with recurrent UTI.

9: *Syndromes of Glomerular Disease*

Diseases of the glomeruli can result in a limited range of clinical abnormalities:
- Proteinuria.
- Haematuria.
- Deranged renal function, i.e. hypertension, oedema or renal failure.

The approach to patients presenting with each of these abnormalities has been discussed in Chapter 7. Before renal biopsy was available it was obvious that certain clinical syndromes existed in which some or all of these abnormalities were present with differing severity. This method of classifying glomerular disease is very useful clinically, since there is a limited number of diseases likely to cause each of them.

The common syndromes are:

1 The nephrotic syndrome.
2 The acute nephritic syndrome.
3 Rapidly progressive nephritis — a particularly severe form of acute nephritic syndrome.
4 Macroscopic haematuria — often recurrent.
5 Chronic glomerulonephritis.

NEPHROTIC SYNDROME

Synonyms include: nephrosis, acute or chronic.

Features of the nephrotic syndrome

The cardinal features are (Table 9.1):
- Heavy proteinuria.
- Hypoalbuminaemia.
- Generalised oedema.
- Hyperlipidaemia.

Hypercoagulability is also commonly present.

Proteinuria

Urinary protein excretion usually exceeds 3.5 g/day in adults or 0.05 g/kg/day in children. This is the fundamental pathophysiological abnormality, and is due to increased glomerular membrane permeability. Albumin (MW 69 000) is the most abundant protein in the urine. There are also smaller amounts of other proteins

Table 9.1 The nephrotic syndrome — a summary

CARDINAL FEATURES
Proteinuria >3.5 g/day
Hypoalbuminaemia <30 g/litre
Generalised oedema
Hyperlipidaemia
(Hypercoagulability)

COMMON CAUSES
Children:
Minimal change glomerulonephritis (GN) — 80%
Focal and segmental glomerulosclerosis (FGS)
Membranoproliferative GN
Poststreptococcal GN

Adults:
Primary GN
    membranous GN
    minimal change GN
    focal and segmental glomerulosclerosis (FGS)
    membranoproliferative GN
Secondary GN
    systemic lupus erythematosus
    drugs (gold, penicillamine, captopril, non-steroidal anti-inflammatory
        drugs)
    neoplasm
Systemic disease affecting glomeruli
    diabetes
    amyloidosis

DIAGNOSIS
Children:
If minimal haematuria and selective proteinuria — trial of steroids
If atypical — renal biopsy

Adults:
Renal biopsy

COMPLICATIONS
Acute renal failure
Thrombosis
Infection
Malnutrition

MANAGEMENT
Determine cause (renal biopsy in all adults)
Treat oedema
Improve nutrition
Prevent infection
Consider anticoagulation
Treat cause

such as IgG (MW 146 000). Very large molecules such as IgM (MW 900 000) and fibrinogen (MW 340 000) are absent.

The enhanced glomerular permeability is the result of abnormalities in the size and charge selective barriers of the glomerular capillary wall (Chapter 3). Fusion or effacement (or spreading) of the foot processes of the epithelial cells is seen with electron microscopy in all causes of the nephrotic syndrome. There is controversy as to whether this is a cause or consequence of increased albumin permeability.

Hypoalbuminaemia

The majority of the protein in the urine is albumin and consequently, once hepatic synthetic rate is exceeded, hypoalbuminaemia results. It is not clear what the actual rate of glomerular loss of albumin is, since some tubular resorption and catabolism takes place. The loss of albumin from plasma therefore exceeds the amount found in the urine. Hepatic synthesis is usually increased, but insufficiently to maintain a normal plasma albumin level.

Generalised oedema

Generalised oedema is the result of salt and water retention. In adults weight gains of 20–30 kg can occur. The mechanisms for oedema in renal disease have been discussed in Chapter 7. At least two mechanisms are important in nephrotic syndrome:
1 There is albumin loss into the glomerular filtrate. Intrarenally this results in a reduction in postglomerular plasma oncotic pressure, with an increase in the albumin concentration and oncotic pressure in the tubule. This then alters glomerulotubular balance with consequent salt and water retention, by poorly understood intrarenal mechanisms.
2 Hypoalbuminaemia results in loss of fluid to the peripheral interstitial spaces. The theory that this usually leads to hypovolaemia with consequent activation of neurohumeral and haemodynamic mechanisms signalling the kidney to retain salt and water is not supported by recent studies which show that usually blood volume is not reduced and plasma renin, aldosterone, antidiuretic hormone and noradrenaline are not elevated in most cases of nephrosis.

Hyperlipidaemia

Richard Bright noted in 1836 that the serum is often milky and opaque in his classic description of patients with renal disease. Accordingly hyperlipidaemia is regarded as constituting one of the essential features of the nephrotic syndrome. Hypercholesteraemia is the most prominent lipid abnormality, though increased phospholipid and triglyceride concentrations also occur.

The mechanism for hyperlipidaemia is complex and poorly understood. It is possible that it contributes to an increased risk of arterial thrombosis in chronic nephrotic syndrome.

Hypercoagulability

There is a greatly increased risk of venous and arterial thrombosis in nephrotic syndrome. Contributing factors include:
• Increased plasma coagulation factors, particularly Factor 8.
• Increased plasma fibrinogen (a large molecule which does not enter the urine).
• Variably increased plasma viscosity.
• Probable accelerated atheroma due to hyperlipidaemia.
This varies with different causes of the nephrotic syndrome. Renal vein thrombosis is particularly common in membranous glomerulonephritis (Chapter 15).

Causes of the nephrotic syndrome

The list of recorded causes of the nephrotic syndrome is enormous and only a few are given in Table 9.2. To put this in context:
• *In the adult* about 80% are due to a glomerulonephritis of unknown cause, and most of the rest are associated with systemic disease, particularly systemic lupus erythematosus, diabetes and amyloidosis. Membranous glomerulonephritis is the single commonest lesion.
• *In the child* about 70% of nephrosis is due to minimal change disease, 15% to primary focal and segmental glomerulosclerosis (FGS) and less than 10% secondary to systemic or other diseases.

Clinical features of the nephrotic syndrome

Severe generalised oedema is characteristic. The legs are most severely affected but truncal and facial oedema is common, and ascites and pleural effusions are sometimes present. The onset can be abrupt, particularly in children. Such patients often notice oliguria with the passage of small amounts of dark urine. A more insidious onset of oedema is common in adults. In children facial oedema and ascites may be prominent, and an occasional child suffers severe abdominal pain perhaps due to liver capsular distention or gut ischaemia. Nowadays primary peritonitis (see below) is rare. In adults the emphasis is usually on oedema of the legs and genitalia, perhaps because they are less likely to be in bed. Frothy urine due to the heavy proteinuria may be noticed.

Complications of the nephrotic syndrome

Complications include:
• Acute renal failure.
• Vascular thrombosis.
• Infection.
• Protein–calorie malnutrition.

Table 9.2 Causes of nephrotic syndrome (common causes in italic)

PRIMARY GLOMERULAR DISEASE
Minimal change disease — 70% of children, 20% of adults
Membranous glomerulonephritis
Focal and segmental glomerulosclerosis (FGS)
Membranoproliferative GN
Diffuse proliferative GN

ASSOCIATED WITH SYSTEMIC DISEASE — 20% of adults
Systemic lupus erythematosus
Diabetic nephropathy
Amyloidosis
Henoch–Schönlein purpura

DRUGS AND TOXINS
Gold
Penicillamine
Captopril
NSAIDs
Phenindione, tridione
Mercurial diuretics
Bee stings
Serum sickness
Heroin

NEOPLASMS — especially in elderly people
Carcinoma — breast, bronchus, colon
Lymphoma
Leukaemia

INFECTIONS — especially in developing countries
Malaria
Poststreptococcal
Hepatitis B
AIDS
Syphilis
Schistosomiasis
Infected ventriculoatrial shunts

PRE-ECLAMPSIA AND ECLAMPSIA

VASCULAR
Malignant hypertension
Renal artery stenosis
Constrictive pericarditis

GENETIC
Congenital nephrosis (Finnish)
Alport's syndrome

Acute renal failure   Although acute renal failure is uncommon it can occur due to:

Reduction in effective plasma volume. If effective plasma volume is reduced, this may cause renal hypoperfusion and prerenal failure or acute tubular necrosis (Chapter 11). This may be precipitated by diuretic therapy, or by the administration of drugs which interfere with intrarenal mechanisms maintaining glomerular and tubular perfusion such as angiotensin-converting enzyme inhibitors (captopril, enalapril) blocking the renin–angiotensin system or non-steroidal anti-inflammatory drugs (NSAIDs) (indomethacin, ibuprofen, etc.) blocking production of vasodilator prostanoids (Chapter 11).

The underlying disease process. Heavy proteinuria can occur in rapidly progressive glomerulonephritis. In such cases macroscopic haematuria is usually present. Another example, becoming increasingly common, is in NSAID-induced nephrotic syndrome where acute nephrosis, with minimal glomerular abnormality, is often associated with acute tubular necrosis due either to acute interstitial nephritis or the concomitant prostaglandin inhibition mentioned above.

Acute renal vascular thrombosis, usually of the renal vein.

Vascular thrombosis   The hypercoagulable state is associated with an increased incidence of:
- Renal vein thrombosis.
- Peripheral renin thrombosis and thromboembolism.
- Peripheral arterial thrombosis.
     The risk of these complications is sufficient to justify oral anti-coagulants in all adult nephrotics presuming no contra-indication is present.

Renal vein thrombosis occurs in 5–50% of cases of membranous GN in different series. It is also seen, but less commonly, in membranoproliferative GN, renal amyloid and minimal change GN. It is now clear that renal vein thrombosis is a consequence, not a cause, of nephrotic syndrome.
     Clinically there are two types of renal vein thrombosis:
1 *Acute renal vein thrombosis.* Severe loin pain, macroscopic haematuria and abrupt decline in renal function occur, signifying partial or complete renal infarction. This usually occurs in the young, and good results have been reported after treatment with anticoagulants or even thrombolytic agents.
2 *Chronic renal vein thrombosis* is usually seen in the adult

with long standing nephrotic syndrome. It may be suggested by increasing proteinuria, perhaps the appearance of haematuria, and decreasing renal function. The insidious character is related to the development of large venous collaterals.

The diagnosis of renal vein thrombosis depends on renal venography, however since thrombosis of only one or more branches rather than the main renal vein is common it is often necessary to combine venography with injection of adrenaline into the renal artery to delay venous washout and allow dye to ascend intrarenal vessels. Renal biopsy may show marginated leucocytes in the glomeruli and interstitial oedema. Rarely a thrombosed vein will be in the biopsy tissue.

Peripheral venous thrombosis particularly affecting the iliac and axillary veins also occurs commonly in the adult, and may be associated with pulmonary thromboembolism.

Peripheral arterial thrombosis — coronary, mesenteric, femoral and other arteries can result in acute infarction.

Infection

Before the widespread use of penicillin, diuretics and effective therapy for minimal change disease, many of the deaths in acute nephrotic syndrome in children were due to primary pneumococcal peritonitis and pneumonia. Cellulitis and pneumonia remain common. The reasons for increased infection include IgG loss in the urine and protein–calorie malnutrition. Prophylactic penicillin, and pneumococcal vaccination may be indicated in the very young and elderly patients with severe or recurrent nephrosis.

Protein-calorie malnutrition

The heavy urinary protein loss places extra demands on a metabolism which already may be quite compromised. Anorexia due to decreased gut perfusion, visceral and hepatic oedema, and a feeling of distention with marked ascites is common and patients, particularly children and elderly people, may eat poorly. Slightly abnormal liver function tests may be present, presumably due to oedema and decreased perfusion.

In prolonged nephrotic syndrome, muscle wasting, loss of hair and development of transverse white lines (Muerke's) on the nails and thin skin with prominent striae attest to the occurrence of malnutrition. The risk of overwhelming infection is greatly increased in the worst cases.

Clinical approach to the nephrotic syndrome

The management of the nephrotic syndrome consists of:
• Diagnosis of nephrotic syndrome.
• Diagnosis of the cause of the nephrotic syndrome.

- Treatment of the cause.
- Treatment of the syndrome.

Diagnosis of the nephrotic syndrome

Diagnosis of nephrotic syndrome depends upon confirming the presence of severe proteinaemia and hypoalbuminaemia. Haematuria or impaired renal function may also be present in some cases; this considerably alters the likely cause (see below).

Proteinuria is virtually always over 3.5 g/day even when plasma albumin has fallen to very low levels. Dipstick testing should show ++++ albuminuria.

Hypoalbuminaemia should be present, but sometimes is only mild. It can be severe, with a plasma albumin concentration as low as 10 to 20 g/litre. Immunoglobulins are also lost, particularly IgG, and there may be a fall in γ-globulins with a relative rise in α and β-globulins.

Plasma calcium is depressed out of proportion to the fall in plasma albumin. This is believed to be due to concurrent depression of 1-hydroxylation of 25-OH vitamin D_3 (Chapter 3).

Hyperlipidaemia is usual, and seems to relate to the severity of hypoproteinaemia.

Diagnosis of the cause of nephrotic syndrome

Urine microscopy. Glomerular haematuria may be present. If red cells are present in large numbers they reduce the chance that the conditions in which haematuria is often not prominent, such as minimal change disease, will occur (Table 9.3). Oval fat bodies are often present.

Renal failure may be present, though not usually in minimal change disease (Chapter 15).

Renal biopsy. In adults, although a likely cause may be apparent virtually all patients with the nephrotic syndrome should have a

Table 9.3 Causes of the nephrotic syndrome in which haematuria may be minimal. In focal and segmental glomerulosclerosis and early membranous glomerulonephritis, nephrosis with minimal haematuria can also occur

Minimal change disease
Diabetic nephropathy
Amyloidosis
Pre-eclampsia

renal biopsy for histological diagnosis, to aid in further investigation, to dictate treatment and to enable a reasonable estimate of prognosis. Investigations to detect diabetes, SLE and other diseases associated with the syndrome (Table 9.2) are usually performed first, but in most cases a renal biopsy will be required eventually.

In children the usual course is to assume the patient has minimal change disease and give a trial of steroid therapy (Chapter 15). Investigation in children should include an assessment of the selectivity of proteinuria, usually comparing the ratio of IgG clearance to that of transferrin. A ratio less than 0.2 usually indicates minimal change disease, one greater than 0.3 is generally inconsistent with this diagnosis. Biopsy is usually only performed if prednisolone fails to produce a remission in 3 weeks, or if significant haematuria, renal functional impairment, hypertension or non-selective proteinuria is present. In frequently relapsing nephrotic syndrome a biopsy is also usually performed.

Treatment of the nephrosis

The aims of treatment of the nephrotic patient are to:
- treat oedema,
- improve nutrition,
- prevent infection, and
- prevent thrombosis,

until the nephrotic state resolves, either spontaneously or because of specific treatment of the glomerular lesion.

Treatment of oedema. Generalised oedema can cause great discomfort, with severe leg swelling, a feeling of bloating and even dyspnoea. Such oedema should be treated. However, there is little to gain in treating mild asymptomatic oedema — the aim of treatment should be only to relieve symptoms, not to improve the appearance. Great care needs to be taken to minimise decrease in intravascular filling, since acute renal failure can be precipitated by over-enthusiastic diuretic therapy in the presence of persisting heavy proteinuria.

Occasionally bed rest or pressure stockings will be required, particularly in the elderly people in whom very gross leg oedema is sometimes seen, presumably due to associated venous insufficiency. In this situation blistering and cellulitis can occur if oedema persists. A close watch should be kept on the indices of intravascular filling — particularly on jugular venous pressure and postural drop in blood pressure.

A weight chart should always be kept, and if the patient is hospitalised there should be a record of fluid balance. A weight and fluid loss of about 0.5–1.0 kg/day is usually aimed for.

Plasma potassium, sodium, creatinine and urea levels should be monitored and potassium supplements may be required.

The usual diuretic regimen is to commence with either a mild diuretic such as a thiazide or a low dose of frusemide. Diuretic therapy can be gradually increased as required. A salt restricted diet is usual and occasionally fluid restriction may be necessary.

There is only a limited place for the use of intravenous albumin in the treatment of oedema. Occasionally it is needed in refractory cases, particularly when intravascular volume is deplete or oliguria is present. Usually 100 ml of 25% albumin is given. This usually results in an increase in urine volume, and a great increase in proteinuria associated with the temporary increase in plasma protein.

Prevention of malnutrition. A high calorie, low salt diet is recommended. There is no evidence that a high protein diet is of value, and it may even be deleterious in the presence of renal failure. A reasonable compromise is to advise 50−60 g/day of good quality protein plus urinary losses.

Prevention and early treatment of infection. Pneumococcal infection is particularly likely. Prophylactic penicillin is given to children, and in relapsing nephrotic syndrome, pneumococcal vaccination should be considered.

Prevention of thromboembolism. It is reasonable to anticoagulate all adults with severe nephrotic syndrome unless a contraindication exists. Most patients should be maintained on such therapy (usually with warfarin) until the nephrotic syndrome has resolved.

Treatment of the cause of the nephrotic syndrome

As mentioned previously a trial of steroid treatment constitutes part of the diagnostic process in children, where a response is regarded as diagnostic of minimal change disease. A similar approach is not generally recommended in adults, where minimal change disease is the cause of only 10−20% of cases of nephrosis. In other cases the treatment is tailored to the diagnosis and its underlying cause.

THE ACUTE NEPHRITIC SYNDROME

Synonyms include: nephritic syndrome and acute nephritis.

Features of the acute nephritic syndrome

The features are (Table 9.4) a sudden onset of:
- Haematuria — often macroscopic.
- Oliguria.

Table 9.4 Acute nephritic syndrome — a summary

Cardinal features
Acute illness characterised by:
  macroscopic haematuria
  oliguria
  hypertension
  oedema — mild to moderate
  mild proteinuria — usually <3.5 g/day

Common causes
usually proliferative glomerulonephritis (GN)
Primary GN
  poststreptococcal GN — particularly in children and developing countries
  idiopathic diffuse proliferative GN
  IgA disease
  membranoproliferative GN
Secondary GN
  Goodpature's syndrome
  Systemic lupus erythematosus
  vasculitis:
    polyarteritis
    Wegener's granulomatosis
    Henoch–Schönlein purpura
Microangiopathic diseases
  haemolytic uraemic syndrome
  thrombotic thrombocytopenia (TTP)

Complications
Hypertension
  encephalopathy, convulsions
  cerebral haemorrhage
Left ventricular failure
Oliguric renal failure — rapidly progressive GN
Progression to chronic renal disease

Management
Determine the cause — usually renal biopsy unless clinically typical
  poststreptococcal GN
Treat hypertension
Prevent salt and water overload
Treat renal failure
Treat the cause

- Hypertension.
- Proteinuria — usually mild.
- Oedema — usually mainly facial.

In some patients one or more of these features may be absent.

Haematuria is due to glomerular membrane damage with leakage of red cells. In most cases a proliferative form of glomerulonephritis is present and glomerular crescents may occur. Occasionally red cells can be seen in Bowman's space but rarely are actual breaks seen in the basement membrane.

Oliguria with less than 400 ml per day of urine is usual. There is usually reduced GFR due to the glomerular disease and increased tubular sodium and water resorption.

Hypertension is mainly the result of sodium retention, though hormonal mechanisms may also be involved.

Oedema results mainly from enhanced tubular fluid resorption. The urine is usually highly concentrated with a high SG and osmolarity and a low sodium concentration. Characteristically the face is mainly involved.

Causes of the acute nephritic syndrome

This is a very recognisable syndrome, the prototype for which is poststreptococcal glomerulonephritis — the commonest cause in children. In adults poststreptococcal disease is less common, and the prognosis is not necessarily as good. Most of the causes (Table 9.5) are associated with some form of proliferative change in the glomeruli. Because this syndrome may lead to rapidly progressive glomerulonephritis (see below) and hence to renal failure, a determined effort to find a treatable cause should always be made, and the patient watched closely until resolution has occurred.

Clinical features of the acute nephritic syndrome

The important clinical features are an acute onset of usually macroscopic haematuria, oliguria, and mild oedema in a patient who is then found to have a high blood pressure and usually mild to moderate proteinuria.

In the worst cases renal failure will be present. Since these represent a medical emergency we have chosen to cover them later under the term 'rapidly progressive glomerulonephritis'. There is a continuum between acute nephritis and rapidly progressive glomerulonephritis, and all patients could potentially belong to the worse group.

Commonly 2 weeks after a sore throat or other infection the patient suffers an acute onset of:

• *Macroscopic haematuria* which may be dark ('Coca-Cola') or smokey. Glomerular red cells (Chapter 8) and red cell casts are present.

• *Oliguria*, with less than 400 ml of urine per day, is usual, although the patient may not have noticed it. In the most severe cases anuria can occur.

• *Oedema* is usually mild and commonly seen in the face and periorbitally.

Table 9.5 Causes of the acute nephritic syndrome

Postinfectious glomerulonephritis (GN)
Poststreptococcal GN
Poststaphylococcal
Bacterial endocarditis
Postviral

Idiopathic proliferative glomerulonephritides
Idiopathic diffuse proliferative GN
IgA disease
Membranoproliferative GN

Systemic lupus erythematosus

Vasculitis
Polyarteritis
Wegener's granulomatosis
Henoch–Schönlein purpura

Goodpastures syndrome

Microangiopathic glomerular disease
Haemolytic–uraemic syndrome
Thrombotic thrombocytopenia (TTP)
Scleroderma
Malignant hypertension
Pre-eclampsia
Radiation nephritis
Renal transplant rejection

Other antigens
Serum sickness
Bee stings

- *Hypertension* can be severe. This, combined with the fluid retention, may cause left ventricular failure with dyspnoea (worse because of associated anaemia), orthopnea and in some cases pulmonary oedema. In children it is critical to remember that the normal blood pressure is quite low and a blood pressure of 120/70 mmHg can represent a severe hypertension. Fundal examination for signs of hypertensive retinopathy (Chapter 12) and cardiovascular examination for left ventricular strain, cardiomegaly and left ventricular failure are important.
- *Proteinuria*, which is usually less than 3.5 g/day, although occasionally in the nephrotic range, when a mixed nephritic–nephrotic illness is said to be present. Rarely proteinuria may be absent.

General symptoms are prominent, with fatigue and malaise. Loin pain, attributed to renal capsular swelling, is present in some cases, and the kidneys may be swollen and tender to palpation.

Complications of the acute nephritic syndrome

The complications are due to severe fluid retention, hypertension, or renal failure (Table 9.6). The renal prognosis depends on the cause (Table 9.5).

In children the prognosis is good, but death may occur (due usually to left heart failure with pulmonary oedema or to cerebral haemorrhage, rather than renal failure). In adults the renal prognosis is not as favourable. In children 90% of cases are followed by complete resolution, while this occurs in only about 50% of adults. The unfavourable outcomes include rapidly progressive glomerulonephritis with rapid progress to renal failure, or the illness may resolve incompletely to a syndrome of persisting hypertension, proteinuria and microscopic haematuria, i.e. chronic glomerulonephritis, with eventual decline in renal function.

Clinical approach to the acute nephritic syndrome

Management of the patient presenting with some or all of the features of the acute nephritic syndrome is based upon:
1 Diagnosis of acute nephritic syndrome.
2 Determination of the cause.
3 Management of the syndrome.
4 Treatment of the cause.

Table 9.6 Complications of the acute nephritic syndrome

Left heart failure
due to hypertension and fluid retention

Cerebral complications of hypertension
Cerebral haemorrhage
Hypertensive encephalopathy
Cerebral oedema
Convulsions

Acute oliguric renal failure
Rapidly progressive GN
Occasionally acute tubular necrosis

Failure of complete resolution
With subsequent:
Hypertension
Chronic glomerulonephritis
Nephrotic syndrome
Chronic renal failure

Complications of the underlying condition
such as complications of SLE or vasculitis

Diagnosis of acute
nephritic syndrome

Urinalysis. Heavy glomerular haematuria is present. Usually with macroscopic haematuria ++++ blood will be found on strip testing. Quantitative phase contrast urine microscopy is invaluable (Chapter 8). Over 10^5/ml glomerular red cells are usually seen in the urine. The cells are of multiple shapes and sizes (Fig. 8.2), and red cell casts are often found (Fig. 8.3).

Proteinuria is almost invariably associated, and may range from only 500 mg/day to nephrotic range proteinuria. Dipstick testing will show + or more. The urine is usually highly concentrated, particularly in the first few days of the disease. A high specific gravity with a low urinary sodium is usual. Should the disease progress to chronic renal failure the ability to concentrate the urine will gradually be lost.

A fluid-balance chart with monitoring of urine output will confirm oliguria. In the worst cases oliguria can be severe, and even anuria can occur. The fluid retention may be also reflected in dilutional hypoproteinaemia and anaemia, though both can occur for other reasons.

Impaired renal function. Although plasma creatinine and urea may not be raised above normal, the GFR or creatinine clearance is always reduced, sometimes drastically as in rapidly progressive disease.

Diagnosis of the
cause of acute
nephritic syndrome

Since poststreptococcal glomerulonephritis is commonly the cause in children and, systemic diseases such as SLE and vasculitis are frequently the cause in adults, special efforts are directed toward these diagnoses. After a full history and examination, in which particular emphasis should be placed on sore throat, skin infections, skin rashes, arthralgia and arthritis (SLE, vasculitis), and bleeding from the lungs or nose (Wegener's granulomatosis, Goodpasture's syndrome), investigations must be immediately pursued to make serological diagnoses (Table 9.7). These will vary with the clinical situation.

In most adults, and in children with atypical features suggesting a diagnosis other than poststreptococcal glomerulonephritis, a renal biopsy should be performed as soon as possible.

Management of the
acute nephritic
syndrome

The clinical features of the syndrome, as well as its cause, should be treated. Complications are usually related to fluid retention, hypertension and renal failure:
• *Fluid retention* is treated by salt and fluid restriction, and by high dose diuretic therapy if necessary. A close watch must be kept on weight, fluid balance and the size of the heart.
• *Hypertension* is controlled by drug therapy (Chapter 12).

Table 9.7 Investigations in the acute nephritic syndrome

Renal function
Urine microscopy (glomerular red cells, red cell casts)
Plasma urea, creatinine and electrolytes
Urine protein
Creatinine clearance

Blood tests seeking a cause
Full blood examination (for microangiopathy)
Antistreptolysin titre, throat swab (for poststreptococcal disease)
ESR (high in SLE and vasculitis)
Antinuclear factor, plasma complement C3 C4 (for SLE)
Antiglomerular basement membrane antibody
Antineutrophil cytoplasmic antibody (for vasculitis)

Chest X-ray
Cardiac size and pulmonary oedema
Lung haemorrhage (vasculitis and Goodpasture's syndrome)

Renal biopsy
in all but clinically typical poststreptococcal GN

Monitor progress
Clinical
  blood pressure chart
  fluid-balance chart
  daily weight
Laboratory
  plasma urea, creatinine, electrolytes
  creatinine clearance
  urine microscopy and protein
  chest X-ray

- *Renal failure* is treated as for other forms of acute renal failure (Chapter 10).

Treatment of the cause of the acute nephritic syndrome

The treatment depends on the cause. Delay in treatment of the cause can allow progression to rapidly progressive disease. Post-streptococcal glomerulonephritis has not been shown to be affected by treatment with penicillin although it is usual to administer this or another antibiotic to kill residual streptococci (Chapter 15). For many other forms of acute nephritis due to systemic diseases, such as SLE and vasculitis, specific therapy is available.

RAPIDLY PROGRESSIVE GLOMERULONEPHRITIS

Definition

Rapidly progressive glomerulonephritis (RPGN) is the most aggressive syndrome of acute glomerulonephritis and is characterised by rapid deterioration to end-stage renal failure in days or weeks unless appropriately treated. Fortunately it is uncommon. Renal biopsy will usually show a high proportion of glomeruli affected by crescents — collections of fibrin, mononuclear cells and later collagen and epithelial cells in Bowman's capsule surrounding the glomerular tuft (Fig. 15.9). The term 'crescentic glomerulonephritis' is used interchangeably with RPGN by some nephrologists, though the syndrome also occurs with thrombotic microangiopathies without glomerular crescents (Chapter 32).

Causes of rapidly progressive glomerulonephritis

Although RPGN can occur with any of the causes of the acute nephritic syndrome (Table 9.5), there are some diseases particularly likely to present in this way (Table 9.8):

• *In the adult* idiopathic diffuse proliferative glomerulonephritis, Goodpasture's syndrome, SLE and Wegener's granulomatosis are particularly likely to cause RPGN.

• *In children* haemolytic–uraemic syndrome is frequently associated with RPGN.

Clinical features of RPGN

The acute nephritic syndrome with heavy haematuria and severe oliguria is usual. Loin pain may be prominent. RPGN should be particularly suspected with:

• *Acute nephritic syndrome in an adult.* All forms of acute nephritis have a worse prognosis in adults than children, and RPGN is more common in adults.

• *Heavy macroscopic haematuria in the acute nephritic syndrome.* The presence of macroscopic haematuria with more than 10^6 glomerular red cells/ml in the urine of a patient

Table 9.8 Common causes of rapidly progressive glomerulonephritis (GN)

Primary proliferative GN	Chapter 15
Diffuse proliferative GN	
IgA disease	
Membranoproliferative GN	
Goodpasture's syndrome (antiglomerular basement membrane antibody-mediated)	Chapter 16
Vasculitis	Chapter 18
Wegener's granulomatosis	
Polyarteritis	
Henoch–Schönlein purpura	
Systemic lupus erythematosus	Chapter 17
Thrombotic microangiopathy	Chapter 32
Thrombotic thrombocytopenic purpura (TTP)	
Haemolytic uraemic syndrome (HUS)	

with acute glomerulonephritis suggests the presence of glomerular crescents.

• *Heavy proteinuria in the acute nephritic syndrome.* Nephrotic range proteinuria in a patient with acute nephritis points to more severe glomerular disease.

• *Severe oliguria or anuria.* Severe oliguria or anuria is common in RPGN. In the worst form anuric renal failure can occur within only a few days. In these cases the prognosis for recovery is poor.

• *Deterioration in function.* It is uncommon for patients with acute nephritis to show a continuing fall in GFR after the first few days of clinical illness. In RPGN a continuous deterioration in function is characteristic.

• *The presence of a systemic disease.* More than 50% of cases of RPGN in adults occur in the presence of an underlying systemic illness (Table 9.8). The presence of haemoptysis, skin rash and joint pain are particularly suggestive.

Clinical approach to RPGN

RPGN is a medical emergency, since delay in treatment can result in permanent renal damage and commonly end-stage renal failure. The most important test is renal biopsy, which should be performed and viewed as quickly as possible, preferably within a few hours of presentation, since delay in treatment can result in further irreversible renal damage. Laboratory tests are as for acute nephritis (Table 9.7).

Treatment of RPGN

Two forms of treatment have been shown to be effective in RPGN:

• *Plasma exchange* — intensive plasma exchange, usually exchanging 4 litre of patients plasma for either albumin or plasma protein solution each day for 1 to 2 weeks, followed by gradual reduction in frequency combined with immunosuppression and antithrombotic therapy (usually prednisolone 1 mg/kg/day, cyclophosphamide 1.5–2.5 mg/kg/day and dipyridamole 400 mg/day). Stabilisation and improvement in renal function occur in virtually all patients who are still passing urine. Patients with complete anuria very rarely recover renal function.

• *Pulse steroid therapy.* Many have reported good results with intravenous 'pulses' of methylprednisolone, given either as 1 g/day for 3 days, or 30 mg/kg given every second day for three doses and repeated 1 week later if the response has been poor.

RECURRENT MACROSCOPIC HAEMATURIA (SYNPHARYNGITIC HAEMATURIA)

One easily recognisable syndrome in glomerulonephritis is recurrent attacks of haematuria, often associated with a concurrent sore throat. This syndrome, which has been also called syn-pharyngitic haematuria, is characteristically caused by mesangial proliferative glomerulonephritis with IgA deposition (Chapter 15). In some cases it seems to be precipitated by other infections, such as of the gastrointestinal tract, or even trauma (e.g. burns or fractures).

Other diseases can cause recurrent macroscopic haematuria, especially non-glomerular disease (Table 7.6). Familial nephritis can also present in this way (Chapter 31).

CHRONIC GLOMERULONEPHRITIS

Most patients with glomerular disease present with a persistent mixture of proteinuria, glomerular haematuria, hypertension and/or impaired renal function. Often these are found on routine examination and the diagnosis is made by renal biopsy, which also often indicates prognosis and therapy.

Many of the patients presenting with the more acute syndromes considered above resolve incompletely, and hence, can then be said to have developed chronic glomerulonephritis.

10: *Acute Renal Failure*

Acute renal failure (ARF) is characterised by a sudden decrease in renal function. It is usually, but not always, reversible. ARF usually occurs on a background of normal renal function, but it can occur in patients with already impaired renal function in which case acute-on-chronic renal failure is said to be present.

CAUSES OF ACUTE RENAL FAILURE

The causes are classified into three groups:
1 *Prerenal or circulatory*. A defect in the perfusion of the kidney is responsible. Repair of the abnormality should result in an immediate return of renal function.
2 *Postrenal or obstructive*. Obstruction to urinary flow is responsible.
3 *Renal or intrinsic*. A disease of the kidney or its vessels is present. There is usually an obvious histological abnormality and recovery does not occur immediately on repair of prerenal factors or obstruction.

Overlap between these groups can occur, e.g. with intrarenal causes of obstruction to blood or urine flow, however, the classification suffices for general purposes. The causes are summarised in Table 10.1.

PRERENAL ACUTE RENAL FAILURE

This is also known as prerenal renal failure, or circulatory acute renal failure. In this condition there is a decrease in glomerular filtration rate secondary to a fall in renal perfusion. Repair of the circulatory problem results in immediate restoration of renal function.

Mechanism of prerenal acute renal failure

Reduced cardiac output, blood volume or blood pressure lead to compensatory responses including activation of the autonomic nervous system, the renin–angiotensin system and release of ADH. The renal response is a drop in urine flow rate with concentration of the urine, hence high urinary urea and creatinine concentrations (ADH effect), and a reduction in urinary sodium

127

Table 10.1 Causes of acute renal failure

Prerenal or circulatory
Hypovolaemia or hypotension
Reduced cardiac output
Increased blood viscosity

Postrenal or obstructive
Bladder outlet or urethral
Both ureters
One ureter or pelvis with:
  single kidney
  opposite kidney damaged

Renal or parenchymal
Tubular and interstitial
  acute tubular necrosis
  acute tubulointerstitial nephritis
  acute tubular obstruction
Acute cortical necrosis
Acute glomerular disease
Acute vascular obstruction
Nephrectomy

concentration (aldosterone effect). The low urinary flow rate produces an increase in tubular passive urea resorption, hence a decrease in urea clearance relative to GFR. The result is a high plasma urea:creatinine ratio (Table 5.1).

The GFR is at first maintained by autoregulatory mechanisms, such that glomerular filtration still continues until the systolic blood pressure falls below about 70 mmHg in otherwise normal adults. The mediators maintaining GFR include the renin–angiotensin system, prostaglandins and other autocoids and neural responses (Chapter 4). With continuation or worsening of the stress ultimately the GFR falls and the plasma creatinine rises.

This critical balance can be upset by drugs interfering with these neurohormonal mechanisms. Important examples include precipitation of ARF by angiotensin-converting enzyme inhibitors (ACE inhibitors) and non-steroidal anti-inflammatory drugs (NSAIDs) in states of renal hypoperfusion such as liver, cardiac or renal failure, nephrotic syndrome, hypovolaemia or bilateral renal artery stenosis. Alternatively urine output can be 'protected' by infusion of low dose dopamine, which causes vascular dilatation and natriuresis, in patients with decreased renal perfusion.

With severe renal hypoperfusion, ischaemic renal damage occurs, with either necrosis and temporary loss of function of renal tubular cells (acute tubular necrosis) or infarction of the renal cortex (renal cortical necrosis). Once this occurs, restoration of the renal perfusion will not restore renal function immediately and renal histological changes can be seen — the condition is no longer prerenal renal failure but instead is classified as ARF with a 'renal' cause.

Causes of prerenal acute renal failure

Prerenal renal failure is usually the result of a decrease in blood pressure, effective blood volume or cardiac output, although increased blood viscosity can have the same effect (Table 10.2).

Hypovolaemia and hypotension

Hypovolaemia and hypotension are the commonest causes of ARF. In most cases the reason is obvious from the history of the patient. Examination may reveal pallor, sweatiness and a cool vasoconstricted periphery with mottled cyanosis. Unfortunately, particularly in healthy young adults, the signs of decompensation, i.e. tachycardia and a fall in blood pressure, can be very late and therefore are unreliable signs of volume depletion. Postural hypotension may be more helpful. In more chronic cases diminished tissue turgor, dry mucous membranes and reduced eyeball pressure may be present. Septicaemia is a common cause of shock, on the other hand in this condition ARF can occur with little obvious fall in blood pressure. Hepatorenal failure is a state of prerenal renal failure where persistent renal functional impairment occurs in the setting of severe liver failure (Chapter 31).

Cardiac failure

Reduced cardiac output is a much less common cause of ARF. In some cases, such as in cardiogenic shock or massive pulmonary

Table 10.2 Prerenal causes of acute renal failure

Decreased intravascular volume
Haemorrhage
Severe gastrointestinal losses
Burns, trauma, pancreatitis

Decreased cardiac output
Severe cardiac failure
Cardiogenic shock
Massive pulmonary embolism

Systemic vasodilatation
Septicaemia
Liver failure (hepatorenal failure)
Drug overdose

Increased blood viscosity
Macroglobulinaemia
Polycythaemia
Myeloma

embolus, hypotension is severe, but in chronic severe heart failure, such as with cardiomyopathy, it may be only mild. The prognosis is very poor if the heart disease is irreversible.

Hyperviscosity-induced prerenal renal failure

Rarely in polycythaemia and macroglobulinaemia or myeloma with production of the large immunoglobulins IgA, IgM and IgD, increased blood viscosity can produce a decrease in renal perfusion and renal function (Chapter 27).

Diagnosis of prerenal renal failure

The diagnosis of prerenal renal failure depends on the demonstration of:
- *Acute renal failure.* Usually oliguria is combined with a rise in plasma creatinine and urea concentrations.
- *Concentrated urine* with retention of sodium and thus a low urinary sodium concentration.
- *Reversal on correction of prerenal factors.*
  Usually the cause is obvious.

Management of prerenal renal failure

The assessment of the patient for the presence of prerenal factors is the first step in the management of both acute and chronic renal failure. A prompt response to correction should occur, although in some patients a lag time of some hours occurs before urine flow is re-established.

POSTRENAL (OBSTRUCTIVE) ACUTE RENAL FAILURE

In these cases ARF is due to obstruction to urine flow (Table 10.3). This obstruction can be partial or complete. Complete ureteral obstruction for a period of only a few weeks can result in permanent renal damage.

Causes of postrenal renal failure

In considering the obstructive causes of ARF (Table 10.3) it is worth remembering the following points:
- If the patient has two normal kidneys the obstruction must involve both ureters or kidneys to cause significant changes in plasma biochemistry.
- Bladder outlet obstruction due to prostatomegaly is by far the commonest cause in adult males.
- Some diseases commonly affect both kidneys and can therefore damage one kidney and obstruct the other (analgesic nephropathy with papillary necrosis, cystine and infection stones).
- Pain and lower tract haematuria are suggestive of obstructive renal failure.
- Absolute anuria is strongly suggestive of obstruction, though

Table 10.3 Obstructive causes of acute renal failure

Bladder outflow obstruction
Bladder — carcinoma, neurogenic
Urethral — valves, stricture
Prostate — hypertrophy, carcinoma

Ureteral obstruction (bilateral, single kidney or opposite kidney diseased)
Intra-ureteral — stone, papilla, tumour, clot
Extra-ureteral — retroperitoneal neoplasm, retroperitoneal fibrosis, surgical
  location

Renal pelvic obstruction (bilateral, single kidney or opposite kidney diseased)
Stone, tumour, detached papilla, clot

Intrarenal obstruction
This is usually regarded as an intrinsic renal cause of ARF (Table 10.4);
  examples include acute urate nephropathy, myeloma cast obstruction and
  papillary necrosis *in situ*

rarely it can occur in rapidly progressive nephritis (Chapter 9).
Non-oliguric renal failure can occur with incomplete obstruction.

Diagnosis of postrenal renal failure

Obstruction must be considered early in all cases of ARF. Accordingly insertion of a urethral catheter and renal ultrasound for pelvic dilatation are among the first investigations in ARF.

Management of postrenal renal failure

Permanent relief of obstruction is required. Obstruction can lead to severe tubular dysfunction. A massive diuresis (postobstructive diuresis) can occur after relief of acute obstruction (Fig. 10.1). If

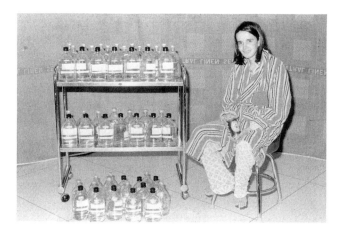

Fig. 10.1 Postobstructive diuresis. A patient with his urine output after relief of obstruction — 50 litre/day

fluid losses are not replaced, severe dehydration or hypernatraemia can occur. Other tubular deficits such as renal tubular acidosis are also common during the postobstructive recovery period, which can last several weeks.

RENAL (INTRINSIC) ACUTE RENAL FAILURE

Also known as parenchymal acute renal failure, acute intrinsic renal failure. In these conditions (Table 10.4) the cause for ARF lies within the kidney itself, and correction of prerenal factors, or relief of obstruction, will not immediately reverse the reduction in GFR.

The most common cause is acute tubular necrosis in which spontaneous recovery without specific therapy can ultimately be expected. With the other causes spontaneous recovery may not occur and specific therapy is often required.

Acute tubular necrosis

Acute tubular necrosis (ATN) is the most common cause of severe ARF and is discussed in detail in Chapter 19. In ATN there is severe but recoverable damage to tubular cells, usually due to shock or nephrotoxins, including drugs such as the amino-glycoside antibiotics, radiocontrast agents and amphotericin (Table 19.1). The usual illness is acute oliguric (20% are not oliguric) renal failure which recovers spontaneously after 1–3 weeks. Once ATN has occurred there is no treatment which will shorten the period of renal failure.

Table 10.4 Intrinsic renal causes of acute renal failure. The common clinical entities are ATN, acute TIN and glomerular diseases

---

Acute tubular necrosis (ATN) and cortical necrosis
Ischaemic
Nephrotoxic

Acute tubular obstruction
Acute urate nephropathy
Acute myeloma kidney
Renal papillary necrosis *in situ*

Acute tubulointerstitial nephritis (TIN)

Glomerular disease (see Table 10.5)
Crescentic glomerulonephritis
Thrombotic glomerulopathy

Vascular disease (see Table 10.6)

Nephrectomy (single kidney)

Acute tubular obstruction

Overlapping with ATN are a group of causes of ARF where the tubules can be seen to be obstructed by casts of various kinds. Examples include acute urate nephropathy (Chapter 24), acute myeloma kidney where the casts contain light chains (Chapter 27) and some instances of crystalluric drug toxicity. The clinical picture is of acute oligoanuric renal failure. If rapid rehydration and diuretic therapy does not lead to an immediate diuresis the course is similar to ATN. Papillary necrosis *in situ* (Chapter 22) can also cause acute intrarenal obstruction.

Acute allergic tubulointerstitial nephritis

Another way in which drugs can cause ARF is by an allergic reaction, with a pathological picture of infiltration of the renal parenchyma by leucocytes. This disease is discussed in Chapter 20. Common causes include antibiotics such as penicillins and sulphonamides (Table 20.1). Diagnosis is by renal biopsy and treatment by cessation of the drug and often a short course of corticosteroids.

Renal cortical necrosis

The most severe type of ischaemic or toxic renal damage is renal cortical necrosis in which patchy or complete infarction of the renal cortex occurs. The process often includes an element of intravascular thrombosis within the kidney, and nowadays usually only occurs in situations where ischaemic and toxic insult is combined, e.g. in acute obstetric haemorrhage, particularly with antepartum haemorrhage or haemorrhage associated with eclampsia. Rarely, toxins (snake-bite or industrial solvents) can cause cortical necrosis.

The clinical picture is of ARF usually with severe oliguria or anuria. Disseminated intravascular coagulation with a bleeding diathesis may be present at the onset. As time passes the kidneys shrink and may develop patchy calcification of the cortex. With dialysis support some slow and incomplete recovery may occur over a period of months.

Glomerular causes of acute renal failure

Several glomerular diseases may cause ARF (Table 10.5), usually with the clinical picture of rapidly progressive glomerulonephritis (Chapter 9). Rapidly progressive glomerulonephritis is a medical emergency. A delay in diagnosis and therapy can result in permanent renal failure. In these diseases macroscopic glomerular haematuria is usually present, with more than 1 million glomerular RBC/ml of urine. Diagnosis is usually by renal biopsy — the pathology is either severe proliferative glomerulonephritis or thrombotic microangiopathy. In children poststreptococcal nephritis and haemolytic—uraemic syndrome are the commonest causes, while in adults systemic diseases should always be considered.

Table 10.5 Glomerular diseases causing acute renal failure

Proliferative glomerulonephritis
Idiopathic
Poststreptococcal
Goodpasture's syndrome
Systemic lupus erythematosus
Polyarteritis, Wegener's arteritis
Henoch–Schönlein purpura

Thrombotic microangiopathy
Haemolytic uraemic syndrome (HUS)
Thrombotic thrombocytopenic purpura (TTP)
Scleroderma crisis
Accelerated (malignant) hypertension
Severe pre-eclampsia and eclampsia

Vascular causes of acute renal failure

Acute obstruction to renal vessels will cause ARF which will not respond to maintenance of the systemic circulation. Causes include vasculitis and renal thrombotic microangiopathies, renal artery atheroma, thrombosis and embolism and renal vein thrombosis (Table 10.6). If the obstruction is sudden the clinical picture is of renal infarction, with loin pain and haematuria, while more gradual or partial obstruction will cause hypertension with gradual deterioration in function.

Inflammatory vascular disease. In a variety of inflammatory and thrombotic microangiopathic diseases involving the

Table 10.6 Vascular causes of acute renal failure

Renal vasculitis

Renal artery embolism
Myocardial infarction
Mitral stenosis
Atrial fibrillation
Subacute bacterial endocarditis

Renal artery thrombosis

Atheroembolic renal failure

Renal artery stenosis
Severe bilateral
  single kidney
  diseased contralateral kidney

Renal vein thrombosis

renal vasculature (Table 10.6) acute deterioration in function can occur. This may be due to a glomerular lesion (microscopic polyarteritis — Chapter 18) but in others there is obliteration of arteriolar lumina by proliferative endothelium and microthrombi (thrombotic microangiopathies — Chapter 32) or vasculitis involving larger renal arteries causing multiple infarcts (classical polyarteritis — Chapter 18).

Renal artery thrombosis and embolism. Renal artery thrombosis usually occurs in the context of renal artery stenosis. Often there is not the clinical picture of renal infarction because of already developed arterial collaterals, but there is an abrupt decline in renal function often associated with worsening of hypertension. In cases of sudden reduction in renal artery flow, as with major thrombosis of a normal or only mildly stenosed artery, or with embolus to the kidney (in atrial fibrillation, mitral stenosis, myocardial infarction and subacute bacterial endocarditis) there may be partial or complete renal infarction with loin pain, haematuria and decline in renal function.

Atheroembolic renal failure. The recently recognised syndrome of atheroembolic renal failure due to microembolisation of the kidney by cholesterol and debris from aortic atheroma is probably far more common than realised. The usual clinical setting is progressive renal failure following aortography or aortic surgery. Microscopic haematuria is usual, and in severe cases petechiae, cyanotic skin mottling or signs of peripheral arterial embolisation are present. Renal biopsy reveals cholesterol emboli in renal vessels and glomeruli. Permanent renal damage is usual. There are anecdotal reports of recovery with the use of prostacyclin, antiplatelet agents, anticoagulation and plasma exchange.

Renal artery stenosis. In severe bilateral renal artery stenosis, ARF can be precipitated by drugs which interfere with the normal compensatory mechanisms for renal hypoperfusion, such as ACE-inhibitors and NSAIDs or by superimposed thrombosis (see above).

Venous thrombosis. Renal vein thrombosis can cause ARF. Common causes include:
- Nephrotic syndrome.
- Infantile dehydration.
- Carcinomatous involvement of renal veins.
  (a) renal carcinoma, and
  (b) retroperitoneal tumours.
- Trauma.

There may be renal infarction (acute renal vein thrombosis) or worsening of proteinuria and deterioration of function in nephrotic syndrome (Chapter 9).

Surgical or traumatic nephrectomy
Occasionally the kidney will be avulsed from its pedicle in high speed trauma, or removed surgically. If the kidney is a single kidney or there is disease affecting the other kidney, ARF (and CRF) will occur. If the opposite kidney is normal there will be a fall in creatinine clearance, but the plasma creatinine will rise by only about 80%, and may not even be above normal limits (Chapters 5 & 6).

COMPLICATIONS OF ACUTE RENAL FAILURE

ARF commonly occurs in very ill patients who are intolerant of the additional problems associated with renal failure. The complications of ARF are similar to those of chronic renal failure outlined in Chapter 11 (Table 10.7). Four complications are more likely to occur with ARF than with CRF.

Table 10.7 Complications of acute renal failure

Cardiovascular
Pulmonary oedema
Cardiac arrythmia
Pericardial effusion

Electrolyte disturbances
Hyperkalaemia
Hyponatraemia
Acidosis

Neurological
Neuromuscular irritability, flap and tremor
Confusion, coma
Convulsions

Gastrointestinal
Nausea, vomiting
Gastritis, peptic ulceration
Gastrointestinal bleeding

Haematological
Anaemia
Haemorrhagic diathesis

Infections
Pneumonia
Septicaemia
Nosocomial infections (urine, chest, wound)

1 *Hyperkalaemia* because of the severe renal failure, associated tissue destruction and tubular dysfunction.

2 *Fluid overload* because of oliguria.

3 *Impaired conscious state* because of the rapidity of development of uraemia and the other illnesses present.

4 *Multi-organ failure* because of the coexistent cause of the ARF.

On the other hand hypertension is uncommon, at least in ATN, and neuropathy and bone disease are absent since they take time to develop.

PROGNOSIS OF ACUTE RENAL FAILURE

The mortality of ARF is about 50% after surgery, 30% medical causes and 15% with obstetric causes. Death usually results from the cause of the ARF rather than the renal failure itself. Prognosis is worst in elderly patients and those with coexistent multi-organ failure.

The common causes of death and their relative frequency are:

- *Infection* particularly septicaemia, pneumonia and peritonitis (30−50%).
- *Haemorrhage* particularly gastrointestinal (10−20%).
- *Cardiovascular* myocardial infarction, arrythmias, pulmonary oedema (10−20%).
- *Respiratory failure* particularly adult respiratory distress syndrome (10%).
- *Multi-organ failure* with combined hypotension, adult respiratory distress, liver failure and septicaemia.

MANAGEMENT OF ACUTE RENAL FAILURE

The management of ARF differs from that of CRF in that the patients are: more likely to have a condition requiring urgent specific therapy, often more ill, more commonly profoundly oliguric, and more prone to acute complications such as hyperkalaemia, and gastrointestinal haemorrhage.

The principles are:

1 To diagnose and treat the cause.

2 To manage the renal failure until function returns.

Diagnosis and treatment of the cause of acute renal failure

Investigation and treatment should proceed together (Table 10.8). It is safer to regard all patients presenting with renal failure as having potentially reversible disease than to make an early decision that the failure is chronic, requiring less urgent management, and thus delay appropriate treatment.

The order of management is to exclude or treat prerenal, obstructive and renal causes in that order.

Clinical assessment

Clinical assessment of the severity of ARF and the presence of complications (Table 10.8) will indicate the urgency of specific therapy (rehydration, treatment of fluid overload, dialysis). The clinical approach should then determine the likelihood of each of the causative groups.

1 *Prerenal.* The commonest causes are often readily apparent (e.g. recent surgery with major blood loss and hypotension). A detailed assessment is made of:
• *Likely precipitating factors*, e.g. trauma, surgery, infections, gastrointestinal fluid or blood loss.
• *Recent fluid balance*, both intake and losses.
• *Fluid status*, including thirst, sweatiness, nausea, shivering, postural hypotension, tachycardia, shock.

2 *Obstruction.* Assessment includes:
• *The bladder* may be full, and detectable by suprapubic percussion if there is bladder outflow obstruction. Prostatomegaly may be found.

Table 10.8 Management of acute renal failure

Diagnose and treat the cause
Prerenal factors
   clinical assessment
   check urinary sodium concentration
   correct blood volume
   administer diuretic
   consider inotropes and dopamine
Postrenal (obstructive) factors
   clinical assessment
   insert urinary catheter
   renal ultrasound
Renal causes
   clinical assessment
   urinalysis
   urine microscopy
   consider renal biopsy, arteriography or other tests.

Treat the renal failure
Idealise and maintain salt and water balance
Provide adequate nutrition
Prevent and treat hyperkalaemia
Prevent and treat infection
Prevent and treat gastrointestinal haemorrhage
Early dialysis or haemofiltration

Treat other organ disease
Most fatalities are in patients with multiorgan (cardiovascular, respiratory, liver, neurological) disease

---

- *Disturbances of micturition* — poor stream, nocturia, dribbling, particularly in adult males.
- *Pain* in the loins or back.

3 *Renal* causes may be suggested by:
- *Drugs* especially those recently commenced, and known direct or allergic nephrotoxins (Tables 19.1 & 20.1).
- *Past and present genitourinary symptoms* especially haematuria, hypertension and proteinuria.
- *Signs of systemic diseases*, such as skin rashes, arthralgia and purpura.

Take blood and urine samples

Plasma creatinine, urea and electrolytes require urgent estimation, particularly the plasma potassium concentration.

It is most important to collect any urine passed for urinalysis and microscopy (Chapter 8).

The value of urine microscopy cannot be overemphasised. In prerenal renal failure there is usually little in the way of urinary cells, casts or protein. Crystals of phosphate or uric acid may be seen. In ATN, tubular cell debris and other casts are usually abundant, and mild proteinuria may be present. In glomerulonephritis and vasculitis it is usual to find large numbers of glomerular red cells and sometimes red cell casts.

Insertion of a urinary catheter

This has three functions:
1 To exclude bladder outlet obstruction.
2 To allow accurate monitoring of urine output during initial assessment.
3 To give a sample of urine if one has not already been obtained.

The catheter should be removed as soon as practicable, since it is a potent source of urine infection.

Assess and correct fluid volume status

A critically important examination is made to determine whether intravascular depletion or overload exists. Blood pressure, jugular venous pressure and the state of the heart and lungs are examined. In ongoing assessment sometimes a central venous catheter, or Swan–Ganz right atrial catheter may be required. If reduced blood volume is apparent it should be rapidly replaced. Even if the patient appears euvolaemic a trial 'fluid-push' consisting of 200–500 ml of intravenous saline over 15 to 30 min should be given and the effect on urine output assessed.

Give a diuretic

Frusemide, in graduated doses from 40 mg to 1 g, given slowly intravenously should be given once the patient is fluid replete (not before). Mannitol (100 ml of 20% over 10 min) can be given instead, particularly if mild hypovolaemia is suspected, however since it is a volume expanding drug that is largely renally excreted it should be avoided in patients with hypervolaemia, and not repeated in established renal failure.

The steps taken to this point should have produced a diuresis in most cases of prerenal renal failure.

Renal imaging

Renal ultrasound has become the mainstay of early renal imaging in ARF, to detect obstruction and to define renal anatomy.

Features to be particularly noted are:
• The presence or absence of pelvic/ureteral dilatation indicating obstruction.
• The presence of two kidneys.
• Renal size to assess the likelihood of chronic renal disease.
A normal renal ultrasound does not exclude obstruction.

Renal radionuclear scanning. Renal scanning (Chapter 2) may be used to confirm the presence of renal blood flow, and to demonstrate delay in renal pelvic emptying in obstruction. In ATN renal blood flow is usually greatly reduced.

Subsequent management of the cause of acute renal failure

Prerenal renal failure. Commonly in very ill patients, usually in intensive care, a delicate balance is achieved where blood pressure can only be maintained by inotropes such as noradrenaline which decrease renal blood flow and GFR. In these situations depamine (0.5 to 3 μg/kg/min by pump infusion) may promote intrarenal vasodilatation and natriuresis. Frusemide may be combined to maintain urine flow. It is not clear whether either of these drugs will prevent ATN but useful fluid loss can be achieved.

Suspected obstruction. If the renal pelvis is dilated percutaneous nephrostomy can be performed to reduce the obstruction and to allow injection of dye thus further defining the level and cause. Cystoscopy and passage of retrograde catheters is still widely employed in areas where the techniques of antegrade nephrostomy are not available. Further investigation in suspected obstruction may include CT scanning of the kidneys and ureters.

Suspected renal cause of ARF. In cases in which the diagnosis is still uncertain a renal biopsy should be performed. Renal biopsy will distinguish ATN and other parenchymal causes of acute renal failure. If ATN is suspected but diuresis has not occurred in 2 weeks, renal biopsy should be considered.

Management of established acute renal failure

The principles are:
• *Idealise and maintain salt and water balance.* Restriction of sodium intake to about 60 mmol/day and limitation of fluid

intake to 500 ml/day in excess of the previous days losses, or 30 ml/hour in excess of the previous hourly urine output will usually maintain body fluid balance. Frequent reassessment and adjustment of the fluid input is required. Assessment includes a careful fluid balance chart, daily weights (if practicable), and frequent observation of blood pressure, pulse and jugular or central venous pressure. In very ill patients right atrial pressure monitoring may be required.

• *Provide adequate nutrition.* A high caloric intake may necessitate oral high calorie supplements or intravenous hyperalimentation. Protein restriction to around 40 g/day is commonly practised in non-catabolic patients to decrease plasma urea but in catabolic patients amino acid supplements are often required in a total parental nutrition regimen. A balance always has to be struck between the load of fluid, potassium, phosphate and nitrogen, and the demands these place on the residual renal function or dialysis needs. In general, it is better to feed more and dialyse early and often rather than to restrict nutrition.

• *Prevent and treat hyperkalaemia.* Hyperkalaemia is common in catabolic patients with minimal renal function. The diagnosis and management is discussed in Chapter 14. Treatment includes correction of acidosis, intravenous glucose and insulin, potassium exchange resins, intravenous calcium in cardiac emergencies and dialysis.

• *Prevention and treatment of infection.* Respiratory and nosocomial (intravenous access, urinary catheter) infection are common causes of death. Chest physiotherapy and scrupulous care of access devices is important. A policy of rapid diagnostic and therapeutic response to fever is important. Urinary catheters should be removed as soon as possible. In conscious patients this is usually once bladder outlet obstruction has been excluded and the patient is stable.

• *Prevention and treatment of gastrointestinal haemorrhage.* Faecal monitoring for blood and early endoscopy if bleeding is suspected is wise. Haemorrhage may present as a rise in the plasma urea/creatinine ratio, with a concomitant fall in haemoglobin. Usually a histamine H_2 antagonist (e.g. ranitidine) is given to patients with ARF as prophylaxis against gastrointestinal bleeding.

• *Dialysis or haemofiltration.* Dialysis or haemofiltration is the mainstay of modern ARF management. It is best not to delay

Table 10.9 Relative advantages of dialysis modalities in acute renal failure

	Advantages	Disadvantages
Peritoneal dialysis	No anticoagulation required Continual dialysis Technically simple Minimal stress to the cardiovascular system	Slow removal of fluid and toxins Need intact peritoneum Peritoneal infection occurs Diaphragmatic splinting occurs
Haemodialysis	Great efficiency in removal of toxins Rapid fluid removal	Intermittent, thus unphysiological Anticoagulation during procedure Staff and equipment intensive
Haemofiltration	Continuous Virtually unlimited fluid removal	Constant anticoagulation Frequent staff supervision Slow removal of toxins

until a high urea, hyperkalaemia or fluid overload force the issue, but to intervene once the immediate irreversibility of the ARF has been established. Plasma urea concentrations should not be allowed to rise above 30 to 40 mmol/litre.

Peritoneal dialysis, haemodialysis and continuous haemofiltration (Chapter 35) each have advantages and disadvantages (Table 10.9). Generally continuous haemofiltration and peritoneal dialysis are best in intensive care, while intermittent haemodialysis using a subclavian catheter for access is used in other patients and as an extra support in catabolic patients not adequately handled by peritoneal dialysis or haemofiltration.

11: *Chronic Renal Failure*

In chronic renal failure there is persistent and irreversible reduction in overall renal function. Some use the term for patients in whom there is an elevated plasma creatinine and/or urea (i.e. azotaemia — see below), while others restrict it to patients who are symptomatic from their renal failure (i.e. uraemia — see below). Because of this confusion there are some other terms that are useful in clinical practice:

• *Renal functional impairment*. This means there is a reduced GFR. It can be qualified as mild, moderate or severe.

• *Azotaemia*. This means that the blood urea nitrogen (BUN) is raised, and is applied if the plasma urea concentration is elevated.

• *Uraemia* is the syndrome resulting from severe renal failure.

• *End-stage renal failure (ESRF)* has occurred once renal function is inadequate to support life (without dialysis or transplantation). The term has replaced 'terminal renal failure'. The medical aspects of dialysis and transplant patients will be dealt with in Chapter 35.

INCIDENCE

In Australia and the UK about 50 new patients per million population per year enter dialysis and transplant programmes, while in parts of the USA rates of over 160 new patients/million per population per year have been reported. This probably represents both difference in disease incidence and socio-economic factors influencing the proportion of patients with ESRF who are dialysed.

CAUSES OF CHRONIC RENAL FAILURE

The causes of renal failure in Australia and the UK are very similar except that Australia has a much higher incidence of analgesic nephropathy. Most common are glomerulonephritis, analgesic nephropathy, reflux nephropathy, polycystic kidney disease and diabetic nephropathy (Table 11.1).

It is worth noting that:

• Glomerulonephritis is by far the commonest cause of ESRF. The commonest form of glomerulonephritis causing ESRF is IgA disease (Chapter 15).

143

Table 11.1 Causes of chronic renal failure*

Glomerulonephritis	35%
Analgesic nephropathy	15%
Reflux nephropathy	10%
Adult polycystic kidneys	5–10%
Diabetic nephropathy	5–10%
Others including hypertensive, obstructive and gouty nephropathy	15%
Unknown	5–10%

* Taken from the numbers of patients entering dialysis and transplant programmes. These vary between countries and centres depending on disease incidence, dialysis acceptance criteria and the effort and indices used to make each diagnosis

- Analgesic nephropathy varies in incidence both within Australasia and worldwide and is now falling in frequency in Australia.
- Diabetic nephropathy varies from 8% in Australia to 25% of all new patients in USA.

CLINICAL FEATURES OF RENAL FAILURE

The functional derangements that occur as renal failure progresses have been discussed in Chapter 6. The clinical features are outlined in Fig. 11.1 & Table 11.2.

General

Patients suffer fatigue, malaise and anorexia. Anaemia is a major contributing factor to fatiguability, while the malaise and anorexia are due to an effect of uraemic toxins on the brain. In children small stature and growth failure is a major problem, particularly if chronic acidosis or renal bone disease are present.

Skin and hands

The sallow skin colour is characteristic of renal failure, due to both anaemia and deposition of 'urochromogens' in the skin. Melanin pigmentation can occur, particularly in patients with 'salt-losing' diseases. The skin is thin and fragile, bruising easily and even spontaneously. Large red-brown subcutaneous ecchymoses are often present as well as long linear scratch mark purpura where the patient has responded to the uraemic pruritus (Fig. 11.2). The skin fragility and bruising are attributed to malnutrition, uraemic toxins and defective platelet function. Rarely, the presence of 'uraemic frost' — white crystals of urea on the skin around the mouth — attests to the high urea content of the sweat.

The nails may show changes of leukonychia. Particularly common is a white nail with the tip discoloured brown (Fig. 11.3).

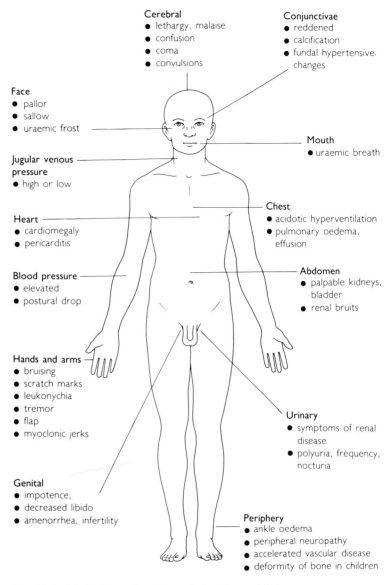

Cerebral
- lethargy, malaise
- confusion
- coma
- convulsions

Conjunctivae
- reddened
- calcification
- fundal hypertensive changes

Face
- pallor
- sallow
- uraemic frost

Mouth
- uraemic breath

Jugular venous pressure
- high or low

Chest
- acidotic hyperventilation
- pulmonary oedema, effusion

Heart
- cardiomegaly
- pericarditis

Blood pressure
- elevated
- postural drop

Abdomen
- palpable kidneys, bladder
- renal bruits

Hands and arms
- bruising
- scratch marks
- leukonychia
- tremor
- flap
- myoclonic jerks

Urinary
- symptoms of renal disease
- polyuria, frequency, nocturia

Genital
- impotence,
- decreased libido
- amenorrhea, infertility

Periphery
- ankle oedema
- peripheral neuropathy
- accelerated vascular disease
- deformity of bone in children

Fig. 11.1 Clinical manifestations of chronic renal failure

Head and neck

Tissue turgor, periorbital oedema or sunken eyes indicate fluid status. A dry mouth and coated tongue may be seen in dehydrated patients or those with acidotic hyperventilation.

Uraemic breath — smelling like urine or ammonia — commonly occurs in patients with a high blood urea, but is variable, presumably depending on bacterial flora degrading salivary urea. Dental caries may be accelerated in the ammoniacal environment.

Table 11.2 The clinical effects of renal failure

General	*Reproductive*
Fatigue, malaise	Decreased libido, impotence
Growth failure	Amenorrhea
Debility	Infertility
	Gynaecomastia
Skin	Galactorrhea
Pale or sallow	
Fragility	*Nervous*
Bruising	Lethargy, malaise
Leukonychia	Anorexia
	Drowsiness
Head and neck	Confusion
Uraemic foetor	Tremor, myoclonus, flap
Dry coated tongue	Convulsions
	Coma
Eyes	
Hypertensive fundi	*Skeletal*
'Red eye'	Hyperparathyroidism
	Vitamin D deficiency
Cardiovascular	
Hypertension	*Joints*
Fluid overload	Gout, pseudogout
Cardiac failure	Extra-osseus
Uraemic pericarditis	calcification
Accelerated vascular disease	
	Haematological
Respiratory	Anaemia
Acidotic hyperventilation	Bleeding tendency
Pulmonary oedema	Immune deficiency
Pleural effusion	
Uraemic pleurisy	*Endocrine*
	Multiple
Gastrointestinal	
Anorexia	*Pharmacological*
Nausea	Renal excreted drugs
Gastritis, peptic ulcers	
Uraemic colitis	
Antibiotic-induced diarrhoea	
Urinary	
Nocturia	
Polyuria	
Thirst	
Proteinuria	
Underlying renal disease	

The conjunctivae Conjunctival pallor occurs with anaemia. On the orbital conjunctiva signs of calcium deposition — conjunctival reddening and irritation (red-eye), scleral calcification or band keratopathy — may be seen. Cataracts and glaucoma are common in diabetics and patients who have had steroid therapy.

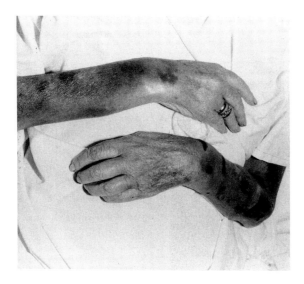

Fig. 11.2 Thin easily bruised skin in severe chronic renal failure

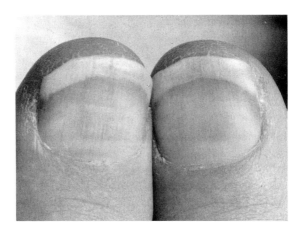

Fig. 11.3 Nail changes (Terry's nails) in chronic renal failure. Pale brittle nails with a brown line across the distal portion

The fundi

The fundi must always be carefully examined. They may show hypertensive changes (Fig. 12.4). It is probable that uraemic haemorrhages and exudates are merely a manifestation of severe hypertension although the uraemic state may make them worse due to capillary 'leakiness'. Diabetes and systemic vasculitis are other diseases that may cause characteristic retinal changes.

Cardiovascular system

A hyperdynamic circulation is usually present, because of the anaemia and acidosis associated with renal failure.

Blood pressure

Hypertension is common, can accelerate renal failure and may cause left ventricular failure. Postural hypotension may occur with salt and water deficiency or antihypertensive therapy, so blood pressure must always be recorded both lying and standing.

Blood and fluid volume

The jugular venous pressure (JVP) must be carefully assessed. Fluid overload, cardiac failure and pericardial effusion with tamponade can all cause elevation of the JVP, while dehydration will produce a low JVP. This may only be appreciated when raised by manual pressure over the liver (hepatojugular reflex). Fluid retention, with generalised oedema, elevation of the JVP, pulmonary crepitations and perhaps pleural effusions, may also occur with cardiac disease. The distinction between fluid overload due to renal and cardiac failure may be difficult.

The heart

Cardiomegaly may reflect fluid overload with cardiac decompensation or left ventricular failure due to hypertensive or atheromatous disease. Cardiac failure may be worsened by severe uraemic anaemia. In some cases with severe overload or hypertension, mitral, tricuspid or aortic valve regurgitation can be present and may resolve after removal of fluid by diuretics or dialysis, or control of hypertension.

Pericarditis is one of the manifestations of severe uraemia attributed to unknown uraemic toxins, and treatable only by intensive dialysis (or transplantation). It can occur quickly, only occasionally causes chest discomfort, and is detected by the characteristic rub. In some cases it can progress rapidly to cardiac tamponade. Elevation of the JVP and an exaggerated swing of blood pressure with respiration are early warning signs, but it can easily be missed and should be considered in any dispoeic or hypotensive uraemic. The fluid is often bloodstained when aspirated.

The blood vessels

Accelerated vascular disease occurs in uraemic patients, particularly manifest as coronary and cerebral vascular disease. Contributing factors are: hypertension, hyperlipidaemia (in chronic renal failure cholesterol and triglycerides are often elevated and HDL decreased) and hyperparathyroidism with vessel calcification. Cigarette smoking and diabetes greatly aggravate this problem.

Respiratory system

Uraemic patients often complain of exertional dyspnoea in the absence of lung disease. Fluid accumulation in the lungs, with pulmonary oedema — the so-called uraemic lung — is the common pulmonary manifestation of uraemia. Pleural effusions can occur with fluid overload or left ventricular failure. Acidotic respiration can cause hyperventilation. In occasional patients a pleural rub may be heard, due to uraemic pleurisy. Usually a pericardial rub is also present.

Gastrointestinal system

Anorexia, vomiting and weight loss are central effects of uraemic toxicity. A metallic taste in the mouth is attributed to urea generation. Peptic ulcer disease and gastritis are common in uraemic patients. Plasma gastrin levels are elevated — whether this is causal is debatable.

Uraemic colitis is manifest by bloody diarrhoea in terminally ill uraemics and is rarely seen nowadays. Instead diarrhoea is most often due to antibiotic treatment. Since renal excretion is minimal, many antibiotics with alternative liver excretion (such as amoxicillin) reach very high concentrations in the gut and predispose to *Clostridium difficile* infection. Aluminium hydroxide and calcium carbonate used to bind phosphate in the gut often cause constipation, as do the calcium-channel blockers used to treat hypertension.

Urinary system

The history often gives a clue to the duration and cause of the renal failure. Nocturia is commonly the first abnormality in patients with renal failure, and may be followed by polyuria and polydipsia, all of which are due to the concentrating defect. Some patients with acute-on-chronic or end-stage renal failure are oliguric. Hypertension is another early manifestation of renal disease. A history of haematuria, proteinuria or other more specific symptoms of renal disease or urinary tract abnormality is of diagnostic importance.

Reproductive system

Loss of libido, amenorrhoea, impotence and infertility all occur with advanced renal failure. Plasma prolactin, FSH and LH are all elevated, and do not cycle as in normal women. In some patients galactorrhoea, and in males, gynaecomastia occur; at least partly related to an elevated plasma prolactin concentration (Chapter 4).

A past history of pregnancy-induced renal disease can be useful in assessing the duration of disease (Chapter 33).

Nervous system

The presence of significant nervous system uraemic toxicity is a sign of severe uraemia and should be treated with dialysis.

Cerebral effects

Lethargy, drowsiness and eventually coma are part of the progression of uraemic encephalopathy. Patients may suffer malaise, anorexia, nausea and vomiting; all cerebral effects of uraemia. A

feeling of coldness is an unexplained symptom frequently present in severe uraemia. With advanced uraemia a variety of abnormal movements occur. These include:
- *Tremor*, best seen in the outstretched hands.
- *Uraemic flap* — an intermittent sudden drop of the hands seen if the arms and hands are held outstretched with the wrists dorsiflexed.
- *Myoclonic jerks* — involuntary jerking movements of the whole body. Often called 'the jumps' by patients this is made worse by sedatives such as opiates or benzodiazepenes.
- *Cramps* can be very troublesome and are attributed to neuro-muscular irritability. They may be made worse by hypocalcaemia or salt depletion.
- *Epileptic seizures* with near terminal uraemia.

Dialysed patients can suffer after rapid dialysis with dialysis disequilibrium, a clinical state that may be difficult to distinguish from uraemic encephalopathy. Dialysis dementia is due to cerebral aluminium toxicity, and is rarely found in patients who are not on maintenance dialysis (Chapter 35).

Peripheral neuropathy

Early symptoms include paraesthesia, 'restless legs' and 'burning feet'. Ultimately numbness and an ascending sensori-motor neuropathy can occur. This disease only occurs in severe protracted uraemia, and is attributed to an unknown toxin.

Musculoskeletal system
Renal bone disease

Most patients with renal bone disease are asymptomatic. Very advanced demineralisation of bone can occur before it is clinically apparent. Bone pain is often the first symptom. Usually vague and deep seated, it is commonly felt in the lower back, hips, knees and legs. Painful spontaneous fractures, often of the vertebrae, ribs and various other bones can occur.

Deformity and growth failure develop quickly in children, particularly in early adolescence when rapid bone turnover is occurring. Severe knock-knees (Fig. 11.4) can result. In adults thoracic kyphosis due to collapse of vertebral bodies may occur.

Skeletal X-rays are the most useful method of assessing renal bone disease though bone biopsy and various densitometry methods are more sensitive. The picture is a mixture of secondary hyperparathyroidism and vitamin D deficiency (Table 11.3). For maximum information a full skeletal survey is required with high resolution films of the hands and the lamina densa of the teeth (Fig. 11.5).

Calcification of other tissues

This is a feature of secondary hyperparathyroidism especially if there is a high calcium-phosphate product. Red irritable eyes occur with conjunctival calcium deposits. Pruritis is partly due

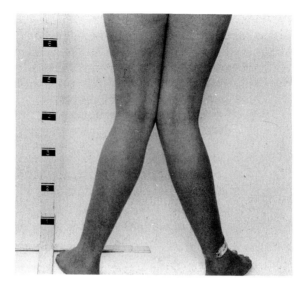

Fig. 11.4 Knock-knees in severe renal bone disease

to skin deposits and sometimes helped by control of hyperphosphataemia or parathyroidectomy. Vessel calcification is seen in plain radiographs and may contribute to accelerated vascular degeneration.

Table 11.3 Radiology of renal bone disease (Fig. 11.5)

Secondary hyperparathyroidism
Generalised decreased bone density
Subperiosteal erosion of bones, best seen as a scalloped edge to the phalanges
Radiolucent bone cysts (Brown tumours) in the neck of the femur, humerus and pelvis
Mottled lucency of the skull ('Pepper-pot skull')
Erosion and lucency of the lateral ends of the clavicles

Osteomalacia
Generalised decrease in bone radiodensity
Looser's zones or pseudofractures, most common in the pubic rami

Rickets, also shows:
Widening and fraying of epiphyseal plates
Bowing of long bones especially the femur and tibia
Slipping of epiphyses

Other features
Areas of increased radiodensity. In the spine the alternation of central radiolucency with subcartilagenous density in the vertebral bodies produces the 'Rugger-jersey spine'
Calcification of vessels best seen in the pelvis and hand
Tissue calcification, particularly in bursae

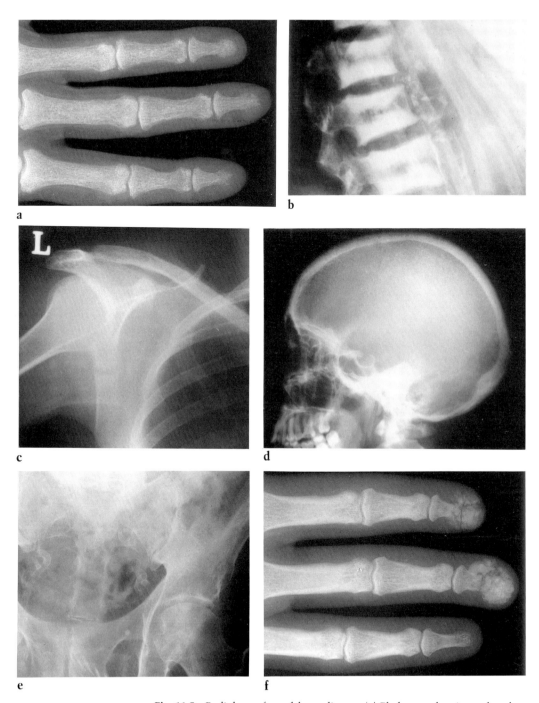

Fig. 11.5 Radiology of renal bone disease. (a) Phalanges showing reduced radiodensity and periosteal erosions. Note the resorption of the tips of the distal phalanges. (b) Spine ('rugger-jersey') in advanced renal osteodystrophy. There is also marked aortic calcification. (c) Pseudofracture ('loosers zone') of the neck of the scapula in severe osteomalacic renal bone disease. (d) 'Pepperpot' skull appearance in hyperparathyroid renal osteodystrophy. Ectopic calcification in renal osteodystrophy (hyperparathyroidism) affecting (e) pelvic vessels and (f) fingertips

Gout and pseudogout These are clinically the same as in non-uraemic patients, though the proportion of acute arthritis due to calcium salts (pseudogout) is much higher in the renal failure patients. Diagnosis is by joint aspiration and microscopy, and treatment is generally with non-steroidal anti-inflammatory drugs (NSAIDs). It must be remembered that NSAIDs can cause abrupt decline in renal function and must be used with great care (Chapter 34). Colchicine can be used safely.

Other musculoskeletal diseases A waddling gait attributed to proximal myopathy affecting the gluteal muscles can occur in patients with osteomalacia or rickets. It responds quickly to vitamin D administration.

In long-term dialysis patients, two new forms of bone disease have come to light. These are:
- Aluminium osteodystrophy.
- Dialysis related amyloid osteoarthropathy.

These are discussed in Chapter 35.

The haematologic system The haematological abnormalities include:
1 Anaemia, generally normochromic, normocytic.
2 Normal white cell count but decreased function.
3 Normal platelet count but decreased function.

Anaemia in renal failure Anaemia is partly responsible for many of the debilitating symptoms of uraemia such as lethargy, tiredness and exertional dyspnoea. Anaemia may be less severe in polycystic disease. Most patients with ESRF have a haemoglobin concentration between 5 and 10 g/dl. The red cells are usually normal in number, size and haemoglobin content, but bizarre shapes such as Burr cells may be seen. The main reasons are erythropoietin deficiency, uraemic marrow depression and mild chronic haemolysis (Table 11.4). It

Table 11.4 Causes of anaemia in renal failure

Erythropoeitin deficiency
Bone marrow depression by uraemic toxins
Low red cell life span
Other factors: Iatrogenic blood loss — tests, haemodialysis Gastrointestinal blood loss — peptic disease Bleeding tendency — menorrhagia, gastrointestinal loss Vitamin deficiency — anorexia Hypersplenism — in multiple transfused patients Marrow fibrosis in hyperparathyroidism Aluminium toxicity

is advisable to look for other causes of anaemia, particularly bleeding, if anaemia is severe. In general blood transfusion should be avoided unless symptoms are severe, as it can cause fluid overload and probably depresses erythropoeitin production. The place of therapy with recombinant human erythropoeitin in uraemic patients not requiring dialysis is not yet clear.

Depressed white cell function in uraemia

Susceptibility to infection is a feature of uraemic patients and is due to widespread defects in granulocyte, lymphocyte and monocyte−macrophage function, though these cells are usually normal in number and appearance. These defects seem to be due to toxins in uraemic serum.

The infections which result are some of the commonest causes of death in renal failure patients, and are particularly likely to occur if another predisposition to infection exists. These include concurrent immunosuppressive drug therapy, debility or invasive procedures.

Defective platelet function and bleeding tendency

A bleeding tendency is present in uraemia despite normal platelet counts and normal or elevated fibrinogen levels. Clinical manifestations include skin bruising, epistaxes, gastrointestinal bleeding or positive faecal occult blood tests and occasional serious bleeding into the brain or other internal organs, especially in hypertensive patients or those given heparin for haemodialysis. The bleeding time may be prolonged but tests of circulating clotting factors are usually normal.

In severe uraemia the bleeding tendency is improved by dialysis. Administration of desamino-D-arginine vasopressin (DDAVP) or oestrogens will temporarily improve the bleeding disorder. Anaemia also contributes to the bleeding tendency, and treatment with transfusion or erythropoetin improves the bleeding time in uraemia.

Endocrine system

A wide variety of endocrine abnormalities occur in renal failure, the majority of which have been dealt with (PTH, 1,25-(OH)$_2$-D3, renin, erythropoeitin, FSH, LH, prolactin, and gastrin). Others are inconstant or not of particular significance given our current level of understanding (thyroid hormones, calcitonin, ACTH, glucagon).

Insulin

Insulin is one hormone that deserves special mention because nearly 2% of the population are diabetic and particularly prone to develop renal failure (Chapter 26). Two opposing effects of renal failure are relevant. First there is reduced renal breakdown of insulin in renal failure. Insulin is filtered by the glomerulus and resorbed and degraded by the tubules. Second the peripheral tissues are insensitive to the effects of insulin, presumably because of the uraemic milieu. The nett outcome is that in most diabetics with renal failure the insulin requirements fall, i.e. the decreased degradation outweighs the tissue resistance.

LABORATORY FEATURES OF RENAL FAILURE

Plasma creatinine and urea

Plasma creatinine is elevated once GFR is less than about 60 ml/min, and rises exponentially with falling GFR (Fig. 5.1). In ESRF the plasma creatinine is usually over 1.0 mmol/litre. The levels in children and elderly people are lower because of their lower muscle bulk. A child may require dialysis when the plasma creatinine is as low as 0.5 mmol/litre. The plasma urea concentration follows renal function less reliably, since it can be reduced by low protein diet and increased by a variety of abnormalities including a high protein diet, saline depletion and a catabolic state (Table 5.1). Plasma urea concentrations of 20−60 mmol/litre are usual in ESRF.

Bicarbonate and pH

Inability to excrete the normal non-volatile acid load leads to a metabolic acidosis with respiratory compensation and a fall in plasma bicarbonate (HCO_3^-), usually to about 15−25 mmol/litre. There is a decrease in plasma pH and an increase in the anion gap such that: plasma sodium − (plasma chloride + bicarbonate) >12 mmol/litre (see Chapter 14).

Sodium and potassium

Plasma sodium concentration is usually normal, but can easily be raised or lowered by inadequate water intake or excessive water loading. Hyperkalaemia is a sign of very severe renal failure unless another cause such as excessive load, renal tubular acidosis or hypoaldosteronism is also present (Chapter 14).

Plasma calcium, phosphate, alkaline phosphatase and parathormone

These are the indices used to assess bone metabolism (Table 11.5). The earliest abnormality is usually elevation of plasma phosphate concentration [P]. The plasma calcium concentration [Ca] falls as [P] rises. Once increased bone turnover commences the alkaline phosphatase begins to rise. An elevated PTH occurs with secondary hyperparathyroidism. Over a long period of time the plasma [Ca] may creep upward, due to the development of 'tertiary' or 'autonomous' hyperparathyroidism.

Blood film

Normochromic normocytic anaemia (5−10 g/dl) is usual. Burr cells may be seen in severe uraemia. White cell and platelet counts are usually within normal limits.

Table 11.5 Disturbances of calcium-phosphate metabolism

	Plasma Ca	Plasma P	Alkaline phosphatase	PTH
Mild to moderate CRF	N	+ to ++	N	N
Protracted CRF	N or −	+++	+	+
Renal osteomalacia or rickets	−	+	+++	+
Severe secondary hyperparathyroidism	− or N	+++	+++	+++
'Tertiary' hyperparathyroidism	+ to ++	N or +	+++	+++
Aluminium osteodystrophy	+ to +++	N or +	N or +	N or +

N, no disturbance; +, slight disturbance to ++++, pronounced disturbance.

Urine microscopy

Broad cell casts may indicate tubular hypertrophy and dilatation. The abnormalities reflecting the underlying disease, such as glomerular haematuria, gradually disappear as less nephrons are present, each making dilute urine.

Urine biochemistry and creatinine clearance

Eventually urine of fixed specific gravity (SG = 1.010) and os-molarity (near 300 mosmol/litre) is passed. The urinary urea and creatinine concentrations are low. The creatinine clearance in-creasingly overestimates GFR, and falls to less than 5 ml/min in ESRF. Proteinuria in the range 200 to 1000 mg/day is usual in ESRF.

DIAGNOSTIC APPROACH IN PATIENTS WITH RENAL FAILURE

There are several questions to be answered in a patient presenting with apparent CRF before treatment can be formulated:
1 What is the cause and is it treatable? Is this acute or chronic renal failure? Are there reversible prerenal or obstructive factors? What is the underlying cause?
2 How severe is the failure and are there complications?

Determination of the cause

Since acute renal failure (ARF) is often severe and in some cases only reversible if the cause is dealt with promptly it is important

Distinction of acute from chronic renal failure

that the distinction from chronic irreversible failure is made quickly.

Clinical assessment. In most cases a strong clinical presumption exists, where a clear cause for ARF may be apparent, or there is a long history of symptoms of renal failure indicating likely CRF. Longstanding nocturia, polyuria and thirst, perhaps with hypertension and a history of renal disease suggests CRF, particularly if the symptoms of advanced uraemia, such as lethargy, nausea and itch have also been present for some time. Occasionally the presence of renal bone disease, or peripheral neuropathy suggests CRF but they can be mimicked by non-renal diseases.

The classical uraemic appearance with sallow atrophic skin with scratch marks and leuconychia takes time to develop and is rarely seen in ARF. In many cases this classical clinical picture is not present. It is therefore safer to regard all azotaemic patients as suffering from acute renal failure until proven otherwise.

Estimation of renal size. Estimation of renal size is the first step in investigation to distinguish acute from chronic renal failure. Renal ultrasound is the most valuable early investigation, since it will not only indicate renal size but also may indicate the cause of renal failure by showing cysts or an obstructed pelvis. Plain X-ray of the renal areas can also be used to indicate renal size and the presence of renal calculi if ultrasound is not available.

If the kidneys are very small then CRF is likely. The size must be adjusted for patient size and age. A normal person over 152 cm (5 ft) in height could be expected to have kidneys at least 10 cm in length by X-ray or 9 cm by ultrasound. If the kidneys are of normal or near normal size this suggests ARF although renal size is relatively preserved in a few causes of CRF, particularly diabetes, amyloid and renal infiltrations (Table 11.6).

Table 11.6 Renal failure with large or normal kidney size

Acute renal failure

Chronic renal failure due to:
Polycystic kidneys
Obstruction   } easily diagnosed by renal ultrasound
Bilateral staghorn calculi
Diabetic nephropathy
Amyloidosis
Infiltrations
  lymphoma
  leukaemia
  sarcoidosis

Detection and treatment of prerenal factors

In many patients presenting with CRF there are reversible prerenal factors (Chapter 10). The commonest are:
- Salt and water saline depletion due to intercurrent infection or gastrointestinal upset.
- Fluid overload with consequent cardiac failure.
- Uncontrolled or accelerated hypertension.

In many cases improvement in renal function can continue over weeks or even months when these prerenal factors have been severe. Usually assessment of tissue turgor, oedema, blood pressure (lying and standing), pulse, jugular venous pressure and cardiovascular status will suffice to determine volume status, but in rare cases with both cardiac and renal disease a central venous or pulmonary wedge pressure measurement may be required.

Exclusion of obstruction

Urinary obstruction must be excluded. Renal ultrasound is usually sufficient, although if obstruction is suspected clinically it cannot be excluded without retrograde pyelography (Chapter 2). Ultrasound will show pelvic dilatation, and will also reveal cysts, calculi and tumours as well as indicating renal size and sometimes the presence of cortical scars.

In the older male and in young children bladder outlet obstruction (prostatic, urethral valves, neurogenic bladder) is an important reversible cause of CRF. Careful palpation and percussion of the bladder may indicate enlargement. Passage of a urinary catheter to measure residual volume and to allow a trial of drainage can be worthwhile. In CRF passage of a urinary catheter is not as much part of the routine management as it is in ARF where the severity of illness, and the need to have continuous accurate monitoring of urine output are usually greater.

Diagnosis of the underlying disease

The procedures followed are very similar in CRF and ARF, though the urgency is less in CRF. Careful history and examination always comes first.

Investigations include:
- Plasma biochemistry, for renal function and electrolyte disturbances (Chapters 5 & 14).
- Urine microscopy and urinalysis (Chapter 8).
- Determination of renal anatomy (Chapter 2).
- Serological tests screening for causes of glomerulonephritis (Chapter 9).
- Tests relevant to infectivity before dialysis (usually hepatitis B and HIV antibody screening).

Consideration of renovascular disease. Renal artery atheromatous disease is an important consideration in the older patient, particularly since it is one of the potentially reversible causes of

CRF. Severe hypertension is usually present. Digital subtraction angiography has increased the ease with which renal artery stenosis can be detected.

Consideration of renal biopsy. If at all possible, renal biopsy should be performed in all patients who do not have a cause clearly demonstrated by renal imaging. The main limitation is renal size, since as the kidneys shrink to less than 10 cm (on ultrasound), the biopsy becomes more difficult and the likelihood of finding a reversible cause becomes less.

Assessment of severity of renal failure

A plan for future treatment is made depending on the severity of renal failure and the prognosis of the underlying disease. Symptoms and complications usually dictate the need for dialysis. Patients vary widely in their tolerance of azotaemia. Renal function is determined by measurement of plasma creatinine and urea concentrations, and determination of the creatinine clearance (Chapters 5 & 6).

These tests, taken together, will help in the assessment of:
- Renal function and 'uraemic status'.
- Protein–calorie intake.
- Prerenal factors.

The plasma creatinine concentration is the most convenient way to follow GFR, remembering that the plasma creatinine and creatinine clearance progressively overestimate GFR with increasing failure. The technique of plotting the reciprocal of plasma creatinine concentration against time (Fig. 5.1) is useful to monitor progress and estimate prognosis. Most patients are very close to ESRF once their plasma creatinine concentration is about 1.0 mmol/litre. In children, elderly people and diabetics the figure is somewhat lower.

Although plasma creatinine gives a better indication of GFR, the plasma urea correlates best with uraemic symptoms. The plasma urea to creatinine ratio is very useful. While normally about 60 (urea 6 mmol/litre : creatinine 0.1 mmol/litre), in near ESRF the usual ratio is about 20 to 40 (urea 20–40 mmol/litre : creatinine 1.0 mmol/litre) in the well-cared-for patient. A high ratio generally indicates excessive protein intake, inadequate caloric intake, salt and water depletion or upper gastrointestinal bleeding (Table 5.1).

MANAGEMENT OF CHRONIC RENAL FAILURE

The principles of CRF management are considered below and in Table 11.7.

Table 11.7 Management of chronic renal failure

Determine and treat the cause
Optimise and maintain salt and water balance
Low protein, high calorie diet
Control hypertension
Control electrolyte imbalance
Prevent and treat renal bone disease
Early detection and treatment of infection
Modify drug therapy with renal function
Detect and treat complications
Prepare for dialysis and transplant programme

Determine and treat the cause

Any possible remediable cause should be excluded (see above).

Optimise and maintain salt and water balance

Optimal salt and water balance in near ESRF usually means that the jugular venous pressure is slightly elevated and there is occasional mild ankle oedema.

In some patients large doses of frusemide (250–1000 mg daily) or other loop diuretics (bumetanide, ethacrynic acid) may be required to prevent fluid overload, while patients with 'salt losing' diseases may require oral sodium chloride or sodium bicarbonate supplements.

• *Body weight* gives a good indication of rapid alterations in fluid status. It should be recorded at each visit and daily if the patient is in hospital.

• *Urine output* should be monitored.

• *A fluid balance chart* should be kept in hospitalised patients so that input can be adjusted, aiming for a constant body weight with input exceeding output by about 500 ml.

Most patients with ESRF are dependent on dialysis for salt and water removal, and are restricted to a sodium chloride intake of about 60 mmol/day, compared with the community norm of 150–200 mmol/day. Because of reduced urine output, water intake is usually reduced, but remains 500 ml/day plus urine output.

Appropriate diet

A low protein (20–40 g/day), high calorie diet ameliorates the anorexia and nausea of advanced uraemia, resulting in a fall in plasma urea and a great improvement in symptoms. Recently it has been suggested that a low protein diet will slow the progression of renal failure (Chapter 6). Excessive intake of potassium and salt should be avoided.

Control hypertension

Uncontrolled hypertension hastens the course of renal failure, is a major factor in the degenerative arterial disease seen in CRF patients, can quickly become accelerated hypertension with the associated risks of encephalopathy and visual disturbances and can result in left heart failure. The management of hypertension in patients with CRF not yet requiring dialysis differs little from that in patients with normal renal function. In renal disease salt and water balance is managed independently of the blood pressure. Diuretic therapy with loop diuretics is often required as well as antihypertensive drugs.

Control electrolyte imbalance

Electrolyte imbalances are discussed in detail in Chapter 14. In CRF the most common are hyperkalaemia and severe acidosis.

Hyperkalaemia can be asymptomatic even when life-threatening. Prevention includes avoidance of:
• High potassium intake (Table 14.5). Usually intake needs to be reduced to about 60 mmol/day in ESRF.
• Potassium-sparing diuretics, including spironolactone, triamterene, amiloride and the compound diuretics in which these or potassium are combined.
• Drugs interfering with potassium excretion such as NSAIDs and ACE inhibitors.
• Severe acidosis or salt depletion which cause potassium release from cells and interfere with kaliuresis.

Detection involves monitoring plasma potassium as symptoms and signs are very late. Electrocardiographic (ECG) abnormalities occur when hyperkalaemia is potentially fatal (Fig. 14.1). Patients with chronic hyperkalaemia are often more resistant to the toxic effects of a raised plasma potassium than those in whom it rises quickly. The urgency of treatment is best assessed by the ECG changes. The treatment of hyperkalaemia is discussed in Chapter 14 and depends on the urgency, the amount of residual function and the presence or absence of dehydration or acidosis.

Acidosis is common and causes symptoms of lethargy, nausea, drowsiness and 'air-hunger' (Chapter 14). It is unusual for symptoms to occur unless the plasma bicarbonate is less than 15 mmol/litre. Most commonly it occurs in very salt-depleted patients and will spontaneously improve with treatment of the dehydration.

Rapid repair of acidosis can be dangerous. In giving sodium bicarbonate there is the risk of fluid overload because of the sodium content (although as has been mentioned most patients are initially salt-depleted), and a rapid rise in pH may precipitate tetany and convulsions by allowing the calcium ions that have been displaced from plasma proteins by hydrogen ions to rebind.

Only in life-threatening situations should rapid repair with intravenous bicarbonate be used, giving increments of 25−50 mmol (25−50 ml of 8.4% i.e. molar) of sodium bicarbonate. Oral sodium bicarbonate is slower and quite effective. The dose can be gradually increased while watching for the effect on plasma bicarbonate and for evidence of fluid overload.

Prevention and treatment of renal bone disease

Prevention of renal bone disease depends on:

Control of hyperphosphataemia. Phosphate binding drugs are taken to bind dietary phosphate and prevent its absorption. Aluminium hydroxide (300 to 1800 mg) is taken with meals. Constipation can be a troublesome side-effect. Evidence that this aluminium load contributes to the development of aluminium toxicity (see below) has led to use of other phosphate binders. Calcium carbonate (500 to 3000 mg) taken with each meal has proved a useful alternative with the added advantage of increasing calcium intake. Hypercalcaemia can occur with high doses, particularly if the patient does not eat well. The search for an ideal phosphate binder continues.

Vitamin D supplementation in the form of $1,25(OH)_2$-D3 (calcitriol) is occasionally required in CRF prior to dialysis. Hypercalcaemia and rapid renal functional deterioration can occur, accordingly plasma calcium and phosphate concentration must be closely monitored.

Parathyroidectomy is indicated if there is bone disease or hypercalcaemia, but is often deferred until the patient commences dialysis since the surgery and subsequent instability of plasma calcium concentration can precipitate ESRF.

Detection and treatment of infection

Urine, chest and other infection increases in frequency with advancing renal failure. Specific localising signs can be vague in the uraemic patient and the febrile response is blunted. For this reason a high index of suspicion must be entertained at all times. The uraemic patient must be recognised as immunosuppressed, and treated more vigorously than non-uraemic patients.

Modify drug therapy

The relationship between drugs and renal disease will be discussed in detail in Chapter 34. Many drugs require reduction in dosage because they or their toxic metabolites are renally excreted. Important examples include digoxin, aminoglycosides, opiate analgesics and allopurinol. Nephrotoxic drugs, such as aminoglycosides, trimethoprim-sulphamethoxazole and amphotericin must be used with great care. Other drugs increase catabolism and hence blood urea; included are tetracyclines, corticosteroids and cytotoxic drugs used in cancer therapy.

Detect and treat complications

With increasing failure the likelihood of severe complications is high, and commonly these constitute an indication for commencing dialysis.

A close watch should be kept to detect:
- Uraemic encephalopathy.
- Pericarditis or pleurisy.
- Peripheral neuropathy.
- Increasing hyperkalaemia.
- Increasing fluid overload.
- Life-threatening infections.
- General failure to thrive; medically, psychologically or socially.

Should these occur, institution of dialysis should be considered.

Preparation for dialysis and transplantation

Preparation for possible future dialysis and transplantation should start immediately CRF is detected, if only in terms of warning the patient that this is a possibility in the distant future. This should allow the patient, his or her family and the medical staff to make appropriate adjustments to minimise the upheavals that accompany commencing a dialysis and transplant program. This includes insertion of an arteriovenous access device when the plasma creatinine is about 0.8 mmol/litre, counselling about live and cadaver transplantation and commencing pretransplant tissue typing and work-up.

The indication for commencing dialysis is usually symptomatic renal failure despite conservative therapy, or the development of a complication as outlined above.

12: *Hypertension and the Kidney*

The relationships between blood pressure and the kidneys are inescapable; renal disease causes high blood pressure and high blood pressure can cause renal disease. Hypertension is thus a common presenting problem in patients with renal disease, and renal disease is the commonest detectable cause of hypertension.

DEFINITIONS

There is no straightforward definition of hypertension, although the World Health Organization has suggested a blood pressure greater than 160/95 mmHg in adults. Mean blood pressure rises with age and is higher in men than women. It is important to refer to tables of normal blood pressure in children, since they have much lower pressures than adults. Similarly in pregnancy much lower pressures are usual. Mortality rises with increasing blood pressure more so in males than females, and particularly in patients with other risk factors such as smoking. The main causes of death are:

- Cerebrovascular accidents, both haemorrhage and infarction.
- Myocardial infarction.
- Renal failure.

CAUSES AND PATHOGENESIS OF HYPERTENSION

The common causes of hypertension are listed in Table 12.1. In the majority of cases a specific abnormality is not detectable, and we are left with the diagnosis 'essential hypertension'. The risk factors for essential hypertension are summarised in Table 12.2.

Accelerated hypertension

Of great relevance to hypertension and the kidney is the entity 'accelerated hypertension', where very high blood pressure (often over 130 mmHg diastolic) is combined with haemorrhages and exudates in the retina and progressive renal damage. Although most cases nowadays occur on a background of renal disease, it can occur with essential and other causes of hypertension.

The mechanism is believed to be a self-perpetuating vicious

164

Table 12.1 Common causes of hypertension

Essential (about 90% of cases)
Genetic influences
  family
  race
  sex
Environmental influences
  salt intake
  stress
  diet, obesity

Secondary
Renal parenchymal disease (7–10% of cases)
Renal artery stenosis (up to 3% of cases)
  atheroma
  fibromuscular hyperplasia
Endocrine ($\ll$1% of cases)
  primary aldosteronism (Conn's syndrome)
  phaeochromocytoma
  pregnancy-induced hypertension (Pre-eclampsia)
Coarctation of the aorta
Drug-induced
  oral contraceptive
  monoamine-oxidase inhibitor (plus adrenergic drug or food)

Table 12.2 Causes of renovascular hypertension

Atheromatous renal artery stenosis

Fibromuscular hyperplasia of the renal artery

Intrarenal vascular disease
Scleroderma (systemic sclerosis)
Polyarteritis
Diabetic vascular disease
Renal transplant rejection
Atheromatous emboli

cycle, with severe hypertension leading to intrarenal vascular changes, including marked intimal hyperplasia of renal arteries (Fig. 12.3). These vascular changes lead in turn to ischaemia and hence activation (or further activation) of the renin–angiotensin system with consequent worsening of the hypertension, further vascular damage and consequent renal functional deterioration.

Renal hypertension Renal diseases are responsible for about 10% of cases of hypertension. The mechanisms are not entirely clear. It is believed that renovascular hypertension (e.g. renal artery stenosis) is mainly mediated by activation of the renin–angiotensin system, and in renal failure salt and water retention is important. In other renal parenchymal diseases without renal failure it is likely that the mechanisms are complex, including these factors as well as aberrations of other intrarenal hormones.

Renovascular hypertension

There are a variety of causes of renovascular hypertension (Table 12.2).

Atheromatous renal artery stenosis. This is commonest in patients over 60 years of age, and those with predisposing factors to accelerated vascular disease including smoking, diabetes, analgesic nephropathy, hypertension and hyperlipidaemia.

The common cause is a plaque usually in the ostium or first 2 cm of the artery (Fig. 12.1). In 25% of cases it is bilateral. Patients often also have clinically apparent cardiac, cerebral, aortic or peripheral vascular disease.

Fibromuscular hyperplasia. This disease, of unknown aetiology, constitutes about 30% of cases of renovascular hypertension, affecting mainly young adult females. Alternating stenosis and dilatation producing a beaded appearance of the arteriogram is characteristic (Fig. 12.2).

Intrarenal vascular disease. In scleroderma, accelerated hypertension and other intrarenal vascular diseases (Table 12.2) renal ischaemia can occur as in extrarenal vascular disease. Atheromatous microemboli from the aorta can obstruct the microvasculature, particularly in patients who have had recent aortic catheters or surgery.

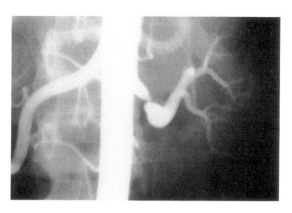

Fig. 12.1 Atheromatous renal artery stenosis (arteriogram). Note the tight stricture and poststenotic dilatation in the renal artery

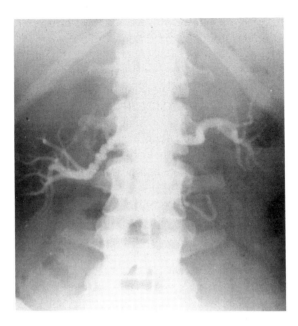

Fig. 12.2 Fibromuscular hyperplasia of the renal artery (digital subtraction angiogram). The beaded appearance of the right renal artery, which is long and supplies a ptosed kidney, is characteristic

PATHOLOGY OF HYPERTENSION

High blood pressure is associated with acute and chronic changes in systemic and renal vasculature.

Accelerated hypertension

In acute severe hypertension the most striking renal abnormality is gross intimal hyperplasia, with near occlusion of the lumen in intralobular and smaller arteries and arterioles (Fig. 12.3). Localised areas of necrosis and fibrinoid degeneration can be seen in the walls as well as luminal occlusion by thrombi — a microangiopathic picture. In severe cases glomerular microthrombosis and necrosis can be seen. This picture, similar in many ways to that seen in other forms of thrombotic microangiopathy (Chapter 32) rapidly results in renal failure if the blood pressure is not controlled.

Chronic hypertension

In the kidney generalised narrowing of arteries by fibroelastic tissue occurs. Related tubulointerstitial change and signs of ischaemia may be present. Despite the histological changes it is very doubtful whether this process, benign nephrosclerosis, by itself leads to sufficient renal damage to cause clinical renal failure. Benign essential hypertension does not, therefore, for

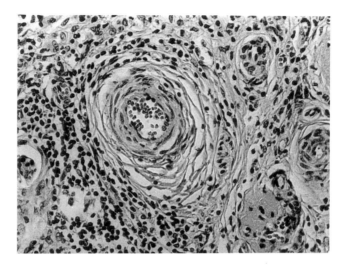

Fig. 12.3 Arterial changes in accelerated hypertension. Renal biopsy showing the severe intimal hyperplasia characterising accelerated hypertension

practical purposes cause end-stage renal failure unless it is complicated by accelerated hypertension or renal artery atheroma. Most cases of impaired renal function attributed to benign nephrosclerosis have underlying renal disease.

CLINICAL FEATURES OF HYPERTENSION

Hypertension is largely an asymptomatic disease, unless acceleration or complications have occurred, mainly in the cardiovascular, renal and neurological systems.

Cardiovascular system. Exertional dyspnoea, orthopnea, pulmonary oedema and angina can occur due to left ventricular hypertrophy, failure and ischaemia due to coronary artery disease. Peripheral vascular disease, including aortic aneurysm and claudication may be present.

Nervous system. Careful examination of the retina is an important part of assessment since the changes give a good indication of the severity of the hypertension (Table 12.3).

Headache, pounding, occipital, worse in the morning and often easing as the day advances, occurs in accelerated hypertension. Nausea and vomiting and confusion may be present. The fundi show haemorrhage, exudates and sometimes papilloedema (Fig. 12.4).

Table 12.3 Hypertensive retinopathy. Grades III and IV occur in accelerated hypertension. Grade IV designates 'malignant' hypertension but the prognosis is the same

Grade	Retinal changes
I	Arterial wall thickening
II	Venous nipping by arteries
III	Haemorrhages and exudates
IV	Papilloedema (Fig. 12.4)

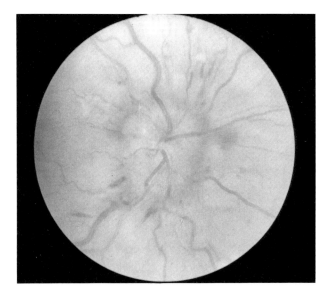

Fig. 12.4 Grade 4 retinal changes in malignant hypertension. Note papilloedema, haemorrhages, soft exudates and extreme arteriolar narrowing

Renal. Since renal disease is the commonest detectable cause of hypertension, and hypertension can cause benign nephrosclerosis and accelerated hypertensive renal disease, a careful renal history and examination is important (Chapter 7). Renal artery bruits may be heard in the subcostal areas or the loins in renovascular hypertension. The presence of proteinuria, haematuria or pyuria and casts suggest a renal cause for hypertension, except in accelerated hypertension when glomerular haematuria and proteinuria often occur prior to adequate control of the blood pressure.

CLINICAL APPROACH TO THE PATIENT WITH HYPERTENSION

The patient should be assessed for:
• Severity of hypertension.

- Complications.
- Other cardiovascular risk factors.
- A cause for the hypertension.

Unless hypertension is severe or there is clear evidence of complications it is unwise to commence therapy on the basis of a single blood pressure reading. A careful examination for complications should be made and the patient reassessed on several occasions before drug treatment is commenced. During this period advice regarding non-pharmacological control of the blood pressure, weight loss, smoking and lipids can be given (see below).

The blood pressure reading, the appearance of the fundi and the presence of cardiomegaly and left ventricular hypertrophy all give an indication as to the severity and chronicity of the hypertension.

The most severe form is accelerated (malignant) hypertension.

Accelerated hypertension is characterised by:
- Very high blood pressure, usually >130 mmHg diastolic in adults. Sudden increases in blood pressure, and in children or pregnant women much lower pressures, can also be associated with accelerated hypertension.
- Haemorrhages, exudates, arterial spasm and papilloedema in the retina (Fig. 12.4). Studies have shown that the renal effects of accelerated hypertension commence with grade III fundal changes.
- Microscopic glomerular haematuria and proteinuria.
- Symptoms of headache, visual blurring, poor concentration or even confusion and convulsions (hypertensive encephalopathy) may be present.

Immediate hospitalisation, and careful reduction of pressure and investigation for a cause is required, since untreated this syndrome leads to death from fulminating progression to renal failure, cerebrovascular accident or left ventricular failure in less than 6 months in most patients.

INVESTIGATION OF THE HYPERTENSIVE PATIENT

The effort to detect a cause is influenced by the severity of the hypertension and the age of the patient. In a young patient with severe hypertension a cause is likely to be found, but in the young if no reversible cause is found the patient faces a long life of drug therapy. All causes other than renal are extremely uncommon. In the examination exclusion of coarctation by careful timing of the femoral pulses, detection of renal masses, auscultation for renal bruits are important, and urinalysis for protein and blood should be routine.

Investigations are aimed at detecting the cause and assessing the degree of end-organ damage from the high blood pressure (Table 12.4).

Minimal investigation includes the following.

Exclusion of renal disease
Urinalysis

Analysis of a urine specimen for blood and protein should be performed in all patients, since up to 10% of hypertension is of renal origin. Microscopy and culture is also performed (Chapter 8).

Plasma creatinine and/or urea

Renal failure must be excluded. It has a bearing on the possible causes, since in practice an elevated plasma creatinine concentration means the patient has primary renal disease or accelerated hypertension.

Plasma electrolytes

Plasma potassium should be measured before starting therapy in all patients. Although the commonest cause overall is diuretic therapy, hypokalaemia in an untreated patient with hypertension suggests that aldosterone secretion is increased (Table 12.5). This can be due to primary hyperaldosteronism, but secondary hyperaldosteronism due to renovascular or accelerated hypertension is far more commonly the cause of hypokalaemia in untreated hypertensive patients.

Further investigations which may be performed in the young patient or those in whom a cause is suspected include creatinine clearance, 24-hour urine protein determination, and if there is an abnormality in the urine or renal function an intravenous

Table 12.4 Investigation of hypertension

Exclude renal parenchymal disease
Urinalysis for blood and protein
Urine microscopy and culture
Plasma creatinine or urea
Plasma electrolytes, especially potassium

Assess complications and other risk factors
Chest X-ray
Electrocardiograph
Fasting blood sugar
Fasting plasma lipids
Plasma uric acid

Consider further investigations
e.g. renal — IVP, arteriography, renal biopsy
Aldosteronism
Phaeochromocytome
Cushing's syndrome

Table 12.5 Causes of hypokalaemia with hypertension

Diuretic therapy (the commonest)
Renovascular hypertension
Accelerated hypertension
Primary aldosteronism (Conn's syndrome)
Glucocorticoid excess (Cushing's syndrome)
Renin-producing tumor
Incidental cause of hypokalaemia (Table 14.7)

pyelogram as a screening test for 'anatomical' renal disease (reflux nephropathy, analgesic nephropathy, hydronephrosis, polycystic kidney disease, etc.). Renal parenchymal disease with a normal IVP usually requires a renal biopsy for accurate diagnosis.

Exclusion of renal artery stenosis

If there is a suggestion of renal artery stenosis, e.g. a bruit, severe hypertension in a young woman, family history of fibromuscular hyperplasia, or rapidly worsening hypertension in a patient with generalised vascular disease, a digital subtraction arteriogram (DSA) should be performed. Isotope renography can be useful in comparing renal blood flow in unilateral renal artery stenosis. A smaller kidney with a delayed and more dense nephrogram and pyelogram may be seen in the IVP. Recently, Doppler ultrasound has also been found useful to screen for renal artery stenosis.

Bilateral renal vein renin estimations may predict response to surgery. If the ratio between the renal vein renin from the affected kidney and the contralateral kidney exceeds 1.5 a good result from repair of the stenosis is likely, although a good response can occur with a lower ratio. Clinical indications are thus the best guide to decisions about surgical or medical treatment.

Assessment of complications and other risk factors

Cardiac size should be assessed and an ECG may indicate left ventricular hypertrophy and ischaemia. Since they influence therapy and prognosis it is usual to screen for:
• Diabetes, with a fasting blood glucose.
• Hyperlipidaemia, with fasting lipid estimations.
• Hyperuricaemia.

TREATMENT OF HYPERTENSION

Since treatment for hypertension is lifelong it is important to ensure that treatment is indicated and that the patient is aware that a lifelong pattern of treatment and review is being undertaken.

Benefits of treatment

Clear increases in survival and decreases in morbid events (mainly cerebrovascular) have been demonstrated in retrospective and prospective studies of the treatment of hypertension, with the benefits being proportional to the severity of the hypertension. In malignant or accelerated hypertension without treatment a 50% 6-month mortality can be expected. Treatment improves this at least five-fold. It has been also shown to result in improvement in renal function, which can continue to improve for over 12 months after control of the blood pressure.

In renal disease poor blood pressure control can result in more rapid deterioration of function. For this reason it is usual to try to keep the blood pressure of patients with renal disease to below about 150/90 mmHg.

Indications for treatment

As a rough guide the following recommendations are made:
- All patients with renal disease, or who have evidence of end-organ damage (cerebrovascular, cardiac, retinal or renal) or diabetes should be treated if blood pressure exceeds 150/90 mmHg.
- All patients with accelerated hypertension should be admitted to hospital for investigation and treatment.
- In other patients a trial of non-drug therapy (see below) can be employed while reviewing the blood pressure, frequently (weekly) if it is greater than 110 diastolic, and monthly if less. During this time relevant investigations (see above) can be performed and may clarify the need for treatment.

In patients without renal disease, diabetes or end-organ damage drug therapy should be introduced if the blood pressure is persistently:
- >160/95 in males <60 years of age.
- >160/100 in females <60 years of age.
- >180/100 in patients >60 years of age.

Non-drug therapy

Time needs to be spent with the patient to discuss the contribution of lifestyle to blood pressure and its complications. Important modifications include:
- Stop smoking.
- Lose weight.
- Increase potassium intake.
- Decrease salt intake to around 100–120 mmol/day unless there is a salt-losing condition. This is helpful in about 50% of cases.
- Regular exercise.
- Reduce alcohol intake.

A vegetarian diet has also been shown to reduce blood pressure. The evidence for calcium supplementation is less convincing.

Methods aimed at reducing the stress component such as hypnosis and relaxation therapy have also been shown to reduce blood pressure.

Drug therapy in benign chronic hypertension

Unfortunately in most patients with renal disease drug therapy eventually becomes necessary. The traditional approach is a stepped approach, where new drugs are added cautiously then increased in dose to a level giving maximum effect with minimal side-effects. It is a mistake to rapidly alter or increase drugs except in urgent situations. It is usual to use only one drug of each class (diuretic, central acting, vasodilator), and to cease any agent which has not been beneficial.

The introduction of very effective new drugs such as the calcium channel blockers and angiotensin-converting enzyme inhibitors, as well as some disquiet about the long-term metabolic side-effects of thiazide diuretics and β-blockers is causing continual reassessment of the traditional approach.

Step 1 drugs

Thiazide diuretics exert their antihypertensive effect both by decreasing body salt and by a vasodilator effect. They amplify the effect of other antihypertensives, many of which promote fluid retention. Common side effects include hypokalaemia, hyperglycaemia and hyperuricaemia. In the elderly hyponatraemia can be a problem, particularly if a thiazide–amiloride combination is used to prevent hypokalaemia. Potassium supplements or adjunctive potassium-sparing diuretics (spironolactone, amiloride, triamterene) should only be added if hypokalaemia develops or the patient is taking digoxin.

Step 2 drugs

In traditional 'stepped care' treatment the second drug has been a β-adrenergic blocking drug.

Beta-adrenergic blocking drugs. A wide variety of β-adrenergic blocking drugs are available, with varying degrees of β_2 selectivity (to avoid bronchoconstrictor effect), intrinsic sympathomimetic effect (to avoid peripheral vasoconstriction and bradycardia) and central nervous system penetration (to avoid sedation and nightmares). It is wise to be familiar with one or two drugs rather than to use the whole gamut, since commonly patients intolerant of one β-blocker are intolerant of all. Beta-blocking drugs also reduce angina.

Side effects are precipitation of asthma (β_1 blockade), vasospasm with Raynaud's syndrome, worsening of claudication and precipitation of cardiac failure (β_2 blockade). They should not be used in patients with asthma or obstructive airways disease, and should only be used with great care in patients with cardiac failure.

Prazosin, a highly selective α-adrenergic blocking drug, is often the third drug introduced. Its vasodilatory effects and resultant tachycardia are a helpful counterbalance to the vasoconstriction and bradycardia that can occur with β-blockers. The main disadvantage is the short duration of action necessitating 2–3 doses per day. Longer acting α-blocking drugs which can be administered daily are becoming available.

Side-effects include a potentially dangerous first dose effect, i.e. a syncopal reaction after first or increased dosage. Prazosin should always be started with a low dose (0.5–1.0 mg) taken at night before going to bed; then increased gradually. The major side effect is postural hypotension.

Calcium-channel blockers. Nifedipine and verapamil have both been widely used for treatment of hypertension. They are particularly useful if the patient also has angina, since they are also effective therapies for this condition.

Side-effects include constipation and cardiac failure with verapamil, and reflex tachycardia, flushing and fluid retention. A variety of long-acting preparations and newer agents could well cause this class of drug to become popular second-line or even first-step antihypertensive agents in the future.

Angiotensin-converting enzyme (ACE) inhibitors. Captopril and enalapril are already being widely used as second-line drugs. Enalapril has the advantage of once daily administration and a slower rate of action, hence less first dose effect. ACE inhibitors should be considered in patients with cardiac failure since they are effective in the treatment of this condition. These drugs can cause an abrupt decrease in blood pressure with the first dose, hyperkalaemia, and decrease in renal function especially if bilateral renal artery stenosis is present. Considerable care is required during the introductory period.

Captopril has been most used, and its most common side effects are rash and loss of taste. Membranous glomerulonephritis with nephrotic syndrome and bone-marrow depression can occur with high doses. Enalapril undergoes hepatic conversion before being active. It is therefore of more gradual onset, and can be used in a once daily dose.

Alpha-methyldopa. This older drug is very effective and can be used in patients with asthma or cardiac failure where some drugs are contraindicated. Side effects include dry mouth, lassitude, somnolence and allergic reactions, including a positive Coomb's test and hepatic toxicity.

Clonidine. This is another effective centrally acting agent, but drowsiness, dry mouth and withdrawal-induced hypertensive crises limit its use.

Hydrallazine. This is a direct vasodilator. Side effects of headache and precipitation of drug-induced SLE, particularly in women who are slow-acetylators and DRw4 positive, (Chapter 17), restrict its use.

Step 3 drugs

Step 3 drugs are only employed once the drugs in the first two classes have been exhausted. This usually only occurs in very severe hypertensives.

Labetolol. This is a combined α- and β-adrenergic blocking drug. It has no particular advantages over a combination of adequate β-blockade and prazosin.

Minoxidil. This direct vasodilator drug is a very powerful anti-hypertensive but causes severe fluid retention, hirsutism (it is now used in creams for baldness!) and pericardial effusion.

Diazoxide. Rarely used nowadays this drug has been useful in hypertensive crises and severe hypertension. Fluid retention, hirsutism and precipitation of diabetes limit its long-term use.

Treatment of accelerated hypertension

Patients with accelerated hypertension should be admitted to hospital. Immediate reduction of blood pressure within minutes is potentially dangerous and indicated in only a very few situations, e.g. hypertensive encephalopathy or arterial bleeding (Table 12.6). In the absence of such an emergency it is preferable to use a rapidly stepped oral regimen.

Sublingual and transcutaneous therapy

Nifedipine, 5–10 mg chewed, or trinitrin, one tablet, is useful for rapid moderate reduction of pressure while awaiting the effect of orally acting drugs. Nitroglycerin paste on the skin can be used with similar effect.

Rapidly active oral agents

Drugs which can be expected to work within hours, and are thus useful initially, include prazosin, nifedipine and captopril.

Table 12.6 Indications for emergency treatment of hypertension

Hypertensive encephalopathy (including eclamptic fitting)

Severe hypertension complicated by
Pulmonary oedema
Intracranial haemorrhage
Aortic dissection
Bleeding

Hypertensive crisis of phaeochomocytoma

Parenteral therapy   This should be reserved for patients in whom oral administration is contraindicated. Suitable agents include intravenous hydralazine, α-methyldopa and, in emergency, diazoxide. Infusion of nitroprusside or nitroglycerin is effective but requires an infusion pump and usually continuous arterial blood pressure monitoring.

13: *Urinary Tract Infection*

Urinary tract infection (UTI) is one of the most common illnesses seen in general medical practice. In most women UTI is a transiently uncomfortable illness with minimal systemic upset and long term sequelae. In a minority of patients UTI reflects underlying urinary tract disease, and can cause serious illness (septicaemia) and renal damage. The clinical approach is based on recognising the few patients in whom the illness is potentially serious among the many who have uncomplicated infection.

DEFINITIONS

Urine infection can be defined as the presence of bacteria in bladder urine, which is normally sterile.

UTI is a term used interchangeably with urine infection. It also includes a variety of infections in the renal tract not necessarily involving bladder urine (prostatitis, urethritis).

Significant bacteriuria. Most of our knowledge of the epidemiology of UTI comes from epidemiological studies which show that more than 10^5 colony forming units (cfu/ml) of bacteria in a midstream urine specimen from an asymptomatic subject has an 85% chance of indicating bladder bacteriuria. In the symptomatic patient UTI with a lower count of organisms is common, though a count of $>10^5$ cfu/ml still indicates probable UTI (see below).

Asymptomatic or covert bacteriuria. If significant bacteriuria is detected by screening subjects not complaining of symptoms, asymptomatic bacteriuria is said to be present. These patients very commonly have past or future symptoms of UTI; accordingly the term covert bacteriuria is preferable.

Acute pyelonephritis is a clinical syndrome of UTI in which loin pain and fever are prominent (see below).

Acute cystitis is a clinical syndrome of UTI in which dysuria and frequency are prominent (see below).

178

Chronic pyelonephritis. It was once thought that renal scarring associated with chronic tubulointerstitial nephritis was mainly due to chronic renal infection. The realisation that the commonest form, reflux nephropathy, was related not only to UTI but also to vesicoureteric reflux in infancy (Chapter 21), and that urinary obstruction, analgesic nephropathy and a variety of other conditions cause chronic tubulointerstitial nephritis (Chapter 20) has lead to the dropping of this term in favour of more specific nomenclature.

INCIDENCE

Symptoms suggesting UTI are responsible for about 0.5 to 1% of consultations in general practice. The vast majority occur in adult women, of whom it has been estimated that about one-third will have symptoms suggestive of UTI at some time in their life.

Significant bacteriuria is found in about 5% of adult women at any time (Fig. 13.1). By contrast only about 1% of children, and under 0.5% of men have bacteriuria. In elderly people, particularly those who are institutionalised and unwell, the frequency of bacteria rises dramatically, with figures as high as 30–50% in the most dependent patients.

The frequency of clinical UTI tends to follow the same age and sex trends. In children with developmental anatomical abnormalities of the urinary tract UTI is likely to occur in the first few years of life. In females UTI is then uncommon until late ado-

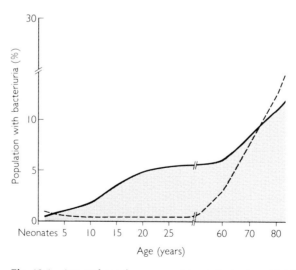

Fig. 13.1 Age and sex frequency of bacteriuria. (---) Males; (——) females

lescence and early adulthood when it becomes common, associated with intercourse and pregnancy. It increases in frequency with old age. In males developmental abnormalities with UTI in infancy are more common than in females but once childhood has passed, UTI, both asymptomatic and clinical, becomes rare until old age.

CAUSES AND PATHOGENESIS

Three aspects will be considered:
1 The organism.
2 The introduction of the organism into the urinary tract.
3 The failure of clearance of the organism from the bladder.

Bacteria causing urine infections

Enteric organisms (derived from the gastrointestinal tract) are the usual cause of UTI, and of these *Escherichia coli* are by far the commonest (Table 13.1). Different strains of *E. coli* vary in their propensity for causing asymptomatic UTI, cystitis or acute pyelo-nephritis, depending on such factors as their surface fimbriae, O and K antigens.

  E. coli are not the only organisms found. While they represent about 90% of the organisms causing UTI in ambulant females, in males and hospital inpatients 30–40% of UTI are due to other organisms such as *Proteus, Staphylococcus* and even *Pseudomonas* spp. (Table 13.1). Their presence is suggestive of an underlying urinary tract abnormality. Multiple organisms usually reflect con-tamination of the specimen, but if not artefactual they strongly suggest a urinary tract abnormality.

Introduction of the organism

UTI is usually an ascending infection (Fig. 13.2). The usual course in women is for the organisms to first colonise the vulva from the anal verge, and then to be introduced into the bladder via the short urethra either spontaneously or by mechanical forces during intercourse. A similar ascending route is suspected but not proven in males, where the long urethra is a barrier. Certainly once the prostate becomes colonised, recurrent ascending infection from this organ is likely (Fig. 13.3).

Table 13.1 Bacteria commonly found in urinary tract infection

Escherichia coli	About 80% of cases
Others*	*Streptococcus faecalis, Klebsiella, Enterobacter, Citrobacter, Staphylococcus albus* and *aureus, Proteus mirabilis, Pseudomonas*

* Isolation of the less common organisms occurs more often in hospitalised patients and those with anatomical abnormalities

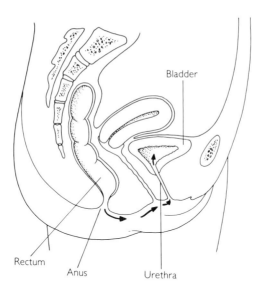

Fig. 13.2 Ascending infection in the female. The usual path of infection is from the rectum via the vulva and urethra

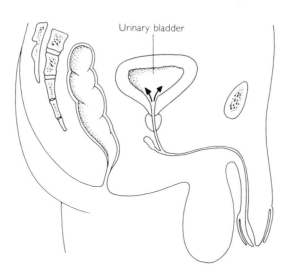

Fig. 13.3 Recurrent infection in the male often is due to chronic prostatic infection

The shorter urethra, intercourse-related introduction of organisms, and perhaps alterations in vulval pH and flora with the menstrual cycle are thought to be the reasons why females are so much more commonly affected by UTI than males. In females prone to UTI it has been shown that pathogenic *E. coli* adhere to the epithelial cells of the vulva and colonise the area, and this constitutes an important initial step in establishing infection.

Other common methods of introduction include urethral instrumentation such as passage of catheters and ascent via indwelling catheters. These are particularly likely to occur in the older population, where prostatomegaly, incontinence and debility are common, and are probably the main reasons for frequent UTI in the institutionalised geriatric population (Fig. 13.1).

Failure of clearance of the organism

Bacteria introduced into the bladder should be rapidly cleared by local defence mechanisms, the most important of which are resistance to bacterial adhesion, the flow of sterile urine from the kidneys, and the frequent emptying of the bladder. Anatomical abnormalities may interfere with these mechanisms by causing stasis of urine or a nidus in which the flow of urine is impeded, such as a stone or renal scar (Table 13.2).

In most women with acute cystitis there is no anatomical abnormality. In these women it is suspected that specific surface characteristics of the patient's uroepithelium and the organism lead to attachment of the organism to the bladder epithelium, preventing clearance. In some women infrequent voiding may also play a role.

The most common predisposing anatomical abnormalities in

Table 13.2 Anatomical abnormalities associated with urinary tract infection

Renal
Scar (reflux nephropathy)
Papillary necrosis
Stone
Cysts

Ureter
Vesicoureteric reflux
Physiological dilatation of pregnancy
Duplex
Stricture

Bladder
Catheter
Prolapse
Neurogenic bladder
Diverticulum

Urethra
Prostatomegaly
Prostatitis
Stricture

women are reflux nephropathy, analgesic nephropathy, stones and pregnancy-induced pelviureteric dilatation with stasis, in men stones and prostatic disease and in children congenital abnormalities.

CLINICAL FEATURES

UTI can be asymptomatic, cause symptoms referable to the lower urinary tract or cause symptoms of renal infection. The infection can be an isolated single attack or recurrent.

Asymptomatic or covert bacteriuria

This is only common in females (Fig. 13.1). These women are likely to have a past and future history of symptomatic UTI. Short courses of treatment for asymptomatic bacteriuria are likely to lead to subsequent symptomatic UTI, presumably due to reinfection with a more virulent organism. In the absence of radiological abnormality there is no evidence that untreated asymptomatic bacteriuria causes any renal damage.

Lower tract symptoms — acute cystitis

Pain or a burning sensation during micturition (dysuria), frequency of micturition, and suprapubic pain (sometimes worse after voiding) are symptoms of bladder irritation. Some patients will complain of foul smelling or cloudy urine, and haematuria may occur. While UTI is by far the commonest cause of dysuria and frequency other causes are listed in Table 13.3.

Upper tract symptoms — acute pyelonephritis

Loin pain and constitutional upset with fever, nausea and rigors indicate renal infection, i.e. acute pyelonephritis. The kidneys may be tender. On the other hand some patients with proven

Table 13.3 Causes of dysuria/frequency

Urinary tract infection

Genital infection
Trichomonas
Gonococcus
Candida

Non-specific urethritis (NSU)
Chlamydial infection

Bladder base irritation
Idiopathic interstitial cystitis
Bladder stone

Unknown — 'The urethral syndrome'

renal infection have only lower tract or no symptoms. The presence of the clinical syndrome of acute pyelonephritis is highly suggestive of an underlying urinary tract abnormality.

DIAGNOSIS OF URINARY TRACT INFECTION

Proof of UTI requires culture of organisms from the urine, though as outlined later in this chapter, it is more cost-effective to treat women with an isolated attack of acute cystitis on a clinical basis and restrict urine culture to the follow-up period. In men, children and women with acute pyelonephritis, urine should be taken for microscopy and culture before therapy commences.

Diagnosis depends on careful urine collection and interpretation of microscopy and culture results.

Collection of urine

The various methods for collecting urine specimens have been described in Chapter 7.

Midstream urine collection

The mainstay of diagnosis of UTI is the midstream specimen of urine (MSU). The urine is best sent immediately to the laboratory, but if this is inconvenient, useful results can be obtained from urine stored for up to 24 hours in a refrigerator (4°C). Patients with recurrent UTI can be taught to collect the urine at home, and bring it to the laboratory next morning. In difficult cases it is preferable to collect the first urine passed in the morning — 'incubation' in the bladder overnight maximising the bacterial concentration.

Catheter specimen of urine

As discussed in Chapter 8, the use of conventional catheters for collection of urine to diagnose UTI should be reserved for patients with indwelling catheters. The recently developed technique of open-ended catheter insertion is very useful in women with difficult to interpret MSU results, since it provides a specimen almost as good as that provided by suprapubic aspiration (see below), with minimal risk of introducing infection.

Suprapubic aspiration of urine

The suprapubic aspirate (SPA) is invaluable in infants and in adults when repeated MSU collections have failed to provide accurate results due to contamination or low bacterial counts. The technique is described in Chapter 8. Under local anaesthetic a needle is inserted suprapubically into the very full bladder and urine aspirated. For practical purposes any organism grown from an SPA indicates infection of bladder urine.

Examination of the urine

Urinary dipsticks should be used to test for proteinuria, haematuria, glycosuria and pH (Chapter 8). Although both haematuria

Urinalysis

and proteinuria can occur with severe lower tract UTI they are more common with upper tract and complicated infection. Glycosuria suggests either diabetes or a renal tubular abnormality.

Microscopy

Microscopy will give information regarding:
- *Contamination* — a large number of squames and debris usually indicates significant vaginal contamination.
- *Pyuria* — significant pyuria ($>$2000 WBC/ml) is usually present when there is symptomatic UTI.
- *Organisms* — organisms may be seen in the urine in UTI but also with contamination.

Culture

If there are greater than 10^5 cfu/ml of bacteria in an MSU from an asymptomatic patient there is an 85% chance that this reflects true bladder infection. This has led to the adoption of the term 'significant bacteriuria' for bacterial counts of $>10^5$ cfu/ml. It is important to realise that this is only a statistical tool, and patients with true UTI often have less than 10^5 cfu/ml in the MSU. Thus $>10^5$ cfu/ml is helpful in making a positive diagnosis of UTI, but not useful in excluding UTI.

Other features to support the diagnosis of UTI include:
1 The presence of pyuria.
2 The growth of a single strain of organism, particularly *E. coli*.
3 The absence of microscopic indications of contamination (vaginal squames).

In urine collected by catheter the presence of lower counts of organisms may be diagnostic, and with SPA the growth of any organisms indicates UTI. Open-ended catheter specimens are very similar to those obtained by needle aspiration.

In women presenting with symptoms of UTI approximately
- 60% will have UTI with $>10^5$ cfu/ml in the urine,
- 20% will have UTI with $10^2 - 10^5$ cfu/ml, and
- over 10% will have organisms which may not be easily cultured (such as anaerobes, ureaplasmas, *Chlamydia*, *Trichomonas* or *Gonococcus*) in the urine or genital tract. A few will have vulval or periurethral diseases causing dysuria (Table 13.3).

The remainder (less than 10%) will have no infection. Although an organic cause, such as interstitial cystitis, may be found, in many of these patients the cause of the symptoms, which are often persistent or recurrent, remain unexplained.

Sterile pyuria

If there is pyuria but no bacterial growth the following possibilities should be considered (Table 13.4):
- *Low bacterial counts* — about 25% of symptomatic women with UTI have $<10^5$ cfu/ml, particularly if the urine is dilute and the organisms are prone to clumping (staphylococci).

Table 13.4 Causes of 'sterile pyuria', defined as pyuria (>2000 pus cells/ml) with less than 10^5 cfu/ml of organisms in the urine

---

UTI with low bacterial count
Diuresis with urinary dilution
Clumping of organisms (e.g. staphylococci)

UTI with inhibition of bacterial growth in vitro
Local soaps, detergents or antiseptics
Recent antibiotic intake

Tuberculosis
Organisms with fastidious growth requirements

Foreign body
Renal papillary necrosis
Infected stone

Non-infectious inflammatory disease
Systemic lupus erythematosus
Acute tubulointerstitial nephritis

• *Antiseptics or antibiotics.* Soaps, detergents or antiseptics may have been used to clean the vulva or glans and contaminated the collection container, killing the microorganisms. The patient may have taken antibiotics which have inhibited bacterial growth.
• *Tuberculosis.* Tuberculosis (Chapter 31) is a rare but most important cause of sterile pyuria.
• *Organisms with fastidious growth requirements.* Ureaplasma are examples of organisms which require special media.
• *Infected stones or foreign body.* These may harbour organisms with minimal bacteriuria.
• *Active tubulointerstitial disease.* In analgesic nephropathy and drug-induced interstitial nephritis there may be many leucocytes in the urine.

CLINICAL APPROACH TO UTI

The clinical approach to patients with suspected or proven UTI depends on the presence or absence of underlying urinary tract abnormality:
• There is little evidence that UTI causes serious renal damage in patients with normal renal function and a normal intravenous pyelogram.
• In patients with abnormal renal tracts UTI can lead to acute pyelonephritis, septicaemia and renal damage.
• UTI is uncommon in males and children with a normal renal tract.

• Acute pyelonephritis is relatively uncommon in patients with a normal renal tract.

The management consists of treating the attack, and investigating further if indicated (Table 13.5).

Screening for bacteriuria

Screening of an asymptomatic population for bacteriuria can only be justified in pregnant women. Bacteriuria is present in 6–8% of pregnant women and these women have a 30–40% chance of developing acute pyelonephritis during the pregnancy (Chapter 33). In patients with known abnormalities of the urinary tract, regular urine culture even when the patient is asymptomatic can be justified because the abnormalities predispose to symptomatic UTI, septicaemia, and severe renal infection with renal damage.

Management of UTI in women

Acute dysuria and/or frequency

At least 80% of women with dysuria and/or frequency have a bacterial UTI. The differential diagnosis includes infection or other irritation of the periurethral or vaginal areas (Table 13.3). If the clinical diagnosis is uncomplicated UTI, immediate treatment should be given with either a single dose or 5-day course of antibiotics (see below), and the only investigation required is an MSU a week later. If this is infected then further investigation is required. In other words, acute cystitis in women should usually only be further investigated if it is recurrent.

Acute pyelonephritis

This should be taken seriously, treated vigorously (see below) and investigated for a cause. A renal tract abnormality is common.

Asymptomatic bacteriuria

If this is found as the result of screening then it should be treated by single-dose therapy (see below) and only investigated if it recurs.

Table 13.5 Patients in whom urinary tract infection should be investigated

All children

All males

Adult females with:
Acute pyelonephritis or upper tract symptoms
UTI which fails to resolve or rapidly recurs after treatment
A history or signs suggestive of underlying renal disease such as:
   History of childhood UTI
   Hypertension
   History of analgesic abuse
   Persistent haematuria
   Persistent proteinuria
   Family history of UTI

Management of UTI in children

All children with any form of UTI should be treated and fully investigated. Over 50% will have an abnormality, the most common being vesicoureteric reflux or scarring (Chapter 21).

Management of UTI in men

Males with UTI should have a 5-day course of antibiotics, and should be investigated (see below). Should the IVP be normal and infection recur a prostatic massage and culture (Stamey 3-specimen test) should be performed to diagnose chronic prostatic infection (Fig. 13.4).

TREATMENT OF URINARY TRACT INFECTION

Treatment consists of encouraging fluid intake to promote diuresis, administering urinary alkalinising agents if there is severe dysuria, and appropriate antibacterial therapy. Antibacterial agents used in UTI should have good gram negative cover and achieve high urine concentrations, i.e. they should be renally excreted. Examples of usual drugs and their doses are given in Table 13.6.

Treatment of acute cystitis

Women with isolated finding of asymptomatic bacteriuria or lower tract symptoms only can be treated with single-dose therapy (Table 13.6), or the more conventional 5-day course of oral therapy.

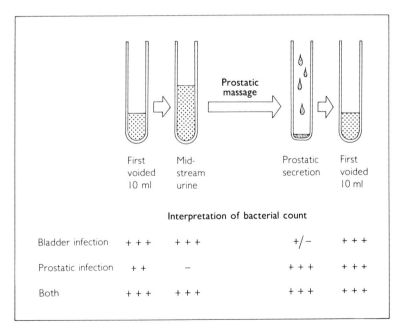

	First voided 10 ml	Mid-stream urine	Prostatic secretion	First voided 10 ml
Interpretation of bacterial count				
Bladder infection	+ + +	+ + +	+/−	+ + +
Prostatic infection	+ +	−	+ + +	+ + +
Both	+ + +	+ + +	+ + +	+ + +

Fig. 13.4 Stamey method for the diagnosis of prostatic infection by culturing before and after prostatic massage

Table 13.6 Drugs used in the treatment of urinary tract infection

	Drug	Dose
Single-dose therapy		
Oral	Amoxicillin	3 g
	Trimethoprim-sulphamethoxazole	320 mg/1600 mg (4 tablets)
	Cephalexin	3 g
Intramuscular	Kanamycin	0.5 g
Conventional therapy (5-day course)		
First line	Amoxicillin	250 mg t.d.s.
	Trimethoprim-sulphamethoxazole	160 mg/800 mg b.d.
	Trimethoprim	300 mg daily
	Nitrofurantoin	100 mg q.i.d.
Second line	Norfloxacin	400 mg b.d.
	Cephalexin	1 g q.i.d.
	Cephalothin	1 g/8 hours/i.m. or i.v.
	Gentamicin	0.8 mg/kg/8 hours/i.m.
	Kanamycin	5 mg/kg/8 hours/i.m.
Prophylactic (at night or postcoital)		
	Nitrofurantoin	50–100 mg
	Trimethoprim	150–300 mg
	Trimethoprim-sulphamethoxazole	40 mg/200 mg

Failure to clear the organisms constitutes an indication for further investigation.

In children and males the likelihood of an underlying abnormality is such that we do not recommend single dose therapy, and believe patients should receive a 5-day course of antibiotic and further investigation for a cause.

Treatment of acute pyelonephritis

Patients with acute pyelonephritis should be admitted to hospital for parenteral antibiotic therapy and investigation. If symptoms do not resolve rapidly renal ultrasound should be employed to exclude renal obstruction.

Treatment of recurrent UTI

There are two types of recurrent UTI. The most common is that of recurrent attacks of UTI with new organisms with each attack. This pattern signifies reinfection, and is the usual pattern in women with recurrent attacks of acute cystitis, and in some patients with anatomical abnormalities. The second pattern is where the infections persistently involve the same organism, i.e. relapse. With the exception of instances where treatment has been inadequate due to antibiotic resistance, persistent infection usually indicates the presence of a nidus of infection such as an infected prostate, stone, papilla or cyst.

Repeated infection. Patients with frequent reinfection are advised to take a high fluid intake and to void often. Further simple measures which are often effective in women are to void, and in some cases to take one dose of antibiotic immediately after intercourse to eliminate any introduced organisms. In difficult cases, long-term prophylactic chemotherapy may be required. The drugs, which are taken in low dose (one-quarter of the normal dose) before going to bed each night, should be excreted in the urine, be effective against a wide range of urinary pathogens, and be unlikely to induce antibiotic resistance or cause side-effects. Usual drugs are nitrofurantoin, trimethoprim and trimethoprim-sulphamethoxazole (Table 13.6). Usually a 3—6-month course is given in the first instance.

Persistent infection. A persistent infection which relapses immediately after treatment usually indicates an infected focus within the urinary tract. A long course of full-dose antibiotic (i.e. suppressive treatment) is required to eliminate infection in such cases.

FURTHER INVESTIGATION OF PATIENTS WITH URINARY TRACT INFECTION

The indications for further investigation of UTI are outlined in Table 13.5. Basically, all but women with isolated attacks of uncomplicated cystitis should undergo investigation aimed at identification of the organism(s) involved and detection of any renal or anatomical abnormality.

The following are the usual investigations:

Repeated urine microscopy and culture. Pyuria between attacks of UTI suggests a nidus such as an infected stone, cyst or papilla (Table 13.7).

Identification of the organisms will often help in suggesting likely causes. Relapsing *Proteus* infection suggests renal infection or stone, multiple organisms in each attack suggests a fistula between the urinary tract and either the intestine or vagina, and persistence of the same organism suggests a nidus harbouring the infection.

Table 13.7 Patterns of recurrent infection

Persistent infection with the same organism
Inadequate treatment
  organism not sensitive
  too short a course in renal infection
  poor compliance

Nidus for persistence
  stone
  papilla
  prostate
  renal cyst

Reinfections with differing organisms
Single organisms in each attack
  women with recurrent cystitis (unknown cause)
  anatomical abnormality:
    vesicoureteric reflux
    obstruction
    duplex ureter
    bladder diverticulum
    inadequate bladder emptying

Multiple organisms
  vesicocolic fistula
  vaginocolic fistula

Intravenous pyelogram. In all patients, other than women with isolated dysuria-frequency responding well to treatment, an IVP should be performed.

Renal function tests. Plasma urea and creatinine should be normal unless there is an anatomical abnormality. Proteinuria and haematuria should be absent between attacks of UTI.

In children UTI is associated with an anatomical abnormality in about 50% of affected children, and the commonest abnormality is vesicoureteric reflux (Chapter 21). In all children <5 years of age a study for reflux is therefore recommended. The IVP may not demonstrate all renal scarring, hence a DMSA isotope scan may be indicated in the very young (Chapter 2).

In men In adult males with a normal IVP, recurrent UTI is virtually always associated with the same organism (i.e. persistence) and this is due to chronic prostatic infection. Prostatic infection can be diagnosed by the Stamey 3-specimen procedure, where prostatic secretion or urethral urine is collected after prostatic massage (Fig. 13.4).

In pregnant women   Renal ultrasound can be used in the place of radiography to exclude calculus and other major anatomical abnormalities. Occasionally with a unilateral dilated tract a single film IVP may be required to exclude obstruction. A formal IVP can then be deferred until after delivery.

In women with   Though investigation is indicated no abnormality will be found
recurrent cystitis   in most cases.

14: *Electrolyte and Acid–Base Disturbances*

DISTURBANCES IN PLASMA SODIUM CONCENTRATION

Sodium is the major cation contributing to plasma osmolality. Disturbances in plasma sodium concentration are more commonly due to disturbances of the mechanisms responsible for maintenance of osmolality and the excretion of water (antidiuretic hormone, ADH, and distal tubule function — Chapter 3), than of the mechanisms controlling sodium excretion. In most cases a change in plasma sodium concentration reflects a reciprocal change in body water.

HYPERNATRAEMIA

Definition. Plasma sodium greater than 145 mmol/litre.

Causes

Hypernatraemia is usually a consequence of water depletion. Since hypernatraemia causes thirst, loss of body water does not usually cause hypernatraemia unless the patient is unable to respond by adequate drinking, as in the very young, the very ill or the very old. The common primary causes are listed in Table 14.1.

A defect in urinary-concentrating ability is the commonest cause of water loss in excess of sodium loss, and can be due to deficiency of ADH (central diabetes insipidus) or to a defect in the renal response to ADH (nephrogenic diabetes insipidus). Nephrogenic diabetes insipidus is usually due to damage to the distal nephron (Chapter 28). In diabetes mellitus with heavy glycosuria osmotic diuresis can lead to hypernatraemia and non-ketotic hyperosmolar coma. Gastrointestinal fluid loss can also result in water depletion and hypernatraemia if water intake is inadequate. Hypernatraemia also occurs in ill patients and infants who are given intravenous or nasogastric fluid of excessive sodium content.

Clinical features of hypernatraemia

The clinical manifestations of severe hypernatraemia are those of cerebral dysfunction with restlessness, tremor, muscular twitching, ataxia, seizures, coma and death. The features are more

193

Table 14.1 Causes of hypernatraemia. Usually hypernatraemia is due to excessive water loss in a patient who is incapable of responding by thirst-induced increased water intake

---

Renal water loss
Osmotic diuresis
    diabetic hyperglycaemia
    hyperosmolar nasogastric or intravenous feeding

Renal tubular concentrating defect (nephrogenic diabetes insipidus)
    toxins:
        drugs (lithium, amphotericin, demeclocycline)
        Bence-Jones protein
    renal diseases particularly affecting tubules:
        postobstructive diuresis
        recovering acute tubular necrosis
        chronic tubulointerstitial nephritis
        polycystic kidney disease
        medullary cystic disease
    congenital nephrogenic diabetes insipidus

Pituitary ADH deficiency (central diabetes insipidus)
    idiopathic (50%), trauma, neoplasm, vincristine

Non-renal water loss
Gastrointestinal loss in confused or comatose patients and infants

Sodium intake in excess of water
Parenteral or nasogastric fluids

---

severe in acute than chronic hypernatraemia. Severe hypernatraemia (plasma sodium exceeding 160 mmol/litre) has a mortality of over 50%. Permanent brain damage may occur due to the sudden shrinkage of brain cells, with tearing of cerebral vessels as well as venous sinus thrombosis. Rapid correction of hypernatraemia can lead to cerebral oedema.

Treatment of hypernatraemia

Acute hypernatraemia may be corrected quickly but chronic hypernatraemia must be treated slowly (plasma sodium falling by about 2 mosmol/litre/hour) to prevent cerebral oedema.

Most patients are hypovolaemic. The volume of the fluid deficit can roughly be calculated by a formula based on a calculated water content of 60% of body weight in adults:

Water deficit (litre) = (plasma Na^+ − 140) mmol/litre
$$\times \ (0.6 \times \text{body weight}) \ \text{kg}$$

e.g. a 70-kg man with a plasma sodium concentration of 160 mmol/litre has a calculated deficit:

$$= (160 - 140) \times 0.6 \times 70$$
$$= 8.4 \ \text{litre.}$$

As always such formulae are only a rough guide and it is best to reassess the situation and adjust therapy frequently. The volume deficit should be repaired first. Once plasma volume is restored, 5% glucose intravenously or water by mouth can be used to further correct osmolarity. In the rare hypervolaemic patient with salt intoxication frusemide followed by 5% dextrose according to urine output should be given.

HYPONATRAEMIA

Definition. Plasma sodium concentration less than 135 mmol/litre.

Causes

This is probably the commonest electrolyte abnormality in hospitalised patients. In most cases there is increased ADH secretion or increased effect of ADH on the kidney, and dilutional hyponatraemia occurs because of water retention. Patients may be hypovolaemic, oedematous or euvolaemic (Table 14.2). A low plasma sodium concentration is also found in pseudohyponatraemia where there is a high concentration of another molecule (e.g. lipid) contributing to plasma osmolarity.

Hypovolaemic states

ADH is secreted in response to stimulation of volume receptors by hypovolaemia. Since volume stimulation overrides osmotic stimulation, plasma osmolarity and hence sodium concentration falls.

Diuretic therapy, particularly with thiazide diuretics and combined thiazide−amiloride combinations, is commonly associated with hyponatraemia. In many cases the diuretic is given for oedema, which can itself lead to hyponatraemia (see below).

Mineralocorticoid deficit, e.g. Addison's disease, can result in a salt-losing state and hypovolaemia.

Salt-losing renal diseases include analgesic nephropathy and other chronic tubulointerstitial diseases (Chapter 20), partial or recovering renal obstruction and recovering acute tubular necrosis (Table 5.2).

Gastrointestinal losses with diarrhoea, vomiting or severe ileus should be obvious clinically.

Concealed losses may occur into the peritoneal cavity, or tissues as in severe burns or crush injury.

Table 14.2 Causes of hyponatraemia

Hypovolaemic
Renal sodium loss (urine Na^+ continues to be >20 mmol/litre)
  diuretic treatment
  mineralocorticoid deficiency
  salt-losing nephropathy (Table 5.2)
  partial or recovering acute tubular necrosis and obstruction
  osmotic diuresis (glucose)
Gastrointestinal sodium losses (urine Na^+ <20 mmol/litre)
  vomiting, diarrhoea
  ileus
Concealed loss (urine Na^+ <20 mmol/litre)
  ascites, peritonitis, pancreatitis
  burns, crush injury

Oedematous
Cirrhosis
Congestive cardiac failure
Nephrotic syndrome
Renal failure with water load

Euvolaemic
Hormonal
  myxoedema
  glucocorticoid deficiency
Massive water load
  compulsive water drinkers
  parenteral fluid
  water infusion during prostatectomy
Syndrome of inappropriate ADH secretion (SIADH — Table 14.3)

Pseudohyponatraemia
Hyperlipidaemia
Hyperproteinaemia

Oedematous states

In congestive cardiac failure, cirrhosis and nephrotic syndrome total body water is increased but it is thought that in these situations there is a fall in 'effective blood volume' and non-osmolar baroceptors in the cardiac atria, aortic arch and carotid sinus respond by stimulating ADH secretion. ADH leads to retention of water out of proportion to sodium. This may be aggravated by diuretic therapy (see above), or an excessive water load, as in beer-drinking cirrhotics.

In severe renal failure an absolute limit to free water clearance is eventually reached where a water load cannot be adequately excreted. In this situation consumption of a large water load can lead to a fall in plasma sodium.

Euvolaemic hyponatraemia

In this group of conditions the diagnosis of hyponatraemia becomes more difficult.

Excessive water intake occurs in compulsive water drinkers or beer drinkers and can cause symptomatic hyponatraemia. This can also occur with parenteral fluid administration.

Glucocorticoid and thyroxine deficiency both can be associated with hyponatraemia since they impair urinary concentrating mechanisms.

The syndrome of inappropriate ADH secretion (SIADH) should only be considered in euvolaemic patients in whom other causes for hyponatraemia have been excluded. A variety of conditions (Table 14.3) have been implicated. Pathophysiological explanations probably include overexcretion of ADH, oversensitivity to ADH and secretion of ADH-like substances by tumours. Drugs that stimulate ADH secretion include nicotine, vincristine, clofibrate and chlorpropamide. Chlorpropamide also increases renal sensitivity to ADH.

Pseudohypo-natraemia

Hyponatraemia can occur in situations where another molecule is contributing sufficiently to plasma osmolarity, so that maintenance of normal total plasma osmolarity requires a fall in plasma sodium concentration. Examples include severe hyperlipidaemia and hyperproteinaemia. In these cases the 'osmolar gap', i.e. the difference between the measured plasma osmolarity and the calculated plasma osmolarity (approximately twice the plasma sodium plus the plasma urea and glucose) will be increased above the usual value of less than 10 mmol/litre. Because effective

Table 14.3 Causes of inappropriate secretion of ADH

Drugs stimulating ADH secretion
Nicotine
Chlorpropamide
Clofibrate
Vincristine

Carcinomas
Lung (oat-cell)
Pancreas, duodenum, bladder

Pulmonary disease
Pneumonia, abscess
Tuberculosis

Neurological diseases
Encephalitis
Cerebral trauma, haemorrhage, infarct
Guillain–Barré syndrome
Delirium tremens, acute psychosis

osmolarity is not reduced, there are no clinical consequences of this hyponatraemia.

Clinical features of hyponatraemia

The effects of hyponatraemia depend greatly on the rate of development. Plasma sodium concentrations above 120 mmol/litre are usually well tolerated, while most patients will have marked cerebral dysfunction once plasma sodium is below 110 mmol/litre. Lethargy, anorexia and nausea are common and vomiting may occur. Irritability and agitation are frequently present, and usually once plasma sodium is below 110 mmol/litre confusion and disorientation occurs, culminating in convulsions and coma.

Treatment of hyponatraemia

In chronic hyponatraemia the first step is to correct the underlying disorder. In the overloaded patient water restriction can be combined with loop diuretics such as frusemide, and sometimes oral salt supplements. In SIADH, lithium or demeclocycline may be given to induce a renal concentrating defect.

In severe hyponatraemia rapid correction with hypertonic saline is contraindicated because of the possibility of inducing the rare condition of central pontine myelinolysis. Water excretion should be promoted by loop-diuretic therapy. Normal saline (Na$^+$ concentration 150 mmol/litre) and in severe cases small amounts (100–200 ml) of hypertonic saline (300 mmol/litre) may be infused. It is wise to aim to increase plasma sodium by only 5–10 mmol/litre per 24 hours.

DISTURBANCES IN PLASMA POTASSIUM CONCENTRATION

Both hyperkalaemia and hypokalaemia are relatively asymptomatic but potently cardiotoxic, hence potentially lethal. Plasma potassium (K$^+$) concentration control largely depends on redistribution of K$^+$ between the intra- and extracellular compartments. Most body K$^+$ is intracellular. The intracellular K$^+$ concentration is about 150 mmol/litre, while the plasma K$^+$ concentration is only 3.5–5.5 mmol/litre. There is a very large renal reserve for K$^+$ excretion but it is relatively slow (30 min or more) in response.

HYPERKALAEMIA

Definition. Plasma potassium concentration greater than 5.5 mmol/litre.

Causes of hyperkalaemia

Because of the resilience of the homeostatic mechanisms protecting against hyperkalaemia it is common for more than one mechanism to be present before clinical hyperkalaemia occurs. The commonest combination is reduced renal excretion combined with another factor such as excessive load or leakage of potassium from cells (Table 14.4).

Increased intake of potassium

Increased intake will only result in hyperkalaemia if it is very rapid, or if there is an associated deficit in renal excretion. These causes of hyperkalaemia are therefore particularly important in patients with renal failure. Intravenous potassium loads can inadvertently be given with stored blood (with red cell-derived potassium free in the plasma), Hartmann's solution (potassium 5 mmol/litre) or potassium-containing antibiotics such as crystalline penicillin. Oral loads occur with dietary excesses (Table 14.5) and potassium containing medications. Most 'salt-substituted' low salt foods contain potassium to replace the 'salty' taste.

Table 14.4 Causes of hyperkalaemia

Acutely increased intake of potassium
Dietary excess
Acute intravenous load
Salt substitutes
Drugs: Potassium penicillin

Shift of intracellular potassium to the circulation
Cell destruction
   incompatible blood transfusion
   crush injury
   cancer chemotherapy
Acidosis
Muscular disease or activity
   excessive exercise
   convulsions
   suxamethonium induction of paralysis
   myositis, myolysis
   periodic paralysis

Decreased excretion of potassium by the kidneys
Renal failure
Drugs acting on the tubules
   cyclosporin
   angiotensin-converting enzyme inhibitors
   non-steroidal anti-inflammatory drugs (NSAIDs)
Sodium deficiency
Mineralocorticoid deficiency

Factitious
Due to leakage from blood cells on the way to the laboratory, with haemolysis, severe leukocytosis or thrombocytosis

Table 14.5 Foods with a high potassium content

Dried fruit
Apricots, peaches, prunes, raisins, sultanas

Nuts
Peanuts, cashew nuts

Chocolate and cocoa

Vegetables
Green leaf vegetables, beans, potatoes, spinach

Fruits
Bananas, tomatoes, citrus fruit

Redistribution of body potassium

Disturbance of the normal intracellular to extracellular potassium balance can quickly result in hyperkalaemia.

Acidosis promotes K^+ efflux from cells, both by the hydrogen ion competing with K^+ for diffusion into the cell, and perhaps by 'poisoning' of the $Na-K-ATPase$ pump upon which the gradient depends. The acute effect on renal tubular cells is similar, resulting in decreased K^+ excretion. The effect on plasma K^+ depends on the severity, rapidity of onset and nature of the acidosis, being most potent with hyperchloraemic metabolic acidosis and minimal with respiratory acidosis.

Cell destruction. When there is massive death of cells as occurs in incompatible blood transfusion, haemolysis, crush injury or occasionally with cancer chemotherapy, large quantities of intracellular potassium are released into the circulation.

Muscular activity. Exercise and convulsions induce release of potassium from cells. Suxamethonium causes potassium to move out of cells and can be a risk to patients with renal impairment undergoing anaesthesia.

Decreased renal excretion of potassium

Normal potassium homeostasis involves about 100 mmol/day oral intake and about 10 mmol/day faecal output, with the balance, about 90 mmol/day being excreted by the kidneys. Because the kidneys have a high reserve for potassium excretion hyperkalaemia usually occurs only when renal failure is severe, or when a defect in tubular excretion is present, as in mineralocorticoid deficiency, salt-depletion or renal tubular disease.

Renal failure. In chronic renal failure adequate potassium excretion is usually preserved until most nephrons are lost, i.e. GFR falls below $5-10$ ml/min. Hyperkalaemia may occur earlier in diseases particularly effecting tubules, and can be precipitated in others by excessive potassium load or saline depletion.

Acute renal failure, on the other hand, is frequently associated with hyperkalaemia, largely because it is usually severe and associated with cell destruction and acidosis.

Drugs interfering with potassium excretion include angiotensin-converting enzyme inhibitors, non-steroidal anti-inflammatory drugs and potassium-conserving diuretics. All may cause hyperkalaemia, especially if renal disease is present.

Adreno-corticoid deficiency. Hyperkalaemia is a major stimulus to aldosterone secretion, which acts in turn on the distal tubule and collecting duct to promote kaliuresis. Mineralocorticoid deficiency can therefore result in hyperkalaemia. Autoimmune, tuberculous or other forms of hypoadrenalism commonly present with volume contraction and hyperkalaemic acidosis.

Hyporeninaemic hypoaldosteronism is a frequent cause of hyperkalaemia in diabetics. Most cases are in elderly diabetics with mild diabetic renal failure. The hyperkalaemia is usually moderate (plasma K^+ 5.5−6.5 mmol/litre) but is aggravated by salt depletion or hyperglycaemia. Usually good control of salt, water balance and diabetes will prevent serious hyperkalaemia.

Factitious hyperkalaemia

Haemolysis due to turbulence with poor venesection technique or storage of the sample is commonly the cause of this laboratory aberration. The plasma or serum will be haemoglobin pigmented. Loss of potassium from platelets or white cells can also be significant when these are present in large numbers, hence leukaemia and thrombocytosis can cause factitious hyperkalaemia.

Clinical features of hyperkalaemia

Hyperkalaemia results in alterations in membrane excitability; particularly important are resultant life threatening cardiotoxicity and neuromuscular disturbances. The severity of the clinical manifestations depends on the severity of the hyperkalaemia and on the rate with which it develops. Patients with chronic renal failure are often remarkably resistant to its toxic effects, presumably as a result of membrane adaptation to chronic hyperkalaemia.

The early symptoms of hyperkalaemia are not remarkable and cardiac toxicity can occur before any are present. Muscle weakness with loss of tendon reflexes can occur. Occasionally tingling, numbness and circumoral paraesthesia are present.

The ECG with hyperkalaemic cardiac toxicity (Fig. 14.1) shows:
• Tall T waves

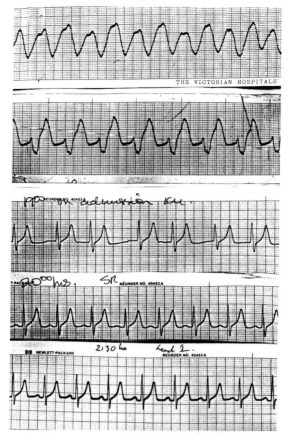

Fig. 14.1 ECG changes in hyperkalaemia. In this dialysis patient with a plasma potassium concentration of 8.7 mmol/litre, the 'sine wave' pattern of severe hyperkalaemia gradually resolves to the picture of tall T waves characterising milder hyperkalaemia

- Widening of the QRS complex.
- Widening of the PR interval.
- Finally cardiac arrest in asystole.

Treatment of hyperkalaemia

The treatment depends on the severity and the degree of renal failure. If ECG abnormalities are present treatment is urgent, and in renal failure excretion in the urine cannot be relied upon. The possible courses of action are considered below and in Table 14.6.

Reduce or eliminate potassium intake

High potassium foods (Table 14.5) should be eliminated, and a restricted oral K^+ intake prescribed. Iatrogenic intake should not be forgotten. Parenteral and nasogastric feeding is often high in K^+, transfused blood and Hartmann's solution also contain K^+.

Table 14.6   Treatment of hyperkalaemia

Emergency
i.v. glucose (25–50 ml of 50% glucose)
insulin (10–20 units soluble) } to shift K^+ into cells

Correct acidosis with i.v.
sodium bicarbonate (25 to 100 ml of 8.4% $NaHCO_3$) } to shift K^+ into cells

i.v. calcium gluconate (5 ml of 10% Ca gluconate
while watching ECG) } to stabilise cardiac rhythm

Increase potassium excretion
Diuresis with saline and frusemide (i.v. 40–1000 mg frusemide followed by normal saline)

Potassium exchange resin. Resonium 25–100 g orally or by enema

Dialysis (preferably haemodialysis)

Encourage urinary potassium excretion

Potassium conserving diuretics (amiloride, spironolactone, triameterene), non-steroidal anti-inflammatory drugs (indomethacin, naproxen, ibuprofen, etc.), angiotensin-converting enzyme inhibitors (captopril, enalapril) all reduce urinary K^+ and should be stopped.

Re-expansion with saline in patients with reduced plasma volume, and administration of loop diuretics (often requiring high dosage in patients with renal failure) will often promote diuresis and kaliuresis. In acute hyperkalaemia in patients with reasonable renal function frusemide–saline forced diuresis is an effective and simple method to reduce plasma K^+.

Repair metabolic acidosis

Plasma K^+ will fall due to movement of K^+ into cells in metabolic acidosis if sodium bicarbonate ($NaHCO_3$) is given. $NaHCO_3$ will also expand plasma volume, increase plasma tonicity and encourage kaliuresis. Acute treatment consists of 25–100 mmol (i.e. 25–100 ml of 8.4 g/dl) of $NaHCO_3$ solution given slowly intravenously.

Administer glucose and insulin

To shift K^+ into cells, intravenous glucose (i.e. 50 ml of 50% glucose) can be given every 15 to 30 min. Usually 10 units of insulin is given with the glucose in urgent situations, otherwise the patients' own insulin production may be depended upon. This will not reduce body K^+, hence other measures are also required. Recently the use of a β-adrenergic drug (e.g. salbutamol) has also been shown to be effective in promoting the movement of K^+ into cells in treating hyperkalaemia.

Stabilise the heart with calcium gluconate

Calcium gluconate (5 ml of 10% solution) is injected slowly intravenously if ECG abnormalities are present. The injections can be repeated while monitoring the ECG pattern, which should respond within minutes.

Exchange resin to promote gastrointestinal potassium excretion

50–100 g of sodium-(Resonium A) or calcium-containing exchange resin can be given as an enema in acute cases, or 25–50 g can be given orally several times a day (it is poorly tolerated) for chronic hyperkalaemia. This will promote gastrointestinal potassium loss but, since there is a one-for-one potassium for sodium exchange, can cause salt and water overload.

Dialysis

In patients with poor renal function acute dialysis may be required to control hyperkalaemia. Haemodialysis is more efficient in K^+ removal than peritoneal dialysis.

HYPOKALAEMIA

Definition. Plasma K^+ concentration less than 3.5 mmol/litre.

Causes of hypokalaemia

Common causes are increased potassium losses from the kidneys or gastrointestinal system (Table 14.7); occasionally there is altered distribution of K^+ or inadequate intake.

Renal potassium loss

If renal potassium excretion continues to exceed about 20 mmol/day in the face of systemic hypokalaemia then excessive renal loss should be suspected.

Diuretic therapy is the commonest cause of hypokalaemia, and is particularly likely if there is also reduced sodium intake.

Renal tubular dysfunction may cause hypokalaemia. Examples often associated with polyuria include the recovery phases of obstructive nephropathy and acute tubular necrosis, some forms of drug-induced tubular damage (amphotericin, cysplatin), and diabetic glycosuria (see below). In renal tubular acidosis, hypokalaemia can be particularly troublesome (Chapter 28).

Recovering diabetic ketoacidosis. In diabetic ketoacidosis severe potassium depletion can occur with the osmotic diuresis, yet not be obvious because the acidosis causes efflux from cells. During treatment dangerous hypokalaemia can result.

Adrenocorticoid excess with primary or secondary aldosteronism (as in renal artery stenosis or accelerated hypertension) or Cushing's syndrome results in kaliuresis and alkalosis.

Table 14.7 Causes of hypokalaemia*

Renal loss
With alkalosis
   diuretic therapy — by far the commonest cause
   mineralocorticoid excess:
      primary aldosteronism (Conn's syndrome)
      secondary aldosteronism (e.g. accelerated hypertension, renal artery
        stenosis)
   glucocorticoid excess (Cushing's syndrome)

With polyuria
   recovering acute tubular necrosis or obstruction
   tubular nephrotoxins — amphotericin, cisplatin
   diabetic glycosuria (also acidotic kaliuresis)

With acidosis
   metabolic acidosis — especially diabetic ketoacidosis during recovery
   renal tubular acidosis, ureterosigmoidostomy, acetazolamide therapy

Gastrointestinal loss
Prolonged or severe diarrhoea
Laxative abuse
Prolonged vomiting
Villous adenoma of the colon
Ileus with massive intestinal dilatation

Redistribution into cells
Metabolic alkalosis
Insulin
Beta-adrenergic agonists
Periodic paralysis

Inadequate intake
Intravenous fluid without potassium

* Common causes are diuretic therapy and gastrointestinal loss

Bartter's syndrome is a rare abnormality with hypokalaemic alkalosis, hyperreninaemic hyperaldosteronism, high urinary prostaglandin E and prostacyclin concentrations and a normal blood pressure. The juxtaglomerular apparatus is hypertrophied on renal biopsy.

Gastrointestinal potassium loss

Here hypokalaemia is associated with a low urinary K^+ excretion (<20 mmol/day). Examples include severe diarrhoea, villous adenoma of the bowel and laxative abuse. The last is often diagnosed by sigmoidoscopy and biopsy where characteristic melanosis coli is seen. Prolonged vomiting may also cause hypokalaemia.

Potassium redistribution

Movement of K into cells occurs in a variety of conditions.

Metabolic alkalosis. In metabolic alkalosis there is movement of K^+ into cells.

Insulin excess and β-adrenergic agonist therapy. Injection of glucose or insulin can acutely lower plasma K^+. Beta-agonists, as used for asthma therapy, e.g. salbutamol, can decrease plasma K^+ by promoting intracellular transport. These drugs are both used to treat hyperkalaemia because of this effect.

Hypokalaemic periodic paralysis is a rare autosomal dominant condition where periodic hypokalaemia causes muscle weakness.

Inadequate potassium intake

Reduced oral intake is rarely the cause of hypokalaemia, though it can contribute when losses are excessive or cannot be reduced appropriately. The normal kidney can reduce potassium excretion to <20 mmol/day. Hypokalaemia is occasionally seen in patients maintained on intravenous fluids with inadequate K^+ replacement.

Clinical features of hypokalaemia

Symptoms usually occur when plasma K^+ is less than 2.5 mmol/litre. Proximal muscle weakness is the most obvious symptom. In severe cases there may be muscle necrosis. Tendon reflexes are depressed. Gastrointestinal hypomotility can occur and lead to paralytic ileus with further K^+ loss into the gut. In chronic hypokalaemia there is tubular damage, with resultant chronic tubulointerstitial nephritis (Chapter 20).

Cardiac arrythmia is the cause of death in severe hypokalaemia.

The ECG changes of hypokalaemia are:
1 Depressed T waves and S–T segments.
2 The appearance of U waves.
3 Widening of the QRS.
4 Finally a variety of arrythmias occur, particularly ventricular ectopic beats and fibrillation.

Treatment of hypokalaemia

Depending on the urgency of the situation K^+ can be given as oral supplements (slow release preparations are not recommended during urgent repletion) or intravenous KCl which generally should not be given faster than 10 mmol/hour.

DISTURBANCES IN ACID–BASE BALANCE

The kidneys, together with the lungs, are responsible for maintenance of normal body acid–base balance (Chapter 3). Plasma pH is normally 7.35 to 7.45 and the concentration of H^+ is normally 36 to 44 mmol/litre. The normal plasma HCO_3^- concentration is 20 to 30 mmol/litre.

Excretion of hydrogen ion load. Daily about 70 mmol of non-volatile acids are produced by body metabolism and must be excreted by the kidneys. The kidneys must also resorb the bicarbonate from normal glomerular filtrate to prevent bicarbonate wastage. The processes of addition of hydrogen ions to the urine (or urinary acidification) and resorption of bicarbonate are linked. Excess hydrogen ion (50–100 mmol/day) is buffered in the urine by ammonium, phosphate and other acids so that urinary pH does not have to fall below its lower limit of about 4.5 pH units (Table 3.5).

Excretion of bicarbonate. If the intake and production of alkali exceeds that of acid the urine is alkalinised by excretion of bicarbonate, to a maximal pH of about 10.0 units.

METABOLIC ACIDOSIS

Metabolic acidosis can result from generation or ingestion of acid, or loss of bicarbonate ion. The acidosis will be in part compensated for by increased ventilation to excrete carbon dioxide, and hence a fall in plasma HCO_3^-.

The features of metabolic acidosis

These are:
- Low plasma HCO_3^- concentration (<20 mmol/litre).
- Low arterial carbon dioxide concentration.
- Low plasma pH (<7.35 mmol/litre).
The pH and carbon dioxide concentration depend on the degree of respiratory compensation.

Causes of metabolic acidosis

Metabolic acidosis results from excessive acid production or intake, or excessive bicarbonate losses (Table 14.8).

Increased load of non-volatile acid

Hypochloraemic acidosis. In most of these cases there is an increased concentration of acid anions other than chloride resulting in depression of the plasma chloride concentration (Table 14.8). The most common causes are diabetic ketoacidosis where the anions are ketoacids, and renal failure where sulphate, phosphate, urate, and creatinine are the major acids retained.

The presence of non-volatile acids present can be deduced by calculation of the 'anion gap'.

Anion gap $= ([Na^+] + [K^+]) - ([Cl^-] + [HCO_3^-])$.

Table 14.8 Causes of metabolic acidosis

Increased load of non-volatile acid
Hypochloraemic
    diabetic ketoacidosis (keto acids)
    renal failure (sulphate, phosphate, urate, creatinine)
    lactic acidosis (lactate)
    poisoning (salicylate, methanol, ethylene glycol, paraldehyde)
    starvation and alcoholic ketoacidosis (keto acids)

Hyperchloraemic
    intake of chloride-liberating acids:
        ammonium chloride in tests of urinary acidification
        lysine and arginine in amino acid preparations

Loss of bicarbonate (hyperchloraemic)
Gastrointestinal losses
    profuse diarrhoea
    pancreatic fistula
    biliary fistula
    ureterosigmoidostomy and ileal conduit

Renal
    renal tubular acidosis
    carbonic anhydrase inhibition — induced with acetazolamide

The anion gap is normally in the range 11 to 19 mmol/litre. In hypochloraemic acidosis the value exceeds 19 mmol/litre. Rarely ingestion of large amounts of chloride-containing acids such as ammonium chloride will lead to hyperchloraemic metabolic acidosis with no increase in the anion gap.

Loss of bicarbonate

Hyperchloraemic metabolic acidosis. If bicarbonate is lost in the urine or from the gastrointestinal tract there is a fall in plasma HCO_3^- and electroneutrality is preserved by a compensatory rise in plasma Cl^-; there is no 'unmeasured acid' — the anion gap will not be increased.
• *Gastrointestinal losses* include profuse diarrhoea, and biliary or pancreatic fistulae.
• *Renal tubular acidosis.* Loss of bicarbonate in the urine can occur as a result of tubular dysfunction in renal tubular acidosis (Chapter 28). The result is hyperchloraemic acidosis, with a normal (<20 mmol/litre) anion gap. By interfering with tubular bicarbonate metabolism, acetazolamide can cause a similar condition.
• *Ureterosigmoidostomy and ileal urinary conduit.* In these conditions exposure of the gastrointestinal mucosa to urine can result in increased mucosal HCO_3^- excretion, with Cl^- resorption from the urine resulting in hyperchloraemic acidosis.

METABOLIC ALKALOSIS

Because of the enormous capacity of the kidney for bicarbonate excretion, a metabolic alkalosis can only be maintained if there is renal dysfunction with either a reduction in HCO_3^- excretion, or enhanced renal generation of HCO_3^-, i.e. renally generated alkalosis.

The features of metabolic alkalosis

These are:
- High plasma HCO_3^- (>30 mmol/litre).
- High plasma pH (>7.45).
- High plasma CO_2 concentration.

The pH and CO_2 concentration depend on the degree of respiratory compensation.

Causes of metabolic alkalosis

A common mediator in metabolic alkalosis is hyperaldosteronism, since aldosterone leads to enhanced K^+ excretion accompanied by H^+ excretion and bicarbonate retention. The result is hypokalaemic metabolic alkalosis. Common causes include diuretic therapy, secondary aldosteronism in cirrhosis, and severe vomiting with both hydrogen chloride loss and volume contraction (Table 14.9).

Unusual causes include primary aldosteronism (Conn's syndrome), glucocorticoid excess (Cushing's syndrome) and liquorice

Table 14.9 Causes of metabolic alkalosis

Renal bicarbonate retention
Adrenocorticoid and similar effects (H and K excretion with bicarbonate retention)
   secondary aldosteronism, e.g. cirrhosis
   primary aldosteronism
   Cushing's syndrome
   Bartter's syndrome
   liquorice, carbenoxolone ingestion
Volume depletion (Cl depletion and bicarbonate resorption)
   diuretic therapy
   others (e.g. chronic diarrhoea, cirrhosis)

Gastrointestinal loss of acid
Vomiting or gastric aspiration

*Ingestion of alkali**
Soluble antacids (usually $NaHCO_3$)
Milk-alkali syndrome

---

* For metabolic alkalosis to be maintained there must be abnormal renal tubular function since the capacity for bicarbonate excretion is enormous

and carbenoloxone ingestion — both of which mimic the effect of aldosterone on the tubule.

RESPIRATORY ACIDOSIS

In respiratory acidosis CO_2 retention occurs. The reaction

$$CO_2 + H_2O \rightarrow H_2CO_3 \rightarrow H^+ + HCO_3^-$$

results in acidosis. The kidneys compensate by excreting acid and resorbing bicarbonate.

The features of respiratory acidosis

These are:
- High plasma carbon dioxide concentration.
- Low plasma pH.
- High plasma bicarbonate concentration.

The plasma pH and bicarbonate concentration depend on the degree of renal compensation, i.e. the amount of acid excreted and bicarbonate resorbed by the kidneys.

Respiratory acidosis occurs with either respiratory disease or central depression of respiratory drive.

RESPIRATORY ALKALOSIS

Excessive respiratory excretion of CO_2 leads to conversion of HCO_3^- to H_2O and CO_2.

Respiratory alkalosis occurs only in very ill patients (e.g. cerebral hypoxia, intracranial disease and a wide variety of poorly explained stimuli such as hypotension, hepatic failure, septicaemia and hyperpyrexia).

DISORDERS OF PLASMA CALCIUM CONCENTRATION

The kidneys, along with the gastrointestinal tract and the skeletal system, play a key role in body calcium and phosphate homeostasis.

Some important disorders relating calcium and the kidney include:
- Renal failure (Chapters 6 & 11).
- Renal stones (Chapter 25).
- Disorders of plasma calcium concentration.
- Disorders of plasma phosphate concentration.

The following are important contributions of the kidneys to calcium and phosphate metabolism (Chapter 3):

Synthesis of 1,25-dihydroxychole-calciferol

Liver derived 25-hydroxycholecalciferol is hydroxylated at the 1-position in the renal cortex. The activated vitamin D ($1,25$-$(OH)_2$-D_3) stimulates:
- Gut calcium absorption.
- Normal calcification of bone.

Renal excretion of calcium

Urinary excretion of calcium (Ca^{2+}) is about 5.5 mmol/day, which represents less than 2% of the filtered load. 85–90% is resorbed in the proximal tubule and the remainder in the distal tubule under the control of parathormone (PTH) which decreases Ca^{2+} excretion.

Renal phosphate excretion

Urinary phosphate excretion varies widely from 5 to 40 mmol/day. 80–95% of the filtered load is resorbed by the proximal tubule (where glucose, amino acid, and low molecular weight protein resorption also occur). Phosphate is a major buffer for hydrogen ion excretion.

HYPERCALCAEMIA

Definition. Total plasma Ca^{2+} concentration greater than 2.6 mmol/litre. The ionised Ca^{2+} (approximately 50% of plasma Ca^{2+}) is the physiologically important moiety, hence the total plasma Ca^{2+} should be 'corrected' for plasma albumin concentration.

Causes of hypercalcaemia

The causes are summarised in Table 14.10. The commonest are malignancy (either involving bone directly or by a humoral mechanism), hyperparathyroidism, sarcoidosis and excessive ingestion of vitamin D or calcium, particularly in the presence of renal failure.

Thiazide diuretics decrease urinary Ca^{2+} excretion, and may cause elevation of plasma Ca^{2+}, particularly if there are other predisposing factors. Loop diuretics, on the other hand, increase Ca^{2+} excretion.

Milk-alkali syndrome is characterised by hypercalcaemia, nephrocalcinosis and alkalosis. It results from ingestion of large amounts of Ca^{2+} and alkali usually in the form of milk and sodium bicarbonate. Renal failure of some degree is almost invariably present and may contribute to this now rare condition.

Clinical features of hypercalcaemia

The mnemonic 'stones, bones, abdominal groans and mental moans' applied to hyperparathyroid symptoms combines the renal, gastrointestinal and central nervous system disturbances common to other forms of hypercalcaemia with the bony manifestations of the primary condition.

Table 14.10 Causes of hypercalcaemia

Malignancy
Multiple myeloma
Bony metastases (lung, breast, prostate, thyroid)
Non-metastatic humoral (breast, lung, renal)

Hyperparathyroidism
Primary
'Tertiary' or 'autonomous'

Sarcoidosis

Bone disease
Immobilisation in Paget's disease
Aluminium osteodystrophy

Endocrine disorders
Thyrotoxicosis
Addison's disease (adrenocortical deficiency)

Ingestion of calcium or vitamin D
Vitamin D intoxication
Milk-alkali syndrome
Renal failure

Raised non-ionised calcium
Hyperproteinaemia

Renal manifestations. Polyuria and polydypsia occur due to the urinary concentrating defect induced by hypercalcaemia, as well as inhibition of distal tubular sodium resorption.

Calcium-containing radiopaque renal calculi commonly occur and may be large or multiple (Chapter 25). Nephrocalcinosis can occur.

Chronic renal failure can be the result of obstruction by stone, nephrocalcinosis or chronic interstitial nephritis secondary to prolonged nephrotoxic effects of hypercalcaemia. Acute renal failure can occur in severe hypercalcaemia due to a combination of reduction in GFR and renal blood flow (a direct effect of hypercalcaemia) and dehydration consequent on polyuria. Usually the acute renal failure resolves on rehydration and treatment of the hypercalcaemia.

Gastrointestinal manifestations. Nausea and vomiting (a central effect) is common and aggravates dehydration. Peptic ulcer disease and pancreatitis may occur.

Nervous system manifestations. Malaise, fatigue and even psychosis, as well as nausea and vomiting, are all central effects of hypercalcaemia.

Metastatic calcification. Nephrocalcinosis, vascular calcification, red conjuctivae ('red eyes'), band keratopathy, conjunctival calcification and generalised pruritis are all attributable to tissue deposition of Ca.

Treatment of hypercalcaemia

The cause of hypercalcaemia should be detected and treated. The hypercalcaemia itself can be treated by the following methods.

Saline diuresis. Replacement of any salt and water deficit is important. If this does not cure the hypercalcaemia a forced diuretic regimen of frusemide and intravenous saline can be effective in patients with reasonable renal function. Plasma potassium and sodium concentrations should be monitored.

Glucocorticoids. These successfully reduce plasma Ca in all conditions other than hyperparathyroidism. In sarcoidosis and vitamin D intoxication 10 mg prednisolone per day may be effective while in malignancy doses as high as 60 mg per day may be required to produce a useful effect.

Other hypocalcaemic agents include:
• *Mithramycin*. This cytotoxic antibiotic is particularly useful in neoplastic hypercalcaemia. The dose is $25-30$ μg/kg and the fall in Ca often occurs within hours and lasts days.
• *Calcitonin*. $50-100$ units $8-12$ hourly has an effect which lasts only a few days.
• *Phosphate*. Intravenous or oral phosphate will bind and reduce plasma Ca but with a risk of causing metastatic calcification.
• *Diphosphonates*. These will suppress hypercalcaemia in hyperparathyroidism.

Dialysis. In renal failure dialysis is an effective rapid way of reducing plasma calcium.

HYPOCALCAEMIA

Definition. Plasma Ca concentration less than 2.20 mmol/litre. Hypoalbuminaemia can reduce total plasma Ca without affecting ionised Ca. Plasma Ca measurements are therefore often 'adjusted' for albumin concentration.

Causes of hypocalcaemia

The most common causes are renal failure, hypoparathyroidism, pancreatitis and hypoalbuminaemia (Table 14.11).

Renal failure. In renal failure a low plasma Ca^{2+} is common, because of hyperphosphataemia causing a reduction in ionised Ca^{2+}, and lack of production of $1,25(OH)_2$-D_3. The acidosis of renal failure may protect the patient from symptoms. Aggressive treatment of acidosis can result in lowering of ionised Ca^{2+} by increased binding to albumin and hence precipitate symptoms of hypocalcaemia, with tetany or convulsions.

Hypoparathyroidism of any cause results in hypocalcaemia.

Vitamin D deficiency. Whether due to dietary deficiency, malabsorption, failure of renal conversion, or lack of sunlight, vitamin D deficiency is associated with hypophosphataemia, hypocalcaemia and elevated PTH levels.

Acute pancreatitis. Many factors, including calcium deposition, result in hypocalcaemia in acute pancreatitis. In other patients with massive tissue destruction (e.g. cellulitis, septicaemia and cytotoxic therapy) complex mechanisms may also result in hypocalcaemia.

Hypoalbuminaemia as occurs in the nephrotic syndrome and cirrhosis is associated with low plasma Ca^{2+} levels that do not reflect low ionised Ca^{2+} levels. In nephrotic syndrome this may be worsened by failure of $1,25(OH)_2$-D_3 production. Many laboratories calculate or measure the ionised Ca^{2+} concentration.

Clinical manifestations of hypocalcaemia

Neuromuscular effects are prominent in acute hypocalcaemia, while chronic hypercalcaemia is often associated with defects in bone calcification, depending on the cause of the hypocalcaemia.

Table 14.11 Causes of hypocalcaemia

Renal failure
Hypoparathyroidism
  idiopathic
  surgical
  pseudohypoparathyroidism

Vitamin D deficiency

Acute pancreatitis and massive tissue injury

Hypoalbuminaemia*

---

* Normal free (ionic) plasma calcium

Neurological effects include tetany, tingling, numbness, paraesthesia and convulsions. Chronic hypocalcaemia can cause depression and irritability. Intracranial calcification and cataracts may occur with chronic hypocalcaemia.

Bone disease includes secondary hyperparathyroidism and osteomalacia in renal failure, and osteomalacia in vitamin D deficiency.

Treatment of hypocalcaemia

The treatment varies with the cause. In renal failure control of hypophosphataemia and vitamin D treatment are important (Chapter 11).

Calcium and vitamin D supplements will increase plasma calcium concentration. In patients with chronic renal failure after parathyroidectomy, huge doses of intravenous Ca^{2+}, even over 40 g/day, may be required initially, particularly if there is severe hyperparathyroid bone disease.

Section 3
Diseases of the Kidney

15: *Primary Glomerular Diseases*

Disorders of glomerular structure and function occur in many diseases (Table 15.1). Those in which the renal glomerulus is the sole or predominant tissue involved are commonly called primary glomerulonephritis (GN). In most cases the cause is unknown.

CLASSIFICATION OF GLOMERULONEPHRITIS

There are three complementary ways of classifying glomerulonephritis:
1 Clinical.
2 Aetiological (including pathogenesis).
3 Pathological.

Clinical classification of GN

As described in detail in Chapter 9 the clinical syndromes resulting from glomerular disease consist of varying features of proteinuria, haematuria, reduced renal function, hypertension and oedema. When a patient is first seen he or she can usually be assigned to one (or occasionally more) of these clinical syndromes. Unfortunately each of these syndromes has a wide variety of possible causes and pathological appearances and therefore the appropriate treatment and prognosis is not obvious.

However, there are a few circumstances, such as in the acute nephrotic syndrome in childhood (Chapter 9) where the clinical syndrome implies a likely pathology, and it is common to proceed on the basis of the clinically apparent diagnosis rather than the result of a renal biopsy.

Aetiological classification of GN

The cause is not known in most cases of GN; moreover, there can be a wide range of clinical and pathological responses to the same causative agent. Poststreptococcal nephritis is one of the few diseases where the cause, clinical and pathological features correlate sufficiently to justify labelling the disease by aetiology. Accordingly an aetiological system for classification is not adequate.

Pathological classification of GN

With the advent of renal biopsy, the histological appearance of the kidney has become the basis of classification of GN. It is important

219

Table 15.1 Classification of glomerular diseases

Clinical
Nephrotic syndrome
Nephritic syndrome
Recurrent macroscopic haematuria
Chronic glomerulonephritis

Aetiological
Inflammatory: glomerulonephritis
  idiopathic
  secondary
    to exogenous antigens (e.g. poststreptococcal, drug-related)
    to endogenous antigens (e.g. systemic lupus erythematosus)
Non-inflammatory: glomerulopathy
  (e.g. diabetic glomerulosclerosis, amyloid glomerulopathy)

Pathological
Glomerulonephritis (see Table 15.2)
Others (e.g. diabetic glomerulosclerosis, amyloid glomerulopathy)

that renal biopsy material be subjected to light microscopy with several stains, immune-labelling for immunoglobulins and often by electron microscopy (EM) (Chapter 2).

A simplified list of the primary glomerular diseases is given in Table 15.2

The terminology employed is dictated by the anatomy of glomeruli.

A disease can be:
- Focal — affecting some glomeruli, or diffuse — affecting all glomeruli.
- Segmental — affecting only part of the glomerulus.
  Within the glomerulus there can be:
- No visible change.
- Proliferation (or infiltration) of cells.
- Basement membrane changes, usually seen as thickening.
- Sclerosis of part or all of the glomerulus.

Often the histology correlates with the broad clinical picture: in particular if there is proliferation then haematuria is usual, membrane changes are associated with heavy proteinuria and extensive crescent formation is the rule in rapidly progressive GN (Table 15.2).

PATHOGENESIS OF GLOMERULONEPHRITIS

Although glomerular injury can be provoked in a wide variety of ways, in the primary glomerular diseases most evidence suggests

Table 15.2 Primary glomerulonephritis GN

	Postulated pathogenesis
Non-proliferative (often associated with heavy proteinuria/nephrotic syndrome)	
Minimal-change GN	Cell mediated
Focal and segmental hyalinosis and sclerosis (FSHS)	Cell mediated
Membranous GN	Immune complex
Proliferative (often associated with haematuria/ nephritic syndrome)	
Diffuse mesangial proliferative GN	Immune complex
Diffuse endocapillary proliferative GN	Immune complex
Focal and segmental proliferative GN	Immune complex
Membranoproliferative GN	Immune complex
Diffuse crescentic (extracapillary) proliferative GN	Immune complex

that the initiating event is immunologically mediated. The disease is a result of at least three variables:

• Genetic predisposition.
• Provoking antigen.
• Immunologically mediated damage to the glomerulus.

Subsequent to the generation of the immune response, glomerular damage results from a variety of interactive mediators which include:

• Antibody-mediated damage (e.g. antiglomerular basement membrane antibodies).
• Cell-mediated injury, by polymorphs, macrophages, and T lymphocytes.
• Mediators of inflammation, including the complement, and coagulation systems.

Based on these concepts, the pathogenesis of various forms of GN is attributed to humoral (antibody–antigen complexes forming or depositing in the glomeruli), cell-mediated, or unknown mechanisms (Table 15.2).

MINIMAL-CHANGE GLOMERULONEPHRITIS

Synonyms. Lipoid nephrosis, foot-process fusion disease.

Definition and pathology

This is a disease characterised by heavy proteinuria in which fusion (or effacement) of the foot processes of glomerular epithelial cells on EM is the only significant glomerular abnormality (Fig. 15.1). Light microscopy is normal or near-normal, and immune

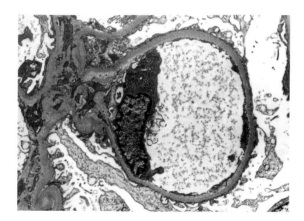

Fig. 15.1 Minimal change glomerulonephritis. Fusion (effacement) of the foot processes of the epithelial cells is he major abnormality (compare with Fig. 1.6)

deposits are usually not found. Associated renal pathology includes lipid droplets in tubular cells as a result of lipid resorption.

Cause and pathogenesis of minimal change GN

The cause and pathogenesis of this disease is unknown. Some intriguing associations include (Table 15.3):

Atopy. There is an association in some patients with eczema, hayfever and asthma.

T-cell function. The disease is thought to result from a disorder of T-cell function. Evidence includes an association with Hodgkin's disease, abnormalities in T-suppressor cell function, and the suggestion that non-steroidal anti-inflammatory drugs (NSAIDs), which may induce the disease, do so by prostacyclin-mediated effects on T cells.

Clinical features of minimal change GN

The clinical features are:

Acute nephrotic syndrome. This disease almost always presents as the acute nephrotic syndrome (Chapter 9). It is the cause of this syndrome in 80% of children and about 20% of adults.

Table 15.3 Causes of minimal-change disease

Idiopathic
Associated with atopy — hayfever, eczema
Hodgkin's lymphoma
Non-steroidal anti-inflammatory drugs

The nephrosis is sudden in onset and usually severe, with gross generalised oedema, heavy proteinuria, hypoalbuminaemia and hyperlipidaemia. Frequently a history of an antecedent respiratory infection, allergy or recent immunisation will be found. In small children severe abdominal pain may be a prominent feature.

Other features suggesting minimal change GN are:

Normal renal function. Most patients have a normal plasma creatinine concentration. When it is raised, this usually can be attributed to prerenal factors.

Absence of hypertension. Hypertension is found in only about 10% of children.

Absence of haematuria. Less than 20% of patients have significant haematuria.

Selective proteinuria in children (see below)

Response to steroids. The diagnosis must be seriously doubted if the proteinuria does not resolve completely with steroid therapy (see below).

Complications of minimal change GN

The complications are those of the nephrotic syndrome (Chapter 9). They include:
- *Infection,* particularly pneumococcal peritonitis and pneumonia.
- *Thrombosis,* including leg and pelvic venous thrombosis and embolism in the adult.
- *Acute tubular necrosis,* which can be provoked by excessive diuretic therapy or concommitant NSAID administration.

Investigations in minimal change GN

Heavy proteinuria (>3.5 g/day), is associated with hypoalbuminaemia and hyperlipidaemia. Urine microscopy often reveals hyaline casts and fat droplets. The urinary erythrocyte count is normal or slightly elevated. Plasma creatinine and urea are usually normal but may be elevated in severe hypovolaemia or when other abnormalities coexist.

Plasma fibrinogen is often increased, and a modest increase in platelet count is common. Haemoglobin may be elevated by haemoconcentration. Plasma complement is normal.

The protein selectivity index is useful in children but not in adults. In children with minimal change nephritis the ratio of the clearance of IgG (MW 150 000) to transferrin (MW 88 000) is virtually always below 0.2.

Renal biopsy is usually performed in adults. In children in whom a clinical diagnosis of likely minimal change nephritis is made it is usual to proceed to a trial of therapy with steroids (see below) and only perform a biopsy in atypical cases or those who do not respond to steroids, since in children 80% of nephrotics will have minimal change GN.

Treatment of minimal change GN

The general care is as for the nephrotic syndrome (Chapter 9). Specific therapy for the glomerular lesion is usually with steroids or cyclophosphamide.

Steroid therapy

Prednisolone (60 mg/day in adults, or 1−2 mg/kg/day in children) is given orally for a maximum 6 week course. The response usually occurs between one and three weeks with an abrupt reduction in proteinuria, accompanied by a diuresis and rapid resolution of oedema. In adults, weight loss of 10−20 kg is not uncommon. Reduction in steroid dosage is rapid and commenced about 1 week after diuresis; reducing the dosage to 40 mg and 20 mg at 2-weekly intervals. Steroids must not be completely withdrawn abruptly since this may be associated with relapse.

Alternative approaches include alternate day steroids to minimise steroid side-effects, particularly in children once remission has occurred, or pulse intravenous doses of prednisolone (e.g. three doses each of 1 g at daily intervals).

Cyclophosphamide

Cyclophosphamide therapy can induce a remission, and more importantly prevents subsequent relapse more effectively than treatment with steroids. In patients with frequent relapse a course of oral cyclophosphamide (100−150 mg/day in adults or 0.2−0.3 mg/kg/day in children) for 6−12 weeks should be considered. The side-effects of bone marrow depression and cystitis can be avoided by close monitoring of white cell count, and administration in the morning. A course of only 3 months is unlikely to affect fertility, however, because of possible long-term effects such as infertility or neoplasia. Most paediatricians prefer to reserve such treatment for the most troublesome recurrent relapsing nephrotic children with steroid side effects such as growth failure.

Course of minimal change GN

In children over 90% respond with complete remission to a short course of prednisolone, and a further 5% to a more protracted course of higher doses, leaving only about 2% of non-responders. Of the responder group, however, 40% have frequent, and 20% infrequent relapses, which again respond to prednisolone. Increasing age is associated with a lower prevalence of early response but also a lower prevalence of frequent relapse.

There is a group of nephrotic patients with renal biopsies showing only foot process fusion with electron microscopy who fail to respond to prednisolone or cyclophosphamide therapy. Some of these will have responded in the past, often incompletely in that they have persisting mild proteinuria. Sometimes poorly selective proteinuria has been documented and occasionally haematuria. It is in this group that later renal biopsy may reveal focal and segmental hyalinosis and sclerosis (FSHS, see below). In some a review of further sections of the original biopsy will show FSHS. Since FSHS is a focal disease it could be that this lesion was present in a minority of glomeruli originally, or alternatively it develops with time. At present we have no way of knowing whether these patients constitute merely a group within minimal-change disease in whom long periods of severe proteinuria results in secondary FSHS, or whether they represent cases of primary FSHS, in some of whom early and partial response to steroid treatment can occur. Suffice it to say that this group has a quite different prognosis, and there are many who regard the presence of steroid-resistance as incompatible with true minimal-change disease.

Prognosis of minimal change GN

The prognosis of minimal-change disease is excellent. Patients who continue to respond to steroids and show no evidence of FSHS do not progress to renal failure.

FOCAL AND SEGMENTAL HYALINOSIS AND SCLEROSIS

Synonyms. FSHS, primary focal and segmental glomerulosclerosis, primary FGS, focal sclerosing glomerulopathy.

Pathology

The characteristic glomerular lesion is sclerosis (capillary collapse and replacement with collagen and mesangial matrix) in segments of some glomeruli, often associated with deposits of glassy eosinophilic material (hyalinosis) in glomerular capillaries (Fig. 15.2).

This pathological appearance can occur in a wide range of diseases (Table 15.4). In some the sclerosis is the result of previous focal and segmental glomerular damage resulting from inflammation or vascular obstruction. Focal and segmental glomerular sclerosis (FGS) also seems to be a final common histological appearance of pathway by which a variety of renal diseases progress to renal failure (Chapter 6).

Primary FSHS is said to be present when no other renal disease is found to explain the glomerular damage. As in minimal-change disease a T-lymphocyte disorder is suspected.

Evidence for a circulating abnormality includes rapid recurrence

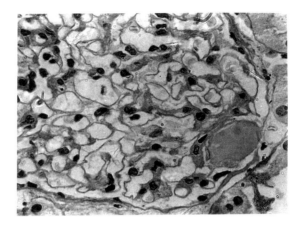

Fig. 15.2 Primary focal and segmental sclerosis and hyalinosis (FSHS)

of nephrotic syndrome in renal allografts of some patients who have gone into chronic renal failure due to primary FSHS. Proteinuria may even be detected as the patient leaves the operating theatre.

Clinical features of primary FSHS

Primary FSHS usually presents as proteinuria, hypertension or renal failure. It is the cause of nephrotic syndrome in about 5% of children and 15% of adults. Although similar to minimal-change disease it differs in several important respects:

Compared with minimal-change disease there is more likely to be:
- Microscopic glomerular haematuria.
- Hypertension.

Table 15.4 Causes of focal and segmental sclerosis

Primary
Secondary Secondary to reduction in renal mass (see Chapter 6); probably complicates all chronic renal diseases, but particularly described in reflux and analgesic nephropathy
Secondary to focal and segmental proliferative GN
Secondary to other focal and segmental glomerular damage 　Heroin addicts 　Atheroembolic disease 　Familial glomerulonephritis (Alport' syndrome)

- Poorly selective proteinuria.
- No response to steroids.

In addition primary FSHS can present with lesser degrees of proteinuria and the clinical picture is one of 'chronic glomerulonephritis' with persistent proteinuria, haematuria and eventual hypertension and renal failure.

Course and treatment of primary FSHS

Primary FSHS is a progressive disease, about 50% of patients reaching end-stage renal failure in 10 years. In patients with nephrotic syndrome the prognosis is worse, with a 10 year renal survival of only about 30% of patients. In patients with asymptomatic proteinuria the prognosis is correspondingly better — as high as 90% at 10 years. This heterogeneity is also seen within the nephrotic group in whom a response to steroids indicates a better prognosis.

There is no specific treatment for FSHS. The clinical effects, particularly nephrotic syndrome, hypertension and renal failure are treated as described earlier (Chapters 9, 11 & 12).

In as many as 30% of cases an improvement in the nephrotic syndrome occurs with steroid administration as for minimal-change disease, though the response is often slower and incomplete, with persisting milder proteinuria. Cyclophosphamide is rarely effective if high dose steroids have failed. Cyclosporin has been used in some resistant cases.

There is some evidence that anticoagulants and antiplatelet agents may improve prognosis, and anticoagulants are indicated in adults with severe hypoalbuminaemia as prophylaxis against thrombosis (Chapter 9).

MEMBRANOUS GLOMERULONEPHRITIS

Synonyms. Membranous glomerulopathy, epimembranous, extra-membranous glomerulonephritis.

Definition and pathology

Membranous GN is characterised by diffuse thickening of the walls of the capillary loop (Fig. 15.3) This thickening can be seen with EM and immunofluorescence to be due to the deposition of multiple immunoglobulin-containing electron-dense deposits between the outside of the glomerular basement membrane (GBM) and the epithelial cell. Basement membrane material extends outward between these deposits and may eventually incorporate them. The foot processes are usually effaced as in all cases of heavy proteinuria. With progression the capillary lumen becomes narrow, capillary loops collapse and the glomerulus becomes fibrosed and functionless.

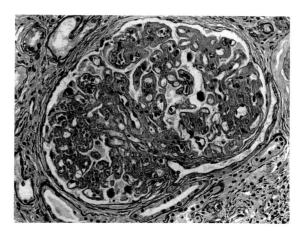

Fig. 15.3 Membranous glomerulonephritis

The extension of the basement membrane around the deposits can be seen as palisades of 'spikes' with silver stains. Immunoglobulin G distributed in a 'granular' pattern along the capillary loops can be demonstrated by immunofluorescent or immunoperoxidase staining.

Causes and pathogenesis of membranous GN

Although in over 80% of cases the cause is unknown there are a wide variety of known causes of membranous GN (Table 15.5). Systemic lupus erythematosus (Chapter 17), drugs (especially gold and penicillamine), and carcinomas are the commonest in Western countries.

The two most accepted explanations for immunoglobulin deposition both depend on a situation of chronic low grade antigenaemia, and eventual formation of immune complexes outside the GBM. These mechanisms are:

● *Circulating immune-complex deposition.* In some diseases immune complexes have been demonstrated in the circulation and in the glomeruli, and it is suggested that these pass through the GBM and form the immune deposits.

● *The 'fixed antigen' theory.* As circulating complexes cannot be detected in many cases an alternate hypothesis is that the antigen itself filters through the GBM and that the immunoglobulin subsequently binds to it.

In gold and penicillamine nephropathy, the drug is not the antigen. Instead it seems that these drugs cause another antigen (presumably of native origin) to be deposited in the complex. An antigen derived from the tubular brush border has been implicated.

Table 15.5 Causes of membranous glomerulonephritis

Common	Rare
Idiopathic — 80% of cases	
Systemic diseases	
Systemic lupus erythematosus	Sarcoidosis
	Thyroiditis
	Guillain–Barré syndrome
Drugs	
Gold	Trimethadione
Penicillamine	Probenecid
Captopril	
Infections	Hepatitis B
	Syphilis
	Schistosmiasis
	Filariasis
	Epstein–Barr virus
Neoplasms	Carcinomas
	lung
	colon
	breast
	Lymphoma
	Leukemia

Clinical features of membranous GN

Nephrotic syndrome (Chapter 9) in the adult is the usual presentation. Over 80% of cases have proteinuria >3.5 g/day. This disease is the commonest cause of nephrotic syndrome in adults, being responsible for over 30% of cases, and an even greater proportion with increasing age. It is unusual in children and adolescents — 80–90% of patients are over 30 years of age.

In those patients in whom nephrotic syndrome is not present the usual abnormality is symptomless proteinuria with or without haematuria. Microscopic haematuria is common, but macroscopic haematuria rare. Hypertension and uraemia occur during the course of the disease and may be the presenting complaint.

Proteinuria is non-selective, and usually heavy. Other laboratory features of the nephrotic syndrome have been discussed already in Chapter 9.

A cause may be found (Table 15.5). SLE and hepatitis B should always be excluded and in patients over 60 years of age a clinical search for an underlying neoplasm should be made. In some series (but not our own) a carcinoma is found in up to 20% of cases.

Complications of membranous GN

Complications of the nephrotic syndrome (Chapter 9) are particularly common in membranous GN. These include:

Renal vein thrombosis

This occurs more often in membranous GN than in any other cause of nephrotic syndrome. It may be suspected because of abrupt increase in proteinuria, haematuria and plasma creatinine, or on renal biopsy where there is interstitial oedema and marginated polymorphs are seen in glomeruli. In some series up to 50% of cases have renal vein thrombosis, and it is particularly likely when plasma albumin falls below 20 g/litre. Diagnosis depends on renal venography (Chapter 2).

Peripheral arterial and venous thrombosis

Leg vein thrombosis, with consequent pulmonary embolism, myocardial and cerebral infarction are common in severely nephrotic adults.

Infection

Pneumonia and cellulitis in the grossly oedematous legs are the commonest infections.

Treatment and prognosis of membranous GN

The nephrotic syndrome in membranous GN tends to be chronic and can be severe, hence careful management is required (Chapter 9).

The treatment of the GN itself depends on the cause. When this is identifiable and removable, as in cases due to drugs, gradual resolution of proteinuria will usually occur once the cause is eliminated, though the immune deposits may persist for many months. The treatment of membranous GN in SLE is discussed in Chapter 17.

Treatment of idiopathic membranous GN

In about 20% of cases of idiopathic membranous nephritis presenting as nephrotic syndrome, spontaneous remission of the nephrotic state occurs during the first 6 months of observation. This relatively high spontaneous remission rate has made assessment of the effects of therapy difficult. Those that do not spontaneously resolve do very badly — about 30% are dead or in renal failure within 10 years. Indications of a likely poor prognosis include persistent nephrosis, impaired renal function and hypertension.

Whether there is an effective treatment for membranous GN is controversial. Proteinuria responds in some patients to a 6 month course of cyclophosphamide, dipyridamole and warfarin. Complete histological resolution may occur in treated cases and is very rare as a spontaneous event. It seems reasonable to first attempt conservative treatment (Chapter 9) and to reserve a trial of therapy for those patients in whom severe nephrotic syndrome persists, impaired renal function is present or deterioration in function occurs.

DIFFUSE MESANGIAL PROLIFERATIVE GLOMERULONEPHRITIS

There is diffuse mesangial proliferation usually with an increase in mesangial matrix and the presence of mesangial deposits. Mesangial IgA deposition, which occurs in over 50% of patients with diffuse mesangial proliferative GN characterises the largest and most important group (see below). Mesangial proliferation can also be seen in a wide variety of other circumstances where it seems to indicate a relatively mild inflammatory process.

We will concentrate on the most important group, mesangial IgA disease. Many of the others with mesangial cell proliferation and no IgA deposits show Thin Basement Membrane Disease (Chapter 31) on EM.

Mesangial IgA disease

Synonyms: IgA disease, Berger's disease. This important disease is the most common form of glomerulonephritis, the commonest cause of haematuria and and the commonest form of glomerulonephritis causing renal failure in our community. Diffuse mesangial IgA deposition is seen in 10–40% of renal biopsies depending on the geographical area.

Cause and pathology of mesangial IgA disease

The main histological feature is diffuse mesangial cell proliferation, with expansion of the mesangial matrix in which granular deposits of IgA are usually accompanied by C_3 and sometimes by IgG are found (Fig. 15.4). This is identical to the glomerular picture seen in Henoch–Schönlein purpura (Chapter 18) which suggests that these may be similar disease processes.

In the more active forms of the disease, focal and segmental proliferation, sometimes with segmental necrosis and crescents, can be found superimposed on the underlying condition.

The pathogenesis is unknown. It has been suggested that circulating IgA-containing complexes of gut or respiratory origin are responsible. IgA deposits have been seen in glomeruli in liver disease, suggesting that in some cases a defect in liver clearance of complexes plays a role. Other causes of mesangial IgA deposition are listed in Table 15.6. However, by far the greatest proportion of cases are of unknown cause.

Clinical features of mesangial IgA disease

Recurrent macroscopic haematuria, usually commencing in late adolescence or early adult life, and far more common in males, is one characteristic presenting feature. The attacks of macroscopic

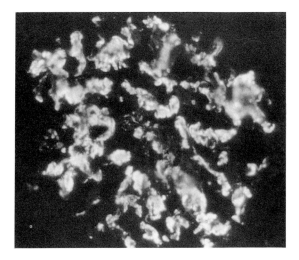

Fig. 15.4 Mesangial IgA disease. Fluorescence of a glomerulus stained with fluoroscein-labelled anti-IgA antibody demoñtrates the mesangial deposition of IgA

haematuria are often associated with an upper respiratory tract infection, sore throat (synpharingitic haematuria) or sometimes a gastrointestinal upset. The haematuria occurs at the height of the illness, rather than 2 weeks later as in poststreptococcal glomerulonephritis. The patients may feel generally unwell, and low grade fever and bilateral loin pain may be present.

A wide variety of other syndromes can occur including:

• *Chronic GN* with persistent haematuria, proteinuria or hypertension.

• *Rapidly progressive GN* with extensive crescent formation.

• *Acute renal failure* at the time of macroscopic haematuria,

Table 15.6 Diseases with predominant mesangial IgA deposition

Primary
IgA
mesangial nephropathy (Berger's disease)

Secondary
Henoch–Schönlein disease
Alcoholic liver disease
Gastrointestinal diseases:
  coeliac disease
  Crohn's disease
Dermatitis herpetiformis

due to acute tubular necrosis.
- *Overlap syndromes with Henoch–Schönlein purpura* in which rash, joint pains or abdominal pain may occur in some but not all attacks of haematuria.
- *Dysuria with loin-pain* in which the diagnosis of haemorrhagic cystitis may be made inappropriately.
- *No clinical abnormality.* IgA is sometimes found in the glomeruli of an apparently healthy living renal transplant donor. It is difficult to say whether this actually represents a 'disease' in this instance.

Laboratory features of mesangial IgA disease

Microscopic or macroscopic haematuria with large numbers of dysmorphic red cells is usual, but a confusing pattern in which there is an admixture of normal-looking red cells in heavy haematuria can be seen. Persistent heavy haematuria has a bad prognosis, since it reflects continuing active glomerular inflammation.

Proteinuria is usually present, but can be quite mild, with over 60% of cases having less than 1.0 g/day. In the uncommon case with persistent heavy proteinuria the prognosis is considerably worse.

Elevated plasma IgA occurs in up to 50% of cases. Plasma C_3 and C_4 are normal.

Skin biopsy reveals pericapillary deposits of IgA and C_3 in 20–50% of cases.

Course and treatment of mesangial IgA disease

The vast majority of patients with mesangial IgA disease do very well. However, the prognosis is extremely variable.
 Clinical features indicating a poor prognosis include:
- Decreased GFR at presentation.
- Persistent heavy proteinuria.
- Persistent heavy haematuria.
- Moderate or severe hypertension.

 There is no proven treatment for IgA disease. Crescentic nephritis may respond to intensive plasma exchange and immunosuppression, and a decrease in the severity of haematuric episodes has been suggested with corticosteroids. Supportive therapy, the most important part of which is blood pressure control, is all that is usually offered. Many of the patients who progress to end-stage renal failure do so because of uncontrolled accelerated hypertension which has occurred because of a lack of medical supervision.

DIFFUSE ENDOCAPILLARY PROLIFERATIVE GLOMERULONEPHRITIS

Synonyms. Postinfectious GN, diffuse exudative proliferative GN.

Pathology

The glomerular lesion is a diffuse proliferative GN, in which the glomerular tufts are swollen and grossly hypercellular with prominent polymorph infiltration (Fig. 15.5). The capillary lumen is often virtually obliterated by infiltrating polymorphs and monocytes, as well as swollen, probably proliferated, endothelial and mesangial cells. Crescent formation can occur, but is uncommon, and if present indicates a poorer prognosis.

A characteristic feature is the presence of large hump-like deposits on the outside of the basement membrane under the epithelial cells. These 'humps' are well seen on EM as electron dense subepithelial deposits. Immunofluorescence is variable, but IgG and C_3 are often found in a granular pattern around capillary loops or in the mesangium in the acute stage.

Causes of diffuse endocapillary GN

Diffuse endocapillary GN is usually secondary to streptococcal infection of the throat. Poststreptococcal glomerulonephritis usually occurs about 10 days after infection with a 'nephritogenic' group A haemolytic streptococcus, particularly type 12. (Rheumatic fever can occur after any Group A streptococcal infection.) In tropical countries the infection is commonly of the skin, and 'epidemics' of poststreptococcal nephritis can occur. Other infections, including staphylococcal and viral infections, can much less commonly be followed by a similar disease.

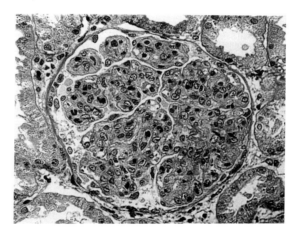

Fig. 15.5 Diffuse proliferative glomerulonephritis (poststreptococcal)

Clinical features of poststreptococcal GN

Males are more commonly affected than females (2 : 1). The disease is more common in children and consists of an attack of acute nephritis (Chapter 9) about 10 days after the precipitating infection which is usually a sore throat. This disease has become quite rare in the adult Western communities. If there are only a few days between the infection and the haematuria, mesangial IgA disease should be suspected.

There is usually a sudden onset of acute nephritic syndrome (Chapter 9) with haematuria (smoky urine or darker), hypertension, oliguria and mild oedema (facial puffiness). Important complications include:

Cardiac failure. Fluid retention and hypertension can result in rapid onset of pulmonary oedema. Rarely patients can have both poststreptococcal nephritis and rheumatic carditis.

Hypertensive encephalopathy or cerebral haemorrhage. These occur as a result of sudden severe hypertension, perhaps aggravated by oedema. Headache, drowsiness, vomiting and convulsions are usual features.

Acute renal failure. Rapidly progressive GN occurs in about 2% of cases, although in most cases there is a rise in plasma urea and often a less impressive rise in plasma creatinine. Anuria or persistent oliguria are ominous signs, and can be associated with diffuse crescentic disease, in which case the prognosis is much worse.

Rare complications include generalised vasculitis, rheumatic fever, and microangiopathic haemolytic anaemia.

Laboratory features of poststreptococcal GN

Glomerular haematuria with large numbers of dysmorphic red cells and red cell casts is usual. Proteinuria is moderate, (1–3 g/day) and rarely of nephrotic range. There is a fall in creatinine clearance. Plasma urea is usually elevated.

Evidence of recent Group A streptococcal infection should be sought. Streptococci may be grown from throat or skin swabs, or a rise in titre of antibodies to streptococcal products (ASOT, antistreptokinase) may be detected. The streptozyme test is often positive.

Plasma-complement abnormalities may occur. Plasma C_3 usually falls early in the disease, while C_4 is less depressed and rises earlier to normal levels. The period of C_3 depression without change in C_4 can cause confusion with type II membranoproliferative GN.

Renal biopsy

Renal biopsy is usually avoided in children, particularly when the disease is classical and mild. Because the disease is uncommon in adults, and seems to have a worse prognosis, renal biopsy should be performed in all adults with acute nephritis.

Course of poststreptococcal GN

The immediate prognosis is excellent, particularly in children. Long-term studies suggest a less favourable outcome in those with severe initial disease, and in adults.

The usual course in children, probably occurring in over 95% of cases, is clinical resolution about 2 weeks after the onset of the disease, with diuresis and clearance of the macroscopic haematuria. Blood pressure falls and oedema resolves, however microscopic haematuria and proteinuria may persist for months or even years. Complete resolution of all laboratory abnormalities should occur in about 6 months, and the prognosis, at least for 10–20 years, is excellent.

In adults both the short and long-term outcome seems less favourable. Although clinical resolution still occurs in most cases renal biopsy reveals continuing abnormalities in about one-third of cases and 40% have proteinuria, hypertension or both at 10 years. Those that progress in this fashion commonly show persistence of mesangial proliferation or development of FGS. A few studies of non-hospitalised adults, with much less severe disease, have reported a better long-term outcome.

Management of poststreptococcal GN

Treatment usually consists of treatment of the infection with penicillin and supportive treatment for the acute nephritis (Chapter 9), particularly control of fluid intake and hypertension.

The severe crescentic disease is treated similarly to other forms of diffuse crescentic nephritis, though there are suggestions that diffuse crescentic disease in poststreptococcal nephritis carries a better prognosis than it does in the idiopathic and other secondary forms.

FOCAL AND SEGMENTAL PROLIFERATIVE GLOMERULONEPHRITIS

This is one of the more common secondary forms of GN.

Causes and pathology

Proliferation of cells affects one or more lobules of some glomeruli, i.e. the proliferation is both segmental and focal (Fig. 15.6). There may be necrosis in some lobules, and crescents in relation to proliferative or necrotic lesions.

This pathological picture has many causes (Table 15.7). About 70% of biopsies also have diffuse mesangial deposits of IgA — the hallmark of IgA nephropathy. Systemic diseases such as SLE

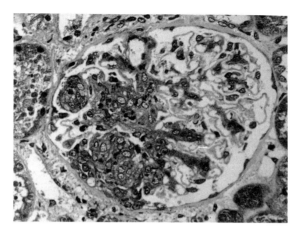

Fig. 15.6 Focal and segmental proliferative glomerulonephritis

(Chapter 17), vasculitis, Henoch–Schönlein purpura (Chapter 18) and Goodpasture's syndrome (Chapter 16) are other important causes.

Clinical features

As most cases of focal and segmental proliferative glomerulonephritis occur as part of some other disease, the clinical picture is heterogeneous, but there is usually moderate to severe haematuria. In some diseases, such as SLE, Goodpasture's syndrome and Wegener's granulomatosis, rapid progression to diffuse crescentic glomerulonephritis can occur, with the concomitant clinical picture of rapidly progressive nephritis (Chapter 9).

Course and treatment

The course and treatment is that of the underlying disease.

Table 15.7 Causes of focal and segmental proliferative glomerulonephritis

Idiopathic
Mesangial-proliferative IgA disease
Idiopathic focal and segmental proliferative GN

Secondary
Systemic lupus erythematosus
Vasculitis:
  polyarteritis
  Henoch–Schönlein purpura
  Wegener's granulomatosis
Antiglomerular basement membrane antibody disease (Goodpasture's syndrome)
Infections
  subacute bacterial endocarditis
Familial nephritis
  Alport's syndrome

MEMBRANOPROLIFERATIVE GLOMERULONEPHRITIS

Synonyms. Mesangiocapillary glomerulonephritis.

Causes and pathology
There is both proliferation of cells in the glomerular tuft and thickening of the glomerular capillary walls (Fig. 15.7). Extra-capillary proliferation with formation of crescents occurs in about 10% of cases and indicates a poor prognosis.

The two main subgroups — Type I and Type II membrano-proliferative glomerulonephritis (Table 15.8) which have different histology and different causes. In addition, extramembranous deposits may be associated. Such cases are usually termed Type III.

Type I membrano-proliferative GN
This is an increasingly uncommon condition in Western countries.

Type 1 membranoproliferative GN is characterised by splitting of the basement membrane, best seen in silver stains (tram-tracks) or on electron microscopy. Subendothelial deposits containing C_3 are found by immunofluorescence and EM in an irregular pattern around the capillary loop. Immunoglobulin deposition is patchy and inconstant. Crescents may be found in up to 30% of cases, and indicate a poor prognosis.

The classical disease is idiopathic, however, the appearance can be mimicked to some degree by a variety of diseases, often characterised by chronic antigenaemia (Table 15.8).

Table 15.8 Membranoproliferative glomerulonephritis: classification

Type I membranoproliferative glomerulonephritis (with subendothelial deposits)
Idiopathic (classical)
Secondary to chronic antigenaemia:
  immune diseases:
    SLE
    Mixed cryoglobulinaemia
  infection:
    quartan malaria
    hepatitis B
    subacute bacterial endocarditis
    infected atrioventricular shunts ('Shunt' nephritis)
  neoplasm
  light chain nephropathy

Type II membranoproliferative glomerulonephritis (dense deposit disease) associated with:
Low plasma C_3 complement
Circulating C_3-nephritic factor
Partial lipodystrophy

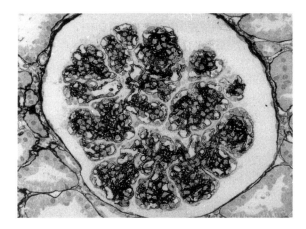

Fig. 15.7 Membranoproliferative glomerulonephritis

Type II membrano-proliferative GN

This is an uncommon disease where long segments of densely staining deposits occur within the basement membrane causing thickening; the alternative name is 'dense-deposit disease'. The dense deposit may be linear or sausage-shaped, and may contain large amounts of C_3. There is no known cause, though there are very specific clinical associations (see below).

Clinical features of membrano-proliferative GN

The clinical presentation is quite varied. The mean age of onset for idiopathic Type I disease is about 25 years, and about 15 years in Type II disease.

Nephrotic syndrome

Nephrosis is the presenting problem in about 50% of cases. About 5% of children and 10% of adults with nephrotic syndrome have membranoproliferative GN. In these cases significant haematuria, hypertension and impaired renal function are common. Patients with persistent heavy proteinuria have a poor prognosis.

Acute nephritis

An acute nephritic illness is the presenting feature in about 25% of cases, particularly children. In some a history of a preceding upper respiratory tract infection is obtained. In the worst case patients can present with rapidly progressive GN.

Chronic proteinuria and haematuria

These are the presenting features in about 25% of cases. Both are usually present together, and coexistence of hypertension and a decreased creatinine clearance is also common. During the course of the disease it is not uncommon for patients to have periods of asymptomatic proteinuria and haematuria interspersed with nephrotic or nephritic illnesses which may be preceded by an intercurrent infection or illness.

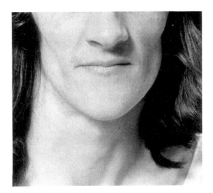
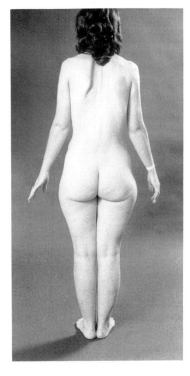

Fig. 15.8 Partial lipodystrophy with loss of fat on face and upper body in a patient with membranoproliferative glomerulonephritis (Type II)

Type II membrano-proliferative GN

There are a few special clinical features in some patients with Type II membranoproliferative GN. These are:
- Partial lipodystrophy, with loss of fat on the face in some patients (Fig. 15.8).
- Persistently depressed plasma C_3.
- C_3 nephritic factor in the plasma (see below).

Laboratory features of membrano-proliferative GN

Proteinuria, haematuria and renal failure are all common.

Proteinuria is virtually always present and exceeds 3.5 g/day in 50% of cases.

Haematuria is also usually found, often with over 10^5 glomerular red cells/ml of urine. A low urinary red cell count is a good prognostic feature. Macroscopic haematuria can occur in acute nephritic illnesses.

Hypocomplementaemia is commonly seen, particularly in Type II disease where there is a persistently low plasma C_3 level. Low plasma C_3 in Type II membranoproliferative GN is associated with the presence in the plasma of C_3-nephritic factor (C_3NeF), an IgG antibody to C_3-convertase, which has the effect of protecting C_3-convertase from enzymatic degradation, with resultant continuous low C_3 levels. It appears that C_3NeF may disappear from plasma with time, and also that C_3NeF is particularly likely to occur in people with partial lipodystrophy. C_3NeF occurs in the plasma of up to 60% of patients with Type II membranoproliferative glomerulonephritis.

Course and treatment of membranoproliferative GN

These are aggressive and progressive diseases, particularly if heavy proteinuria, hypertension and an elevated plasma creatinine are present. Type I membranoproliferative GN has a 10-year renal survival of only 40% if nephrosis is present, and 85% if not nephrotic. Type II membranoproliferative GN has an even worse prognosis.

Other than some reports of benefit from antiplatelet agents there is no proven treatment, other than of the hypertension and other clinical features.

DIFFUSE CRESCENTIC GLOMERULONEPHRITIS

Synonyms. Diffuse extracapillary GN, rapidly progressive nephritis with glomerular crescents.

Cause and pathology

Crescents are accumulations of cells, fibrin and collagen in Bowman's space, where they may compress the capillary tuft (Fig. 15.9). Eventually the tuft is irreversibly obliterated. Formation of crescents commences with severe damage to the glomerular capillary wall. Leakage of fibrin from the glomerular tuft into Bowman's space is followed by macrophage infiltration and subsequent organisation by fibroblasts and collagen.

The presence of crescents in a large proportion (80% or more) of glomeruli is usually associated with a rapidly progressive course, regardless of the lesion in the underlying glomerular tufts. The underlying glomerular pathology is almost invariably a severe proliferative lesion with necrosis and fibrin deposition.

The causes include all those of severe proliferative GN and an idiopathic group (Table 15.9). Goodpasture's syndrome, polyarteritis, Wegener's granulomatosis and SLE are likely to be complicated by diffuse crescentic GN.

Clinical features of diffuse crescentic GN

In diffuse crescentic nephritis the usual picture is rapidly progressive GN (Chapter 9) with macroscopic haematuria and rapidly deteriorating renal function. Proteinuria is usually over 1 g/day.

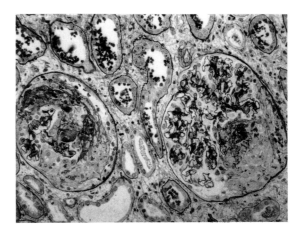

Fig. 15.9 Crescentic glomerulonephritis, with a crescent-shaped accumulation of fibrin, macrophages, fibroblasts and proliferated capsular epithelial cells in Bowman's space, compressing the glomerular capillary tuft

Hypertension is often absent. Progression to oliguric or even anuric renal failure can occur in days or weeks. Profound oligo-anuria often means damage is irreversible.

The syndrome is more common in adults. A systemic disease is present in as many as 30–50% of cases, commonly Good-pasture's syndrome, systemic lupus erythematosus or necrotising vasculitis. These all have characteristic clinical features of their own. For this reason a very careful clinical and laboratory search for such diseases is important in every case.

Idiopathic diffuse crescentic GN

A small group of patients exist in whom no underlying cause can be found. Usually middle-aged or older these patients may have

Table 15.9 Causes of diffuse crescentic glomerulonephritis

Idiopathic

Superimposed on other primary GN
Membranoproliferative
Mesangial IgA
Diffuse endocapillary proliferative (poststreptococcal)

Associated with systemic disease
Goodpasture's syndrome (Chapter 16)
SLE (Chapter 17)
Necrotising arteritis (Chapter 18)
  Wegener's granulomatosis
  polyarteritis
Henoch–Schönlein purpura (Chapter 18)

vague constitutional systems suggesting vasculitis, or a history of infection. Renal biopsy reveals a diffuse crescentic GN with extensive proliferation and necrosis in the glomerular tufts. Granular deposits of IgG and C_3 may be found, suggesting immune-complex disease, but in others no such deposits are seen. This group appears to have a particularly poor prognosis.

Prognosis and management of diffuse crescentic GN

Patients presenting with macroscopic haematuria, proteinuria and failing renal function represent a medical emergency. Delay in diagnosis can result in end-stage renal failure.

In all adults renal biopsy should be performed as an emergency. If crescentic disease is present there are two regimens that have been shown to result in improvement in renal function, but only if instituted before the patients become anuric. These are repeated plasma exchange combined with immunosuppression, and treatment with 'pulse-dose' steroid (three doses each of 2 g of i.v. methylprednisolone every second day).

Despite treatment the outcome is still poor overall, with a significant proportion of patients dying or developing end-stage renal failure.

16: *Anti-Glomerular Basement Membrane Antibody-Mediated Glomerulonephritis: Goodpasture's Syndrome*

Goodpasture described a fatal syndrome of pulmonary haemorrhage and nephritis in 1919. Common usage has generally equated this syndrome with a disease mediated by antibodies to glomerular and pulmonary basement membrane. Although there is no evidence that this was the case in the original description, and there are many other causes of pulmonary haemorrhage, haematuria and acute renal failure (Table 16.1), the term Goodpasture's syndrome is usually used for an uncommon disease characterised by:

- Acute glomerulonephritis.
- Pulmonary alveolar haemorrhage.
- Circulating antibodies to glomerular basement membrane (anti-GBM antibodies).

Since cases of acute glomerulonephritis (GN) with circulating anti-GBM antibodies can occur without pulmonary haemorrhage these can be included under the general heading 'anti-GBM antibody-mediated GN' or anti-GBM disease.

The natural history of untreated anti-GBM disease is usually one of rapid progression to death from either fatal pulmonary haemorrhage or renal failure.

CAUSES AND PATHOGENESIS OF ANTI-GBM DISEASE

This disease is characterised by the presence of circulating antibodies to GBM resulting in a severe crescentic GN. Immunofluorescent staining demonstrates IgG and C_3 in a linear distribution along the GBM (Fig. 16.1). The antibodies also may react with pulmonary alveolar basement membrane, producing alveolar haemorrhage and haemoptysis in most cases. Why some patients may have predominant renal disease with little lung involvement, while others have the reverse, is unclear.

Antibody production seems to depend on both genetic and environmental factors.

Genetic factors. HLA DRw2 is linked with predisposition to the disease.

Table 16.1 Common causes of pulmonary haemorrhage with haematuria

	Chapter
Anti-GBM antibody-mediated disease	16
Systemic vasculitis	
Wegener's granulomatosis	18
Polyarteritis	18
Systemic lupus erythematosus	17
Others	
Legionnaire's disease	
Renal vein thrombosis with pulmonary embolus	
Renal failure with acute pulmonary oedema	

Environmental factors. Inhalation of petrochemicals has been documented to precede the disease in many cases. There is some evidence that cigarette smoking increases the risk of lung haemorrhage.

CLINICAL FEATURES OF ANTI-GBM DISEASE

Anti-GBM disease occurs most commonly in young adult males, although no age group is exempt and this male preponderance is lost with increasing age. The major clinical features are haemoptysis and haematuria.

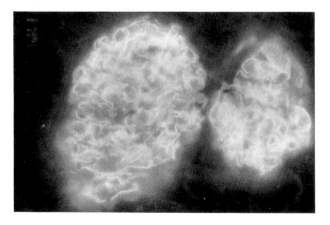

Fig. 16.1 Linear immunofluorescence with anti-IgG along the basement membrane in Goodpasture's syndrome (anti-GBM antibody-mediated glomerulonephritis)

Haemoptysis occurs in 70% of cases. It can vary from only a few flecks of blood to massive life-threatening bleeding, with respiratory failure due to intra-alveolar blood. In some patients mild haemoptysis has occurred over several months before the onset of haematuria. In some patients without haemoptysis profound anaemia and patchy opacities on chest X-ray indicate that alveolar bleeding is occurring. A small proportion of cases have no evidence of pulmonary involvement.

Haematuria is invariable, and usually macroscopic. Proteinuria is usually present (averaging about 2.5 g/day) but hypertension and oedema are uncommon.

Impaired renal function is usually apparent on presentation and rapidly progresses. In some patients oliguria and anuria can occur within one week of onset.

LABORATORY FINDINGS IN ANTI-GBM DISEASE

Anaemia is often severe and out of proportion to the haemoptysis or haematuria. Circulating antiglomerular basement membrane antibody is usually detectable. Urinary red cells and red cell casts are seen. Complement C_3 and C_4 are normal. Chest X-ray shows fluffy opacities which wax and wane with episodes of intra-alveolar haemorrhage.

Renal biopsy

The most important test is immediate renal biopsy, although this may be deferred in cases where immediate treatment is required (see below). A diffuse segmental proliferative GN with extensive crescents, segmental necrosis and diagnostic linear immunofluorescence with IgG is found (Fig. 16.1). Fibrin is seen in necrotic loops and in the crescents.

Linear fluorescence for IgG is occasionally seen in a few other diseases where the IgG is believed to be adsorbed to an abnormal GBM (Table 16.2)

COURSE AND MANAGEMENT OF ANTI-GBM DISEASE

This disease constitutes a medical emergency, since in the worst cases irreversible anuric renal failure or fatal haemoptysis can occur within a week of onset. In other cases a grumbling course over several months leads to chronic renal failure. Severely impaired renal function, oliguria and anuria are the most ominous signs from a renal point of view.

Table 16.2 Causes of linear immunofluorescence with anti-IgG

Anti-GBM antibody-mediated disease

IgG deposition
Pregnancy (pre-eclampsia)
Systemic lupus erythematosus
Diabetic nephropathy

Autofluorescence of GBM
Old age

Treatment

Immediate treatment is with intensive plasma exchange, high dose prednisolone and cyclophosphamide. In the more advanced and clinically obvious cases it is safer to commence this therapy while awaiting the result of the anti-GBM antibody assay because of the risk of renal bleeding after biopsy. Renal biopsy can then be deferred until the situation stabilises. In most cases, however, a renal biopsy is performed before embarking on this expensive and dangerous therapy.

If the patient is treated before irreversible damage has occurred, the disease can be controlled with preservation of renal function. This is usually a 'single hit' disease so that most patients do not require more than 3 to 12 months of immunosuppression. Very rarely recurrence can occur, even in transplanted kidneys.

17: *Systemic Lupus Erythematosus, Scleroderma and Rheumatoid Arthritis*

SYSTEMIC LUPUS ERYTHEMATOSUS

Systemic lupus erythematosus (SLE) is a multisystem disease characterised by circulating autoantibodies to DNA. Renal involvement is a major cause of morbidity in patients with SLE, and although with modern treatment renal failure is becoming less common, in many series of patients with lupus nephritis 10–30% eventually develop renal failure.

Cause and pathogenesis

SLE is an autoimmune disease, which seems to occur in predisposed individuals with a variety of precipitating factors.

Genetic predisposition

Sex. Females outnumber males 10:1.
Race. The disease is more common and severe in non-white races.
HLA type. HLA A1, B8 and DRw3 are associated with an increased risk of SLE.
Complement deficiency. Lupus-like syndromes occur with a variety of congenital complement deficiencies.

Precipitating factors

Viral infection. Virus infection has been postulated as a common precipitating factor.
Sunburn may aggravate or precipitate SLE.
Trauma. Physical or psychological trauma may precede the illness.
Drugs. A variety of drugs (Table 17.1) can precipitate or cause a similar disease (see below).

Pathogenesis of renal involvement in SLE

The renal lesion in SLE is believed to be due to the deposition of circulating immune complexes in the glomeruli. Subepithelial, subendothelial and intramembranous immune deposits of IgG, IgM, IgA, C_3 and C1q are found, and DNA and anti-DNA antibodies have been shown to be present.

Renal pathology in SLE

The usual feature is glomerulonephritis (GN), though interstitial nephritis and vasculitis can occur.

Lupus GN

The glomeruli can be normal on light microscopy, but more

248

Table 17.1 Drugs causing lupus-like syndrome

Common	Uncommon
Hydrallazine	Anticonvulsants (e.g. phenytoin)
Procainamide	Sulphonamide
Isoniazid	Dapsone
	Many others

commonly there are proliferative changes (commonly segmental), and/or membrane thickening with immune deposits along the basement membrane. The immune deposits may be so dense that the basement membrane has thickened segments with a dense bright appearance with eosin stain — the 'wire loop' lesion. Haematoxyphil bodies may be present. A feature common to all forms of lupus nephritis is granular deposition of IgG, IgA, IgM, C_3 and C1q in glomeruli.

It is usual to classify the lesions into five major groups:

1 *No histological abnormality* (less than 10% of patients).

2 *Mesangial proliferative* (10–20%).

3 *Focal and segmental proliferative* (15–20%), often associated with local fibrin deposition and necrosis. Overlying crescents may occur.

4 *Diffuse proliferative* (50% of patients). This is the most common lesion. Most glomeruli are affected by proliferation which may have segmental accentuation. Fibrin and crescents are commonly found.

5 *Membranous* (15% of patients). Here there is dense deposition of immune deposits along the GBM, and varying amounts of associated proliferation. The appearance can be indistinguishable from idiopathic membranous GN (Chapter 15).

Lupus arteritis

Rarely lupus can be associated with renal arteritis, with ischaemia and renal cortical infarction. This form of lupus is usually associated with circulating 'lupus anticoagulant'.

Lupus interstitial nephritis

Tubulointerstitial damage in lupus nephritis can be out of proportion to the glomerular lesions, and in rare cases immune complexes may be demonstrable along the tubular basement membrane.

Clinical features of SLE

SLE usually occurs in young women, and has a variety of features (Table 17.2), of which skin rashes (Fig. 17.1), Raynaud's syndrome, polyarthralgia, anaemia and renal involvement are the most common.

Table 17.2 Features of systemic lupus erythematosus

Clinical
Skin rashes (malar, discoid, photosensitive)
Raynaud's syndrome
Arthritis
Serositis (pleurisy/pericarditis)
Renal disease
Neurologic disorder (seizure/psychosis)
Haematologic disorder — part or all of a pancytopenia
  Coombs positive haemolytic anaemia
  thrombocytopenia
Oral ulcers
Hair loss

Laboratory
Positive antinuclear factor (homogeneous)
Positive anti-DNA antibodies
LE cells
Positive VDRL (false)
Positive Coombs test
Lupus anticoagulant
Anticardiolipin antibodies

Clinical features of lupus nephritis

Lupus nephritis can cause any of the clinical syndromes of GN (Chapter 9). Acute nephritis, the nephrotic syndrome and rapidly progressive nephritis are all common. Although there is some correlation between proliferative change and haematuria, and membranous change and proteinuria, the parallel between clinical picture and pathological lesion is insufficient to rely upon in the individual case. It is therefore wise to perform a renal biopsy on any patient presenting with active SLE if any suspicion of renal involvement is present.

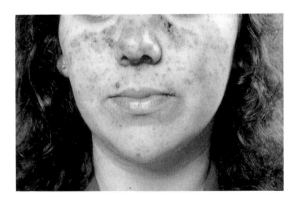

Fig. 17.1 Typical 'butterfly' distribution facial rash in systemic lupus erythematosus

Investigations in lupus nephritis

The diagnosis of SLE is confirmed by positive tests for antinuclear factor (ANF) — a useful screening test, and DNA-binding antibodies — the confirmatory test.

The activity of SLE can be monitored by ESR, ANF titre, DNA binding antibody titre and plasma complement since C_3 and C_4 often fall in severe active lupus. Unfortunately none of these indices are reliable indicators of renal involvement, where the degree of proteinuria and microscopic haematuria better reflect activity.

Renal involvement can only be accurately diagnosed by renal biopsy, however other important findings include:
- The presence of proteinuria.
- Urine microscopy. The so-called 'telescoped' urine sediment where red cell casts, oval fat bodies and broad casts are all seen along with glomerular red cells occurs in active lupus nephritis.
- Renal functional impairment.

Course and management of renal SLE

Untreated lupus nephritis has a very poor prognosis. In older series:
- Diffuse proliferative GN had only a 25% 5-year survival.
- Focal proliferative GN had a 65% 5-year survival.
- Membranous GN had an 85% 5-year survival.

Treatment is based on the renal biopsy appearance. Proliferative glomerulonephritis should be treated with high dose prednisolone (60 mg/day for 3 months) with gradual reduction of steroid dosage and consideration of introduction of azathioprine as a steroid-sparing drug once prednisolone dosage is below about 30 mg/day. In crescentic disease even more aggressive therapy may be used, including intensive plasma exchange, pulse steroid therapy and oral or intravenous cyclophosphamide therapy. In this group of patients there is a difficult balance between immunosuppressive control of lupus activity, and the risk of death due to infection.

There is often no need for specific treatment of membranous GN, since the untreated course is usually good. In patients with nephrotic syndrome a course of steroids will reduce proteinuria.

The tendency of SLE to remit and relapse must not be forgotten. All patients with renal SLE must be watched closely for evidence of exacerbation, particularly if they have ever had severe renal lupus.

Drug-induced SLE

A variety of drugs can cause an SLE-like syndrome (Table 17.1). Commonly the ANF is speckled in appearance and the antibodies are not to DNA, but to other nuclear proteins. Usually arthralgia and rash are present and renal involvement mild, though severe crescentic nephritis can occur.

Subjects likely to develop SLE with hydralazine are:
- Taking high doses (>200 mg/day).
- Female.
- HLA DRw4.
- Slow drug acetylators.

Drug-induced SLE usually reverts on cessation of the drug.

SCLERODERMA

Synonym. Progressive systemic sclerosis.

Causes and pathogenesis

Scleroderma is a generalised immunologically mediated vascular disorder. Most patients have a positive speckled ANF and other autoantibodies. The mechanism for the vascular disease is unknown, however, vasoconstriction (as evidenced by Raynaud's syndrome), collagen proliferation and intravascular thrombosis all occur, resulting in reduced renal perfusion. Renal ischaemia causes renin secretion. A vicious cycle with angiotensin-induced vasoconstriction leading to further ischaemia can then occur.

Pathology

The main lesion is of severe arterial intimal hyperplasia with deposition of mucinous material or collagen occurring in the interlobular and smaller arteries (Fig. 17.2). Similar 'onion-skin' changes can be seen in a variety of other diseases (Table 17.3). Fibrinoid necrosis and intraluminal fibrin thrombi may be found

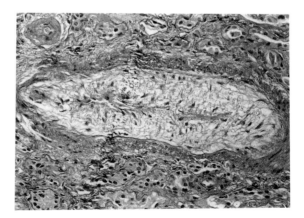

Fig. 17.2 Renal biopsy in scleroderma showing typical 'onion skin' intimal hyperplasia

Table 17.3 Diseases with severe renal arterial intimal hyperplasia ('onion-skinning')

Scleroderma
Malignant hypertension.
Thrombotic microangiopathy (HUS and TTP)
Pre-eclampsia and eclampsia
Renal transplant rejection
Radiation nephritis
Arteritis
Circulating 'lupus anticoagulant'

in afferent arterioles, and this process may extend into the glomerular tuft itself.

General features of scleroderma

Scleroderma occurs three times as commonly in females as in males, usually between 20 and 50 years of age. Common features include:
- *Skin.* Skin thickening and tightness occurs, especially on the fingers and periorally. Raynaud's syndrome can be severe, and digital pulp atrophy can occur. Multiple facial telangiectasia is common. Calcinosis occurs in 10% of cases.
- *Gastrointestinal tract.* Dysphagia due to oesopheal involvement occurs in 50% of cases, symptoms of oesopheal reflux are common, and diffuse gastrointestinal disease can cause malabsorption.
- *Lung.* Pulmonary fibrosis occurs in 30% of cases and can be a major disability.

Renal involvement in scleroderma

Renal involvement in scleroderma occurs usually several years after diagnosis with the abrupt onset of severe hypertension and rising plasma creatinine concentration, sometimes with oliguria, left heart failure and convulsions. This 'scleroderma crisis' is a common cause of death in scleroderma, with an average survival of less than one year once the plasma creatinine is first noted to be elevated (in the untreated case).

Associated proteinuria is rarely severe, and only mild microscopic haematuria is found. The renal biopsy is diagnostic (Fig. 17.2).

Treatment of renal scleroderma

Stabilisation of renal function has been demonstrated with a variety of procedures. The most important is control of blood pressure. The widespread use of ACE-inhibitors has the advantage of specifically interrupting the intrarenal cycle (see above). Steroids and immunosuppressives are not of proven benefit. Scleroderma is a systemic disease, and even if the renal manifestations are controlled the overall prognosis is still dismal.

Table 17.4 Renal disease in rheumatoid arthritis

Drug toxicity
Analgesic nephropathy (Chapter 22)
Other side-effects of non-steroidal anti-inflammatory drugs (Chapter 34)
Gold and penicillamine reactions (e.g. nephrotic syndrome) (Chapter 9)

Secondary amyloidosis (Chapter 27)

Overlap syndromes
SLE
Scleroderma

Specific involvement (rare)
Vasculitis
Glomerular changes
   mesangial proliferation
   membranous glomerulonephritis

MIXED CONNECTIVE TISSUE DISEASE

This disease, which is clinically a mixture of SLE, polymyositis and scleroderma, is associated with circulating antibodies to ribonucleoprotein (RNP), a non-DNA nuclear antigen. The ANF is positive but speckled in appearance. Patients can have renal involvement similar to SLE, though it tends to be less common and usually mild.

RHEUMATOID ARTHRITIS

Renal disease in patients with rheumatoid arthritis is more commonly due to secondary amyloidosis or side effects of drugs than specific renal involvement in the disease (Table 17.4).

18: *Renal Vasculitis (including Henoch–Schönlein Purpura)*

In vasculitis there is inflammation (cellular infiltration and necrosis) of vessel walls.

Systemically there may be:

- *Small vessel vasculitis* with purpuric skin rash, polyarthralgia, peripheral neuropathy or other organ involvement (e.g. lung, brain, gastrointestinal tract).
- *Larger vessel disease* with multiple larger infarcts. Myocardial, cerebral and distal limb infarction are typical.

In the kidney vasculitis can involve:

- *The glomerular tuft*, where it produces a necrotising proliferative glomerulonephritis (GN).
- *The extraglomerular vessels* where it produces renal ischaemia, renal infarcts and hypertension.

Though there are many possible syndromes resulting from mixtures of renal and extrarenal vasculitis, the most important to the kidney are:

1 Polyarteritis: (a) polyarteritis nodosa (classical polyarteritis), and (b) microscopic polyarteritis.
2 Wegener's granulomatosis (granulomatous arteritis).
3 Henoch–Schönlein purpura (anaphylactoid purpura).

POLYARTERITIS

The two major forms of polyarteritis are distinguished by the size of the vessels involved, though there is some overlap.

Though in most cases the cause is unknown, polyarteritis can occur as a complication of a variety of autoimmune diseases, infections and antigens (Table 18.1).

Polyarteritis nodosa

Synonym. Classical polyarteritis. This disease is most common in middle-aged males. It is rare. Features include:

- *Systematic illness* with fever and malaise.
- *Infarction* of non-renal organs, including cerebral, myocardial digital or gastrointestinal infarcts.
- *Renal disease* resulting from ischaemia. Renal infarction, with loin pain and haematuria and severe hypertension are common. Progression to renal failure may occur.

Table 18.1 Secondary forms of vasculitis

Autoimmune disease
Systemic lupus erythematosus (SLE)
Rheumatoid arthritis
Takayasu's disease
Anti-GBM disease

Miscellaneous antigens
Hepatitis B infection*
Drugs — co-trimoxazole, sulphonamides, penicillin
Poststreptococcal nephritis
Carcinoma

* This is often present in patients with polyarteritis in the USA, but rarely so in the UK and Australasia.

The diagnosis can often be made by arteriography demonstrating aneurysms (Fig. 18.1) and obstruction in renal, splenic, hepatic or gastrointestinal vasculature. Nuclear scans of kidneys, liver or spleen may demonstrate infarcted areas.

Pathology of classical polyarteritis

There is a necrotising arteritis involving segments of medium sized arteries (Fig. 18.2). Because only short segments of some vessels are involved, a biopsy may be unhelpful if it misses the diseased segments. Sometimes glomeruli are also involved, as in microscopic polyarteritis (see below).

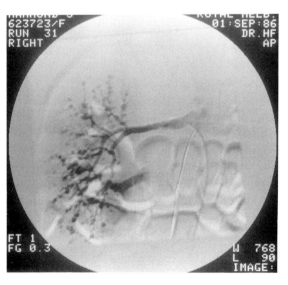

Fig. 18.1 Classical polyarteritis nodosa, showing multiple aneurysms in digital subtraction angiogram

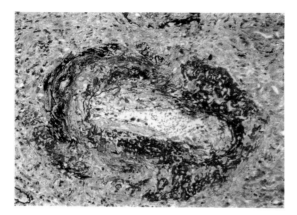

Fig. 18.2   Medium-sized artery affected by vasculitis

Microscopic polyarteritis

This is far more common than classical polyarteritis. Features include:

• *Systemic illness* with fever and weight loss.

• *Generalised small vessel vasculitis* with clinical features including polyarthralgia, skin rash (Fig. 18.3), polyneuritis, or lung involvement with asthma or haemoptysis.

• *Glomerular disease* — haematuria, mild or severe is usual. In the most severe cases rapidly progressive nephritis can occur. Proteinuria is usually mild.

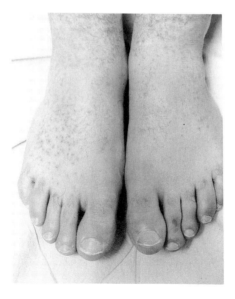

Fig. 18.3   Vasculitic skin rash in microscopic polyarteritis

Pathology of microscopic polyarteritis

Renal biopsy shows a focal and segmental proliferative GN (Fig. 15.6), usually with fibrinoid necrosis of one or more lobules of affected glomeruli, often associated with crescent formation (Fig. 15.9). In cases with a rapidly progressive course, diffuse proliferation and crescent formation is usual. Immunofluorescence studies show little or no evidence of glomerular immunoglobulin deposition, which helps to distinguish this lesion from many other causes of focal and segmental proliferative nephritis (e.g. SLE, IgA disease, Henoch-Schönlein purpura and Goodpasture's syndrome — Table 15.7).

Occasionally there will be a larger vessel showing vasculitis in the renal biopsy, otherwise the diagnosis depends on demonstrating affected vessels elsewhere in the body, e.g. in skin, nerve or muscle.

Laboratory features in polyarteritis

Recently, circulating antibody to polymorph cytoplasm (anti-neutrophil cytoplasm antibody) has been shown to be present in polyarteritis and Wegener's granulomatosis and this may be of diagnostic use. The erythrocyte sedimentation rate (ESR) and C-reactive protein concentration are usually elevated.

Haematuria and impairment of renal function occur with renal involvement. Urine microscopy and renal function tests are those of severe proliferative GN.

Diagnosis is based on the clinical picture, and biopsy of involved tissues. Renal biopsy is not always diagnostic, since an inflamed artery may not be included in the specimen, but it is likely to show the glomerular lesion when there is glomerular haematuria.

Course and treatment of polyarteritis

The prognosis of the untreated disease is very poor, while the response to treatment is good if irreversible tissue damage has not already occurred.

Treatment is based on steroids, immunosuppressive agents (cyclophosphamide or azathioprine) and plasma exchange. The response to high-dose steroids (prednisolone 60 mg/day) is usually rapid and impressive with resolution of systemic and renal manifestation over days or weeks. In patients with severe disease, e.g. severe crescentic nephritis, intravenous pulse doses of prednisolone or plasma exchange may be given.

In some cases the disease proves to have a 'one hit' nature and on slow withdrawal of steroids over 6–12 months the disease remains quiescent. In others, particularly the more severe cases, lifelong therapy is required. A general rule is that steroids should not be completely withdrawn if the initial illness was severe and led to permanent impairment of renal function.

WEGENER'S GRANULOMATOSIS

Synonym. Systemic granulomatous arteritis. This particularly aggressive form of generalised vasculitis affects the nasal passages, lungs, and kidneys.

Clinical features

The disease mainly affects middle-aged or older men.

Nasal involvement

This is prominent in about 60% of cases. Purulent nasal discharge, epistaxis and nasal obstruction are common, due to vasculitic involvement of the mucosa. In time, erosion and collapse of the nasal bridge can occur ('saddle nose' Fig. 18.4). Nasal mucosal biopsy is usually not helpful, showing only necrosis. CT scanning of the nasopharynx is sometimes diagnostic, showing erosion of bone by soft tissue masses.

Pulmonary involvement

Cough, haemoptysis and sometimes chest pain occur. Chest X-ray may show nodular cavitating pulmonary infiltrates, or migratory fluffy patches.

Renal disease

Acute nephritis or rapidly progressive GN are the usual clinical syndromes (Chapter 9).

General symptoms

Fever and weight loss are usually present. Arthralgia is frequent, but arthritis and skin rash are less common than in polyarteritis or Henoch–Schönlein purpura.

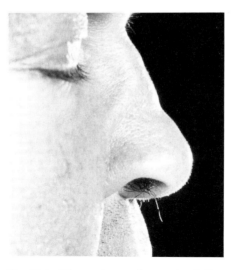

Fig. 18.4 Wegener's granulomatosis. Collapse of the nasal cartilage can lead to a 'saddle nose' deformity

Other organs

There may be evidence of more widespread vasculitis, affecting particularly the liver and the neurological system.

Renal pathology

There is a segmental necrotising proliferative glomerulonephritis with crescent formation. This very quickly develops to a diffuse crescentic necrotising GN. Immunofluorescence is unimpressive, though granular IgG and C_3 may be found. Fibrin is prominent in crescents and necrotic tufts. The diagnostic feature is granulomatous arteritis affecting small and medium sized arteries in the kidney and lungs. This may not be found in biopsy material, since an affected segment of the artery may not be included.

Investigations in Wegener's granulomatosis

The ESR is usually over 100 mm/hour and leucocytosis is common.

Antineutrophil cytoplasmic antibody

An important recent discovery has been that most patients have circulating antibodies to neutrophil cytoplasm. This has become an important diagnostic test.

Tissue biopsy

A biopsy taken from the lung, kidney or uncommonly the nasal passages may show granulomatous vasculitis. Most cases are diagnosed on the basis of a consistent clinical picture, with involvement of the respiratory system and kidney, along with a consistent (but not diagnostic) renal biopsy picture of focal and segmental necrotising GN.

Course and treatment of Wegener's granulomatosis

Without treatment of Wegener's granulomatosis death within 6 months is usual. Nowadays therapy with high-dose steroids and cyclophosphamide, and possibly plasma exchange in the patients with extensive crescents, has produced a remarkable improvement in prognosis.

All patients should be treated with oral cyclophosphamide and steroids. If cyclophosphamide is withdrawn the likelihood of relapse is high.

HENOCH–SCHÖNLEIN PURPURA

Synonym. Anaphylactoid purpura. Features of this disease are:
• *Purpuric skin lesions* particularly involving the buttocks and lower limbs (anaphylactoid purpura).
• *Polyarthritis* usually involving large joints.
• *Abdominal pain* due to gastrointestinal vasculitis.
• *Acute GN.* Clinically significant nephritis occurs in only a minority of children with the disease but is more common and more severe in adults.

Renal pathology in Henoch–Schönlein purpura

There is a focal and segmental proliferative GN. In the worst cases a diffuse crescentic nephritis can occur. A distinguishing feature from other forms of vasculitic nephritis is the presence of granular deposits of IgA in the mesangium (Fig. 15.4). The renal lesion is indistinguishable from focal and segmental nephritis due to IgA disease (Chapter 15).

Aetiology of Henoch–Schönlein purpura

An 'allergic' basis is assumed, particularly since the disease may follow antigenic stimuli with infections, insect bites and various drugs including penicillin.

Clinical features of Henoch–Schönlein purpura

The disease is far more common in children than adults.

Skin lesions

These are the real clue to diagnosis. These commence as urticarial lesions resembling insect bites on the buttocks and exterior surfaces of the legs and arms, progress to pink maculopapules in a few hours, then become red-purple purpuric macules that do not blanche on pressure. Smaller punctate purpuric spots may also be seen, particularly around the ankles. Biopsy reveals a vasculitis with perivascular polymorphs and mononuclear cells ('leucocytoclastic vasculitis'). IgA, C_3 and often other immunoglobulins are found in a granular perivascular distribution in affected and seemingly normal skin.

Joint manifestations

Acute large joint polyarthralgia, often with painful swelling, and commonly affecting the knees and ankles develops over several hours and can persist for weeks. Joint destruction and deformity do not occur.

Gastrointestinal manifestations

Purpuric lesions in the gastrointestinal tract can cause severe abdominal pain, colic and even melaena or bowel bleeding. On occasions the picture is of an acute abdomen. Usually, however, the gastrointestinal symptoms are mild, and they are often absent.

Renal manifestations of Henoch– Schönlein disease

Renal involvement, detectable as haematuria or proteinuria, occurs in almost 50% of cases, although it is likely that renal biopsy would reveal mesangial IgA in virtually all patients. Clinically, haematuria, acute nephritis or occasionally nephrotic syndrome (Chapter 9) are usual.

Laboratory findings in Henoch– Schönlein disease

There are no diagnostic laboratory tests. The renal function and urinary sediment reflect the glomerular disease. In about 50% of cases plasma IgA is elevated.

Course of Henoch–Schönlein nephritis

The patients with mild haematuria or proteinuria do well. In patients with nephritic syndrome or rapidly progressive GN, both of which tend to occur in the more severe cases associated with extensive crescent formation, the outlook is less good.

Particular signs of a poor prognosis include:
- Renal insufficiency at onset.
- Extensive crescents on renal biopsy.
- Persistence of urinary abnormalities.

Occasional patients have a relapsing course over several months or even years, with new episodes of purpura, arthralgia, and renal involvement.

Treatment of Henoch–Schönlein nephritis

As with IgA disease, no treatment of renal involvement has been proven to be effective. Steroids often are helpful for the abdominal pain but have no unproven effect on the renal lesions. Currently severe renal involvement is usually treated with high-dose steroids, often combined with immunosuppression (e.g. cyclophosphamide). Severe crescentic disease is managed as with other forms of diffuse crescentic nephritis (Chapter 15).

SECONDARY FORMS OF VASCULITIS

Polyarteritis-like syndromes can occur after exposure to a wide range of antigens and in a variety of autoimmune diseases (Table 18.1). In the cases in which the antigen can be removed there is usually subsequent remission. In the autoimmune diseases there is commonly a poor prognosis.

19: *Acute Tubular Necrosis*

Acute tubular necrosis (ATN) is the most important cause of acute renal failure (Chapter 10). It can be due to tubular ischaemia or nephrotoxins (Table 19.1). The usual illness is acute oliguric renal failure which recovers spontaneously after 1–3 weeks.

PATHOLOGY AND PATHOGENESIS OF ACUTE TUBULAR NECROSIS

There is renal tubular damage with tubule cell necrosis, loss of brush borders, increased numbers of casts in tubules, and interstitial oedema and cell infiltration (Fig. 19.1). Mitoses may be seen in tubular cells. This relatively minor pathological abnor-

Table 19.1 Common causes of acute tubular necrosis

Ischaemic
Septicaemic shock
Pancreatitis
Drug overdose
Haemorrhage (usually major obstetric, surgical or traumatic)
Renal artery or aortic trauma or surgery
Renal transplantation

Nephrotoxic
Exogenous nephrotoxins
  Drugs:
    antibiotics — aminoglycosides, amphotericin
    cyclosporin
    radiological contrast media
    methoxyfluorane
  Industrial poisons:
    carbon tetrachloride
    polyethylene glycol (radiator antifreeze)
    heavy metal salts — mercury, arsenic
    insecticides — paraquat

Endogenous nephrotoxins
  Myoglobinuria
  Haemoglobinuria
  Acute urate nephropathy
  Acute myeloma kidney

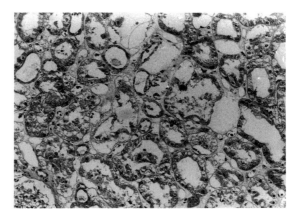

Fig. 19.1 Acute tubular necrosis

mality is, however, accompanied by severe functional abnormality with a grossly decreased GFR, and in 80% of cases reduced urine volume.

Similar necrosis of tubular cells is often also seen in acute interstitial nephritis (Chapter 20), and occasionally in glomerulonephritis (GN) and vasculitis. In such cases the tubular damage probably contributes to associated acute renal failure.

Mechanism of renal failure in ATN

Multiple factors coexist to produce ARF in ATN, and it is likely that these vary in severity and impact with different causes of ATN. They include:

Reduction in renal blood flow

Reduction in renal blood flow to 60% of normal occurs, with concurrent diversion of blood from the cortex to the medulla. This reduction in blood flow would not be sufficient to cause severe renal failure by itself, though it may contribute. Proposed mediators include the renal–angiotensin, prostaglandin and adrenergic systems.

Alterations in glomerular hydrodynamics

The fall in GFR is disproportionately greater than the fall in renal blood flow. This may be due to enhanced activity of the renin–angiotensin system. Roles for other substances such as prostaglandins, adenosine, bradykinins and adenosine have also been suggested.

Tubular back-leak

In severe ATN back-leak of up to 50% of filtered dextran from the tubular lumen to the interstitium has been shown to occur. It is less prominent in mild or non-oliguric ATN, and most prominent in severe toxic or ischaemic ATN.

Tubular obstruction

Obstruction by casts of Tamm–Horsfall protein and tubular cell debris has been suggested in some patients with ATN. In situations where intratubular casts of crystals (e.g. urate, sulphonamides, ethacrynic acid) or other abnormal constituents (e.g. radiocontrast agents, myoglobin, haemoglobin, Bence-Jones proteins) are present this is very likely to be the case, and there is therefore overlap between ATN and ARF due to tubular obstruction. In tubular obstruction oligoanuria is usual, and recovery often poor or delayed.

CAUSES OF ACUTE TUBULAR NECROSIS

There are two main groups of causes, ischaemic and nephrotoxic (Table 19.1), though they often coexist.

Renal ischaemia

The mechanisms for maintaining GFR in the face of renal hypoperfusion have been discussed in Chapter 10. These not only maintain GFR but also provide blood to the renal tubular cells which are consuming large amounts of energy in resorbing sodium and other solutes. Should the hypoperfusion be severe, as in protracted shock, the tubular cells suffer ischaemic damage.

In many cases there is not only hypoperfusion but also a toxic insult and in these cases ATN is more likely to occur than in situations of pure blood loss. Most of these are characterised by tissue injury, e.g. obstetric blood loss, major trauma or surgery, pancreatitis and septicaemia.

The list of common causes of ischaemic ATN (Table 19.1) therefore tends to accentuate causes of prerenal ARF in which major tissue damage or circulating toxins are present.

Nephrotoxins

These cause ATN by direct toxic effects on tubular cells. The list of tubular toxins is long, and only selected common examples are given in Table 19.1.

Predisposing factors

Predisposing factors to direct tubular nephrotoxicity include:
- High plasma levels of the toxin.
- Dehydration or salt depletion.
- Pre-existing renal functional impairment.
- Old age.

Exogenous nephrotoxins

The most common are nephrotoxic drugs, such as aminoglycoside antibiotics, radiocontrast agents, amphotericin and cyclosporin.

Endogenous nephrotoxins

A variety of endogenous substances are nephrotoxic when present in the circulation in abnormal amounts. In many of these cases tubular obstruction and direct tubular cell toxicity may both play an important role.

Myoglobinuria. Myoglobin (MW 14000) can circulate in large amounts after massive rhabdomyolysis (Table 19.2).

Features of myoglobinuric renal failure include:

- Oliguric renal failure with red-brown urine which tests positive for haemoglobin with dipstick tests but is actually coloured by myoglobin.
- Acidosis and hypovolaemia which probably also contribute to the ATN, hence early treatment includes saline repletion and the use of bicarbonate to decrease urinary acidity.
- Hyperkalaemia, hyperphosphataemia and hypocalcaemia are more pronounced than in other forms of ATN because of altered balance across muscle cell membranes.
- Dialysis is often required to be both early and intensive.

Haemoglobinuria. Release of haemoglobin (MW 68000) from haemolysed blood, particularly in the presence of hypotension and saline depletion, can cause ATN by both obstructive and toxic tubular effects. Massive intravascular haemolysis is usually responsible (Table 19.3). Early treatment is with saline and bicarbonate as in myoglobinuria.

Hyperuricaemic acute renal failure. This complication of leukaemia or lymphoma occurs with massive tumor lysis associated with treatment, and is discussed in Chapter 24. Renal failure is probably caused by acute obstruction of tubules by uric acid crystals.

Table 19.2 Causes of myoglobinuric renal failure

Crush injury	Muscle ischaemia
Ethanol intoxication	Epileptic seizures
Sedative overdose	Severe infection
Snake bite	

Table 19.3 Causes of haemoglobinuric renal failure

Incompatible blood transfusion
Intravenous water injection (during transurethral prostatic resection)
Snake bite
Infections — Blackwater fever (malaria), gas gangrene

DIAGNOSIS OF ATN

ATN is often a diagnosis of exclusion. If ARF occurs in a clinical setting compatible with ATN, and prerenal, obstructive and other renal causes of ARF have been excluded (Chapter 10), then it is assumed that the ARF is due to ATN. If there is any doubt, a renal biopsy should be performed.

Distinction of ATN
from prerenal failure

It has been common to use certain diagnostic tests to distinguish established ATN from prerenal renal failure. These are all based on the distinction of the highly concentrated urine in prerenal renal failure from the poorly concentrated urine once tubular necrosis has occurred. Thus in prerenal renal failure the urine should have a high specific gravity, a low (<20 mmol/litre) sodium concentration and there should be a high urine to plasma urea and creatinine concentration ratio, while the opposite occurs in ATN. These tests are not sufficiently reliable to justify management based entirely on their results.

First, the abnormalities can be mimicked by disease processes other than ATN or prerenal renal failure. For instance in early acute GN the urine is concentrated, while in chronic renal failure dilute urine is still found even when prerenal events have lead to sudden deterioration in function.

Second, each can be misleading either in the presence of partial ATN or non-oliguric renal failure, or when diuretic substances are present in the urine. Since diuretics are often given when oliguria is noted, and before urine is collected for laboratory estimates, this particularly reduces the clinical value of these tests.

Accordingly the best test to determine whether prerenal renal failure is present is to correct prerenal factors and then to administer a diuretic as described in Chapter 10.

COURSE OF ACUTE TUBULAR NECROSIS

The course of ATN is divided into three phases: the oliguric, polyuric, and recovery phases (Fig. 19.2).

The oliguric phase
of ATN
Oliguric ATN

About 80% of patients are oliguric, with urine volumes of 50–400 ml/day. Plasma creatinine concentrations rise by about 0.2 mmol/litre each day and the GFR is less than 5 ml/min. The oliguria usually lasts from 10–14 days, with a range of a few days to even months. A prolonged course is more likely in elderly patients and with severe insults. During this phase all of the risks of renal failure are present, particularly those of fluid overload

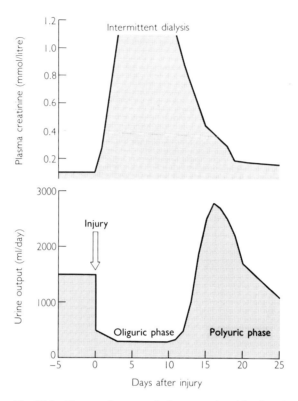

Fig. 19.2 Course of acute tubular necrosis with oliguric renal failure — prerenal, oliguric and polyuric phases. This is followed by a 'recovery' phase with minor tubular dysfunction which can last months

and hyperkalaemia with cardiac arrythmia. The normal accompaniments of renal failure occur, i.e. elevated plasma creatinine, urea, phosphate and uric acid levels, as does a fall in haemoglobin, plasma pH and bicarbonate concentration. Hypocalcaemia is usual and attributable to hyperphosphataemia, inefficient 1-hydroxylation of 25-hydroxycalciferol and in many cases concurrent hypoproteinaemia. Hypertension is usually absent.

Non-oliguric ATN   A urine output of 500–1500 ml/day is maintained in about 20% of patients with ATN. This appears to represent a less severe form of ATN rather than a separate disease. There is a higher GFR, a lower urinary sodium concentration and the maximum plasma creatinine concentration reached is lower. The time to recovery is shorter than in oliguric ATN and the prognosis is much better with about a 20% mortality compared with 50% in oliguric ATN. Non-oliguric ATN appears to occur more commonly in aminoglycoside nephrotoxicity and perhaps when high dose diuretics have been given early in the course.

Polyuric phase of ATN

Recovery from oliguric ATN is heralded by an increase in urine volume which may rise to levels greatly above normal. The reasons for polyuria include:

- Salt and water overload acquired during the oliguric phase.
- Osmotic diuresis from retained osmotic products such as urea.
- Residual tubular defects with decreased concentrating capacity.

Severe polyuria (>10 litre/day) can occur but usually results from either gross fluid overload during the oliguric phase, or overenthusiastic replacement during the diuretic phase. Rarely some patients are polyuric from the commencement of ATN.

Soon after the commencement of diuresis plasma creatinine and urea concentrations stabilise, then fall. The urine in the first few days is poor in urea and creatinine, as tubular function is slowly recovering. Plasma creatinine and urea usually reach normal levels within 2 weeks, although full recovery of GFR and tubular functions may take 3−12 months.

The polyuric phase is very reassuring to both patient and doctor, but is a period where complications are common, due to both the debilitating effects of the previous illness and the abrupt changes in fluid and electrolyte balance that may occur.

Recovery phase of ATN

Most patients recover normal renal function, however GFR may remain 20−40% below normal for periods of a year or more, and recovery of subtle tubular functions, such as acidifying and concentrating ability may be even more delayed.

Irreversible ATN does seem to occur in a small proportion of cases. It is most likely when ATN occurs in the setting of:

- Old age.
- Diabetes.
- Multiple myeloma.
- Pre-existing renal disease.
- Nephrotoxic renal failure.

In some cases partial recovery to a new but lesser renal function occurs, in others, though renal biopsy shows no evidence of cortical necrosis, recovery of useful function never occurs.

MANAGEMENT OF ACUTE TUBULAR NECROSIS

There is nothing which will hasten the recovery of ATN. The management is therefore supportive (see Management of ARF — Chapter 10).

20: *Tubulointerstitial Nephritis: Acute and Chronic*

The term tubulointerstitial nephritis (TIN) covers a group of diseases in which the major histological abnormality is inflammation of the renal interstitium and tubules. There are many causes, most covered elsewhere in this book. TIN can be acute or chronic.

ACUTE TUBULOINTERSTITIAL NEPHRITIS

Synonyms. Acute interstitial nephritis, acute allergic interstitial nephritis. Acute TIN is a common cause of acute renal failure (ARF — Chapter 10). It is most commonly a drug reaction (Table 20.1).

Table 20.1 Causes of acute tubulointerstitial nephritis

Drugs
Antibiotics
    penicillins — amoxicillin, methicillin
    sulphonamides, co-trimoxazole
    cephalosporins
    rifampicin
Non-steroidal anti-inflammatory drugs
Diuretics
    thiazides
    frusemide
Others
    cimetidine
    allopurinol
    diphenylhydantoin
    phenindione
    radiocontrast agents

Systemic diseases
Systemic lupus erythematosus
Sarcoidosis

Postinfectious
Bacterial, viral, protozoal

Idiopathic

Renal transplant rejection

Pathology

The predominant feature is patchy or dense infiltration of the interstitium with leucocytes, mainly lymphocytes, with varying numbers of plasma cells, macrophages and eosinophils (Fig. 20.1). There are usually tubular changes suggestive of tubular necrosis. In some cases, particularly if the cause is not removed, the disease progresses to chronic TIN with collagen infiltration, glomerular sclerosis and sometimes inflammatory granulomas.

Causes of ATN

Though drug reactions are the usual cause, occasionally a systemic disease or a recent infection is responsible. In some cases no cause can be found (Table 20.1).

Drug-induced acute TIN

This is an allergic drug reaction. In some cases there is an associated rash, fever, eosinophilia and eosinophiluria. However, these are commonly absent, hence acute TIN should be suspected in any patient who has an unexplained deterioration in renal function while taking a drug, particularly if that drug is a common cause of acute TIN (e.g. penicillins, sulphonamides, and non-steroidal anti-inflammatory drugs — Table 20.1).

Systemic immune-mediated diseases causing acute TIN

Rarely renal sarcoidosis causes ARF with acute TIN, often with giant cells and granulomata (Chapter 31). Severe hypercalcaemia with dehydration is a more common cause of ARF in sarcoidosis. In SLE there is commonly TIN and in rare cases this can dominate the histological picture.

Infection-induced acute TIN

Acute TIN can be associated with septicaemia (particularly streptococcal) or following a wide variety of infections — bacterial, viral and protozoal. This should be distinguished from acute pyelonephritis in which intense polymorph infiltration may be

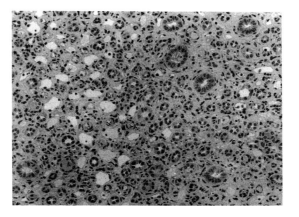

Fig. 20.1 Acute tubulointerstitial nephritis

found secondary to bacterial infection of the kidney, but ARF does not occur unless prerenal factors or urinary obstruction is present (Chapter 13).

Idiopathic acute TIN   Occasionally acute TIN can occur with no apparent cause. In some cases it may have an autoimmune aetiology.

Diagnosis of acute TIN   The diagnosis is based on a high index of clinical suspicion and renal biopsy. Urine microscopy may show large numbers of eosinophils, and usually granular casts, tubular cell debris and fat are present.

Treatment of acute TIN   Treatment involves management of the ARF (Chapter 10) and withdrawal of the causative agent (it is wise to withdraw all the drugs the patient is taking, if possible, since so many drugs can cause this syndrome). The role of a short course of corticosteroid therapy (prednisolone 40–60 mg/day) is controversial. Complete recovery is expected, but it can take many weeks, and incomplete recovery with permanent renal impairment may occur.

CHRONIC TUBULOINTERSTITIAL NEPHRITIS

Chronic TIN is a histological picture found in a wide range of chronic renal diseases (Table 20.2).

Pathology   Chronic TIN is characterised histologically (Fig. 20.2) by:
• Patchy infiltration of the interstitium by mononuclear cells (mainly lymphocytes and macrophages).

Table 20.2 Common causes of chronic tubulointerstitial nephritis

	Chapter
Macroscopically abnormal kidneys	
Renal scarring	
reflux nephropathy	21
analgesic nephropathy	22
obstructive nephropathy	23
Cystic renal diseases	29
Without macroscopic abnormality	
Urate (gouty) nephropathy	24
Myeloma kidney	27
Chronic hypercalcaemia	
Renal sarcoidosis	
Chronic nephrotoxins (e.g. lithium, lead)	
Chronic renal transplant rejection	

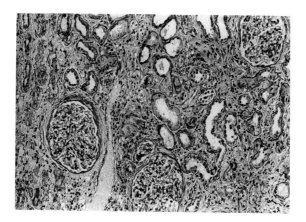

Fig. 20.2 Chronic tubulointerstitial nephritis

• Interstitial fibrosis with collagen infiltration; periglomerular fibrosis may be prominent.
• Tubular atrophy, including in some cases tubular dilatation, with pink casts filling tubules (thyroidaceous change).
There is global sclerosis of the glomeruli attached to atrophic tubules and in some cases secondary focal glomerulosclerosis (FGS) occurs in residual glomeruli, with consequent proteinuria and progressive renal failure as discussed in Chapter 6.

Causes and manifestations

There are a wide variety of causes of chronic TIN (Table 20.2). The most common are reflux nephropathy (Chapter 21), analgesic nephropathy (Chapter 22) and obstructive nephropathy (Chapter 23). In these diseases the diagnosis is usually made on radiological grounds, since macroscopic scarring involving the renal cortex or papilla is usually obvious. Cystic diseases of the kidney can cause similar histological changes. With other causes, such as gouty nephropathy and chronic tubular nephrotoxicity there is no detectable macroscopic anatomical abnormality.

Most patients with chronic TIN have hypertension or impaired renal function. Since there is tubular damage, features such as a concentrating defect and salt loss are common. Sometimes renal tubular acidosis, glycosuria or other signs of severe tubular dysfunction may be present. Unless there is secondary FGS, proteinuria is normally only mild and oedema and haematuria are much less common than in glomerular diseases. Urine microscopy may show granular and broad casts. Pyuria may be seen, particularly if there is an ongoing toxic cause, such as continued analgesic intake in analgesic nephropathy, or there is associated urine infection.

21: *Reflux Nephropathy*

DEFINITION

Reflux nephropathy is characterised by coarse renal cortical scars overlying clubbed calyces (Fig. 21.1), occurring as a result of primary vesicoureteric reflux in infancy. The term chronic atrophic pyelonephritis is equally acceptable. It is preferable not to use the older term 'chronic pyelonephritis' since this term is non-specific, having been also applied to other diseases causing chronic interstitial nephritis (Chapter 20).

INCIDENCE

Reflux nephropathy is one of the commonest renal diseases. It is the cause of 5–10% of end-stage renal failure (ESRF) in patients entering dialysis programmes; and 25% in those under 20 years of age.

Vesicoureteric reflux occurs in about 0.5% of neonates, and reflux nephropathy is present in at least 0.2–0.5% of adult women. In infancy equal numbers of boys and girls have reflux nephropathy, but in older clinical series females outnumber males by about 6:1 probably because of the role of urine infection.

CAUSE AND PATHOGENESIS

Development of renal scars

Three factors contribute to the development of renal scars in infancy:
1 Vesicoureteric reflux (VUR).
2 Intrarenal reflux due to refluxing papillary orifices.
3 Urinary infection.

VUR in infancy

VUR is the result of a developmental abnormality of the ureteric entrance into the bladder, such that the normal one-way valve mechanism is incompetent. The anatomical abnormality is a less oblique and shorter ureteric tunnel through the bladder wall (Fig. 21.2). VUR allows urine to pass up the ureter during voiding, carrying bacteria toward the pelvis if the urine is infected. Primary VUR is often familial, and some evidence suggests an autosomal

274

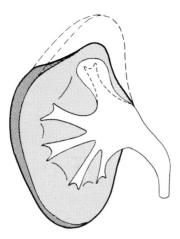

Fig. 21.1 Typical focal reflux scarring. There is a dilated polar calyx and an overlying cortical scar

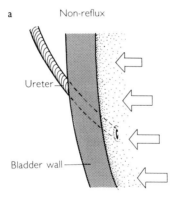

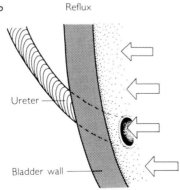

Fig. 21.2 Vesicoureteric reflux occurs due to a congenitally short and less oblique ureteric tunnel in the bladder wall

dominant inheritance. Other congenital malformations, especially duplex ureters, are sometimes present.

In about 90% of cases VUR in infancy spontaneously resolves by adolescence due to further maturation of the vesicoureteric junction. Accordingly over 50% of adults with reflux nephropathy no longer exhibit VUR.

Intrarenal reflux due to refluxing papillary ducts

The openings of papillary ducts are normally slit-like and will not allow reflux of urine from the pelvis into the ducts. Some papillae, particularly those found at the upper and lower poles of the kidney, are compound, draining two or more renal pyramids, and thus having a blunter tip than the more simple papillae. In compound papillae the ducts are more open and may allow reflux of urine into the papilla (Fig. 21.3). It has been shown in infants that intrarenal reflux can occur with severe VUR, and that the areas into which intrarenal reflux occurs are the areas which subsequently scar.

Urine infection

While sterile reflux can cause renal damage there is overwhelming evidence that most scars in children occur as a consequence of UTI. VUR and intrarenal reflux deliver bacteria into the renal substance, leading to acute pyelonephritis in the juvenile kidney.

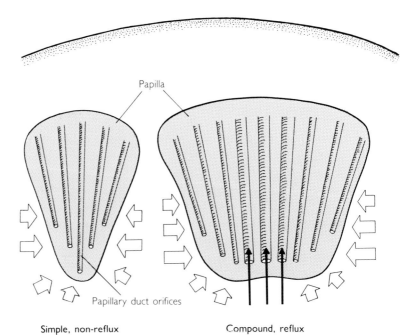

Papilla

Papillary duct orifices

Simple, non-reflux   Compound, reflux

Fig. 21.3 Intrarenal reflux occurs into the open duct orifices of the compound papillae, most commonly found at the poles of the kidney

That portion of the kidney becomes scarred and fails to grow, and the scar is made more evident by the growth and hypertrophy of the surrounding renal tissue.

Progression to end-stage renal failure

In only the minority of cases does the disease progress to end-stage renal failure. This is occasionally because the kidneys are so grossly scarred in infancy that there is little or no functioning residual tissue, and renal failure occurs in early childhood.

More commonly the patient is left with renal scars affecting part or all of one or both kidneys. In some patients slow progression to renal failure occurs over the next 21–50 years, and this can occur despite spontaneous resolution of VUR, absence of UTI, and control of hypertension. The hallmark of deterioration is the appearance of proteinuria. This proteinuria reflects the presence of a glomerular lesion — focal and segmental glomerular sclerosis (FGS) (Fig. 6.1). The pathogenesis of FGS in residual glomeruli of damaged kidneys is discussed in detail in Chapter 6. One hypothesis is that the damage is a consequence of hyper-perfusion, hyperfiltration, and hypertrophy in these 'overworked' glomeruli.

CLINICAL FEATURES

In adults the disease is usually diagnosed in women. The common presenting complaints are urinary tract infection (UTI), hypertension, proteinuria and renal functional impairment.

UTI

In infancy this is commonly manifest as fever and failure to thrive. In older patients the more usual symptoms of UTI (Chapter 13) such as dysuria, frequency, and acute pyelonephritis occur. The first detected UTI commonly occurs in childhood, or in early adulthood with sexual activity or pregnancy. Reflux nephropathy is the commonest renal abnormality found in females with UTI. In adult males UTI is a less common presenting complaint than hypertension or features of impaired function.

Hypertension

About 40% of all patients with reflux nephropathy become hypertensive. It is the commonest cause of severe hypertension in childhood. Accelerated hypertension can occur and lead to rapid deterioration in renal function.

Proteinuria and renal failure

The development of albuminuria in reflux nephropathy is a sign that future deterioration in function is likely. While early in the disease tubular resorption may be a problem, resulting in low molecular weight proteinuria, and sometimes renal glycosuria or other markers of renal tubular damage, in the later stages glomerular albuminuria occurs due to the development of FGS (Chapter 6).

Older patients, particularly males, may thus present with a history of hypertension and proteinuria and impaired function or even ESRF. In others this deterioration is noticed on the more typical background of recurrent UTI.

There are a variety of other clinical features which may suggest a diagnosis of reflux nephropathy. Childhood bed wetting (nocturnal enuresis) is rarely due to an anatomical abnormality, but there is a history of nocturnal enuresis in about 20% of patients with reflux nephropathy. Since the scarring is present from infancy the disease antedates any pregnancy, hence renal complications of pregnancy are common, including acute pyelonephritis, hypertension and pre-eclampsia. About 20% of women with the disease first present because of pregnancy-related symptoms, and about half develop such complications during pregnancy. A much less common complaint is of loin pain on voiding, a symptom attributed to distension of the pelvis by refluxing urine.

DIAGNOSIS

The diagnosis is usually made on the IVP appearance of the kidney, where marked focal scarring overlying clubbed calyces is characteristic (Fig. 21.4). This may affect only one pole, most frequently an upper pole, or the whole of one or both kidneys.

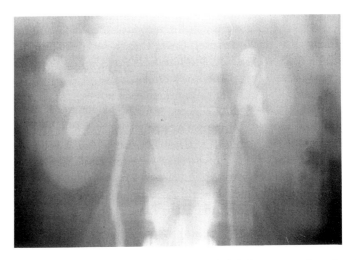

Fig. 21.4 Reflux nephropathy (IVP). The left kidney is grossly reduced in size, with clubbed calyces and overlying scars seen at the upper poles of both kidneys. The right kidney is hypertrophic

Marked disparity of renal size is common when only one kidney is severely affected, since there is compensatory hypertrophy of the other.

In cases where the diagnosis is unclear, a micturating cysto-urethrogram (MCU) may show vesicoureteric reflux (Fig. 21.5). Only about 50% of adults with reflux nephropathy still have VUR.

Cystoscopy can be helpful since the refluxing ureters commonly insert more laterally into the bladder base and may have an open 'golf-hole' appearance.

MANAGEMENT

The major efforts are directed at control of UTI and hypertension.

Urine infection   Control of UTI in infancy and childhood has been shown to reduce renal scarring. In children in whom VUR has been diagnosed it is recommended that prophylactic antibiotics be given, and the urine regularly monitored for UTI until adolescence or until VUR disappears spontaneously as it does in about 80% of cases, particularly those with lower grades of reflux. In adults there is

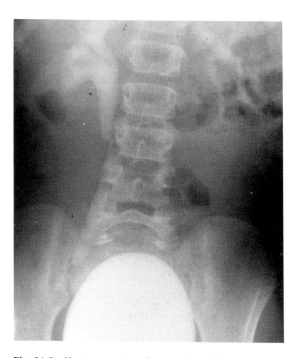

Fig. 21.5 Vesicoureteric reflux on the right in the micturating cystogram of a woman with severe bilateral reflux nephropathy

no evidence that control of UTI alters the rate of progression of the disease but it does reduce the morbidity, hence either early treatment or prophylaxis for UTI is recommended, depending on the frequency of infections. Methods for prevention and treatment of UTI are outlined in Chapter 13.

Hypertension

Poorly controlled hypertension can lead to rapid deterioration in function, as well as increasing the risks of stroke and myocardial infarction. The control of hypertension is discussed in Chapter 12.

Repair of reflux

VUR can be eradicated by operations in which the ureter is led through a new oblique tunnel in the bladder wall. In adults repair of VUR does not affect the course of the disease, although it will occasionally reduce the frequency of attacks of acute pyelonephritis in women in whom the response to prophylactic antibiotics has been poor.

In children there is more controversy. A large controlled trial has shown that surgery does not improve the outcome in children in whom UTI is prevented by antibiotic therapy. Surgery may reduce future scarring in children who receive no special care relating to UTI. There are therefore still some who recommend repair of severe VUR in the very young, on the basis that failure of prophylactic therapy to prevent UTI might be expected. It certainly can be justified in young children in whom poor compliance with medical care can be predicted. Recently repair of reflux using the less traumatic technique of endoscopic injection of synthetic material around the ureteric orifice has been shown to be effective. The role of this less traumatic procedure is being evaluated.

22: *Analgesic Nephropathy*

DEFINITION

Analgesic nephropathy is a chronic renal disease characterised by renal papillary necrosis (RPN) and chronic tubulointerstitial nephritis (Chapter 20) which occurs in patients who have taken large amounts of analgesics, particularly compounds containing aspirin with phenacetin, or paracetamol, but also other non-steroidal anti-inflammatory drugs (NSAIDs).

INCIDENCE

The prevalence of analgesic nephropathy varies widely between countries and regions within countries. In Australia analgesic nephropathy has decreased from being the cause of 20% of new patients entering dialysis programmes in 1982 to 13% in 1987, though Australia has still among the world's highest incidences of analgesic nephropathy. Other countries particularly afflicted by this condition include Switzerland, Belgium and Denmark. In New Zealand and the UK 1–2% of end-stage renal failure (ESRF) patients have analgesic nephropathy.

Factors responsible for this geographic variation include community analgesic intake and climate, where a warmer climate seems to predispose to the disease. There may be also a variation in physician awareness and hence diagnosis of the disease.

CAUSES AND PATHOGENESIS

Most patients have taken large amounts of 'compound APC' analgesic tablets or powders for many years. Aspirin, phenacetin (not in Australia since 1975) or paracetamol, and caffeine or codeine (hence APC tablets or powders) are the usual constituents of these agents.

It is rare for patients who have only taken one NSAID such as aspirin or indomethacin in large amounts, e.g. for chronic arthritis, to present with typical analgesic nephropathy. It seems therefore that APC compounds are more toxic than the analgesics taken alone.

281

PATHOLOGY

The kidneys are small and scarred but not so coarsely scarred as in reflux nephropathy (Chapter 21). When cross-sectioned the kidneys have a characteristic appearance with pigmented necrotic papillae and overlying cortical atrophy alternating with areas of hypertrophy in Bertin's columns (Fig. 22.1). Histologically there is chronic tubulointerstitial nephritis (Chapter 20).

RPN does not only occur in analgesic nephropathy. It can be seen in a variety of other conditions where papillary ischaemia or infection are believed to be responsible (Table 22.1).

CLINICAL FEATURES

The usual patients are middle-aged or older women. The female to male ratio is about 4 : 1.

Analgesic intake

Typically the patient will admit to taking 5–10 tablets or powders per day for 5–20 years, often starting in adolescence or in early adult life with premenstrual headaches. On occasion backache or other chronic pain is responsible, often without a proven organic cause. The patients may say they got a 'lift' out of the analgesics, or a headache if they tried to stop taking them (caffeine withdrawal). There may be a familial tendency to analgesic abuse. A psychopathology similar to other forms of dependence is described and many patients are also dependent on laxatives and/or cigarettes.

Renal manifestations

Renal manifestations include:
- *Renal colic and haematuria* due to passage of sloughed papillae. The patient may recall passing 'a piece of flesh'.
- *Recurrent urinary tract infection*, particularly acute pyelonephritis where there is a risk of septicaemia since there may also be sloughed obstructing papillae.

Table 22.1 Causes of renal papillary necrosis

Analgesic nephropathy

Papillary ischaemia
Diabetes mellitus
Renal transplant rejection
Sickle cell anaemia

Papillary infection
  (usually in combination with diabetes or obstruction)

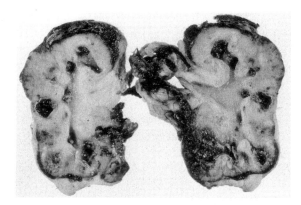

Fig. 22.1 Renal papillary necrosis in analgesic nephropathy. Cut section shows shrunken kidneys with necrotic pigmented papillae

- *Hypertension* which can be severe and sometimes improves with salt repletion. Renal artery stenosis may also occur.
- *Chronic renal failure*, often of the 'salt wasting' type associated with prominent skin pigmentation and tendency to dehydration.
- *Uroepithelial malignancy*. Transitional cell carcinoma of the kidney, ureter or bladder can occur as a late manifestation.

Non-renal manifestations

A wide variety of non-renal manifestations of analgesic abuse are associated, and the term 'analgesic syndrome' has been coined to cover the clinical picture (Table 22.2). Some are explicable as known side-effects of NSAIDs such as gastrointestinal ulceration and bleeding while others may be related to the reason for analgesic intake, such as migraine, dependent personality and cigarette abuse. However, some, such as accelerated atheromatous disease, and premature ageing (Fig. 22.2) are not well explained.

DIAGNOSIS OF ANALGESIC NEPHROPATHY

Investigations include:

Proof of analgesic intake

A careful history, concentrating on the reason (e.g. headache) for taking the analgesics rather than the analgesics themselves will commonly allow the patient to admit to an analgesic intake which they would not reveal if directly asked about analgesic abuse. Urine testing for phenylketone (Phenistix) will be positive if aspirin products are present, as will the plasma salicylate level. Similarly on occasions the family will often give evidence of the intake denied by the patient.

Table 22.2 Analgesic syndrome

Analgesic nephropathy
Renal papillary necrosis (colic, haematuria)
Acute pyelonephritis
Renal failure
Salt-losing nephritis
Hypertension
Papillary adenocarcinoma of pelvis, ureter, or bladder
Renal artery stenosis

Gastrointestinal
Gastric bleeding
Gastric ulcers

Haematological
Iron deficiency anaemia
Met- and sulph-haemoglobinaemia

Cardiovascular
Accelerated atherosclerosis
   cardiac
   renal artery
   peripheral vascular
   cerebral

Neuropsychiatric
Dependency
Cigarette and laxative abuse

Gynaecological
Menorrhagia
Dysmenorrhea
Miscarriage

Premature ageing
Wrinkled skin
Grey hair

Analgesic intake
Headache, migraine
Backache
Psychological 'lift'
Occasionally rheumatoid or other arthritis

Demonstration of RPN

Rarely a papilla is passed and is available for histological identification to prove RPN. More commonly the diagnosis is made radiologically (see below).

Radiological appearance

In the IVP the kidneys are usually diffusely decreased in size, since the technique is not sufficiently sensitive to demonstrate the irregular surface. Occasionally an irregular outline can be

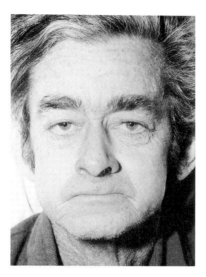

Fig. 22.2 Prematurely aged facial appearance of a 53-year-old man with analgesic nephropathy

seen. The major IVP abnormalities involve the papillae, where a variety of appearances can occur (Fig. 22.3). These include:
• Papillary sloughing, leaving an irregular cavity, or an intrapelvic radiolucent opacity.

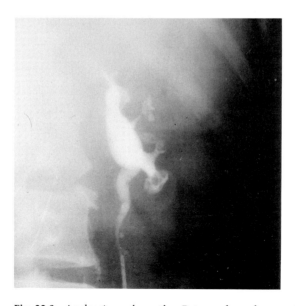

Fig. 22.3 Analgesic nephropathy. Retrograde pyelogram shows shrunken kidney with necrotic papillae lying in calyces

- Papillary calcification which may be seen in plain X-ray films.
- The 'ring-shadow', where the dead papilla is seen in a cavity in the medulla.
- Uroepithelial cancer, usually of the renal pelvis.

The absence of radiological manifestations of papillary necrosis does not exclude this diagnosis because papillae may remain *in situ* for years after necrosis occurs.

MANAGEMENT

The principles of management are:
- Cease analgesic intake.
- Repair salt deficit.
- Control urine infection.
- Control hypertension.
- Relieve obstruction due to sloughed papillae.
- Management of the 'analgesic syndrome'.

The most important step is to ensure that the patient never takes analgesics again. It is more difficult to withdraw NSAIDs in a patient with chronic painful arthritis and such patients commonly have RPN at autopsy. If withdrawal of analgesics can be achieved dramatic and persistent improvement in renal function can occur. Acute deterioration in a patient with analgesic nephropathy may occur with recurrence of analgesic intake, obstruction by sloughed papillae, urine infection, uncontrolled hypertension, renal artery stenosis and development of transitional cell carcinoma. In chronic cases slow deterioration with proteinuria occasionally occurs with the development of glomerulosclerosis (Chapter 6).

In the long term it is often the other manifestations of the syndrome, particularly premature vascular disease, that eventually cause the death of these patients.

23: Obstructive Nephropathy

DEFINITION

Obstructive nephropathy is a renal disease secondary to prolonged partial or complete obstruction to urine flow. The disease can be unilateral or bilateral. There is usually dilatation of the pelvis with blunting of papillae (Fig. 23.1) and histologically there is chronic tubulointerstitial nephritis (Chapter 20). If urine infection is also present the renal damage progresses far more rapidly and the interstitial inflammation is greater.

CAUSES

The common causes are listed in Table 23.1. The details of each are mainly covered in other chapters, or in urological texts. Bladder outlet obstruction leads to bilateral obstructive nephropathy, while renal and ureteral obstruction can cause unilateral or bilateral disease.

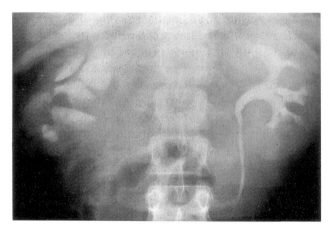

Fig. 23.1 Obstructive nephropathy. IVP showing postobstructive changes in the right kidney. Note the grossly diminished cortical width and dilated calyces

Table 23.1 Causes of obstructive nephropathy

	Chapter
Renal pelvic Obstruction	
Congenital hydronephrosis	31
Renal calculi	25
Renal pelvic carcinoma	30
Ureteral obstruction	
Renal calculi	25
Retroperitoneal neoplasm	
Retroperitoneal fibrosis	
Bladder	
Neurogenic bladder	
Bladder outlet obstruction	
urethral valves	
prostatomegaly	
urethral stricture	

CLINICAL FEATURES

Loin pain, urine infection and haematuria are common, depending on the cause of obstruction. Acute or chronic renal failure can occur. Distal tubular dysfunction can occur with partial obstruction and can also be a problem after relief of obstruction, particularly massive diuresis and hypokalaemia.

DIAGNOSIS

Usually dilatation of the renal pelvis is obvious with renal ultrasound (Fig. 23.2). The IVP shows dilatation of the pelvis and in

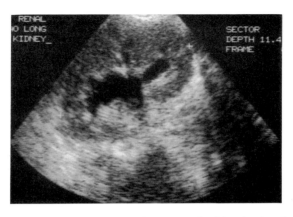

Fig. 23.2 Renal ultrasound showing the dilated pelvicalyceal system (dark area) in an obstructed kidney

more severe obstruction blunting of all papillae (Fig. 23.1). The cause may be apparent on IVP. Other useful investigations include cystoscopy and retrograde ureteric catheter studies, percutaneous antegrade pyelography and pressure studies of the urinary tract. When extrinsic ureteric obstruction (e.g. neoplasm or retroperitoneal fibrosis) is suspected a CT scan of the abdomen should be performed.

TREATMENT

The treatment is relief of the obstruction. During the recovery phase distal tubular function is often impaired, and polyuria is usual. Care must be taken that postobstructive diuresis does not lead to dehydration or hypokalemia. Permanent renal damage occurs after six or more weeks of obstruction and far more rapidly if infection accompanies obstruction.

24: *Gout, Uric Acid and the Kidney*

Uric acid is the end product of breakdown of endogenous and exogenous purines found in nucleic acids — RNA and DNA. Filtered urate is virtually completely resorbed in the proximal tubule, consequently almost all uric acid in the urine is the result of active distal tubular secretion.

The normal plasma urate concentration is less than 0.47 mmol/litre and the 24-hour urine excretion less than 3.6 mmol/day. Both are higher in males than females. The excretion increases with a high purine intake — generally foods with a high proportion of nucleoproteins such as organ meats (liver, kidney) and yeast (as in some beers). Allopurinol (a xanthine oxidase inhibitor) interferes with the production of urate from xanthine, while sulphinpyrazone and probenecid increase the urinary excretion of urate.

EFFECTS OF HYPERURICAEMIA ON THE KIDNEY

Uric acid deposits can occur in the pelvis and ureters as calculi, in the interstitium where they are accompanied by chronic tubulointerstitial nephritis and chronic renal failure. Deposits can also occur acutely in tubules where crystals can cause obstruction and renal failure.

Uric acid stones

About 20% of patients with primary gout develop radiolucent urate stones (Chapter 25).

Chronic urate (gouty) nephropathy

Chronic tubulointerstitial nephritis (Chapter 20) may complicate chronic hyperuricaemia and lead to hypertension and renal failure. There are many other reasons why hyperuricaemia and renal failure may coexist (Table 24.1), and these should be considered in the differential diagnosis.

Clinical features

The features are of chronic progressive renal failure with hypertension and mild proteinuria. The kidneys are smooth and decrease in size as the disease progresses. Usually the patient has a long history of tophaceous gout (Fig. 24.1), and in some cases the disorder is familial.

290

Table 24.1 Causes of chronic renal failure with hyperuricaemia

Gouty nephropathy
Obstructive nephropathy secondary to urate calculi
Renal failure with secondary hyperuricaemia

Non-steroidal anti-inflammatory drug treatment of gout
  analgesic nephropathy
  chronic allergic reaction

Lead nephropathy

Diagnosis

Although a history of familial or tophaceous gout and con-firmation of hyperuricaemia and hyperuricosuria are helpful, the diagnosis depends on the renal biopsy showing chronic tubulo-interstitial nephritis (Chapter 20). Uric acid crystals may be found in the interstitium surrounded by a chronic inflammatory infilt-rate, in which case the biopsy is diagnostic (Fig. 24.2).

Treatment

In familial gout early treatment with allopurinol seems to prevent the disorder. Treatment of advanced cases (i.e. those with estab-lished renal functional impairment) is disappointing though renal function may remain stable for years.

Acute urate nephropathy

In a variety of conditions causing massive breakdown of cell nuclei, acute severe hyperuricaemia can result and lead to acute renal failure, particularly if the patient is also dehydrated. The commonest situation is in the chemotherapy of myeloproliferative disorders (lymphoma, leukaemia, polycythaemia), though it can occur with spontaneous or radiation-induced tumour necrosis.

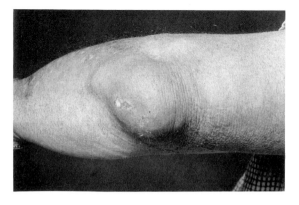

Fig. 24.1 Gouty tophus on the elbow of a patient with recurrent uric acid calculi

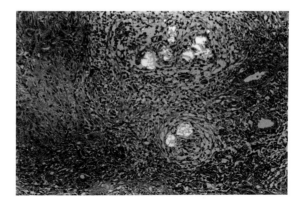

Fig. 24.2 Chronic urate nephropathy showing chronic tubulointerstitial nephritis. Urate crystals are seen in the interstitium with polarised light

The condition is due to tubular obstruction by uric acid crystals, and is characterised by the abrupt onset of oliguric renal failure.

Prevention is most important, and a high fluid intake, urinary alkalinization and administration of allopurinol is now routine in patients receiving chemotherapy. Similar treatment may avert the condition if administered early in the course.

EFFECT OF RENAL DISEASE ON PLASMA URIC ACID

Uric acid in chronic renal failure

Hyperuricaemia is a late manifestation of CRF, occurring only with GFR below about 20 ml/min. Secondary gout can occur but is commonly confused with pseudogout due to calcium pyrophosphate deposition which also commonly complicates chronic renal failure. They can be distinguished by examination of joint fluid under polarised light — urate crystals are strongly negatively birefringent while pyrophosphate is weakly negatively birefringent.

Allopurinol must be given with great care in renal failure since it has renally excreted nephrotoxic metabolites. Rarely, a generalised potentially fatal vasculitic disease, with rash, hepatitis and renal failure can occur. In severe renal failure 100 mg on alternate days is the maximum dose allowable.

Uric acid in hypertension

The coincidence of essential hypertension and hyperuricaemia is greater than would be expected by chance, and the combination appears to be associated with increased risks of cerebrovascular and cardiovascular disease. In some cases there is an elevated haematocrit. The mechanism is poorly understood.

Uric acid in pregnancy

In pre-eclampsia (Chapter 33) an early abnormality is a decrease in the clearance of uric acid, which may occur weeks before the clinical syndrome appears. Accordingly the monitoring of plasma urate levels is particularly important in the management of pregnancy in women with renal disease.

25: *Urinary Calculi*

Urinary tract calculi occur in over 0.5% of the population, most commonly in men.

CAUSES AND PATHOGENESIS

Urinary stones are formed by precipitation of urinary solutes. In most cases an increase in the urinary excretion of precipitable chemicals, such as calcium salts, uric acid or cystine, can be demonstrated.

Other factors contributing to stone formation include:
- Urinary stasis due to local obstruction.
- A 'nidus' or focus for crystal formation.
- Dehydration, as in hot climates, with consequent concentration and decreased flow rates of urine.
- Urine infection.
- Effects of urinary pH on solubility of urinary constituents.
- Variations in the presence of poorly understood inhibitors of stone formation such as citrate.

TYPES OF STONES

There are four main types of stones (Fig. 25.1).

Calcium oxalate and phosphate stones

Sixty to 80% of stones are formed of calcium oxalate or a mixture of oxalate and phosphate (hydroxyapatite). They are hard, and densely radiopaque due to their calcium content (Fig. 25.2). Stone recurrence is usual — at least 50% of patients experience recurrence within 5 years.

Pathogenesis

A cause for urinary tract calculi can be found in at least 80% of patients (Table 25.1).

Hypercalciuria is present if urinary calcium excretion exceeds 6.3 mmol/day. Hypercalciuria is usually idiopathic but may be secondary to other diseases, particularly primary hyperparathyroidism (Table 25.2).

294

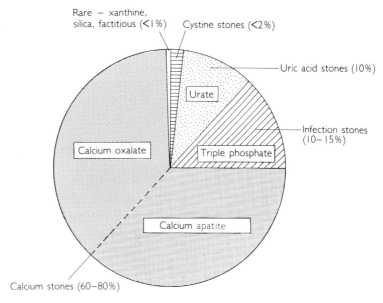

Fig. 25.1 Types of renal stones and their frequency

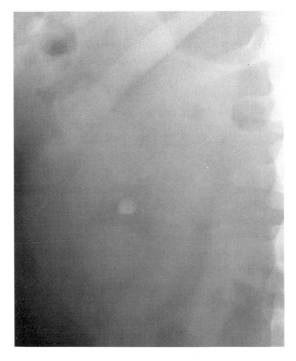

Fig. 25.2 Calcium oxalate renal stone. Typically densely radiopaque with an irregular surface (plain radiograph)

Table 25.1 Causes of calcium stone formation

	Percentage of cases
Hypercalciuria	50
Idiopathic	>40
Primary hyperparathyroidism	5
Renal tubular acidosis	3
Hyperuricosuria	25
Hyperoxaluria	<1
Primary	
Secondary (steatorrhea, diet)	
Stasis due to anatomical abnormality	<5
Unknown	10–20

Table 25.2 Common causes of hypercalciuria

Normocalcaemic
Idiopathic hypercalciuria
Renal tubular acidosis
Medullary sponge kidney
Immobilisation (paraplegia, quadriplegia)

Hypercalcaemic
Primary hyperparathyroidism
Neoplasms
  Bone
    multiple myeloma
    metastases: breast, bronchus, prostate
  Non-metastatic hypercalcaemia
Sarcoidosis
Excessive vitamin D ingestion

Idiopathic hypercalciuria. This is by far the commonest cause of urinary stones, being found in 40% of calcium stone formers and about 25% of all patients with stones. Patients have hypercalciuria but are normocalcaemic and have no other biochemical abnormalities. 2–4% of the population have idiopathic hypercalciuria, but only about 10% of these develop stones.

Both increased gastrointestinal absorption and decreased renal tubular resorption (i.e. hyperexcretion) of calcium have been demonstrated. There are probably several genetic influences involved, and familial stone disease is common.

Stone formers are mainly males who present in the third or fourth decade. Other causes of hypercalciuria (Table 25.2) and anatomical abnormalities causing stasis should be excluded.

Other causes of normocalcaemic hypercalciuria. Chronic calcium loss into the urine can occur in immobilisation such as is common with paraplegia, quadriplegia and other conditions where prolonged bed rest occurs. Renal stones commonly complicate these conditions.

Classical, distal Type 2 renal tubular acidosis is characterised by mild chronic acidosis, osteomalacia, and the presence of nephrocalcinosis or multiple renal stones (Chapter 28).

Hypercalcaemia with hypercalciuria. Primary hyperparathyroidism and sarcoidosis are two causes of chronic hypercalcaemia often associated with calcium stones.

Hyperuricosuria. About 25% of calcium stone formers have hyperuricosuria. It is possible that the uric acid crystals form a nidus for calcium phosphate deposition, and remarkable reductions in stone recurrence can be achieved with allopurinol treatment (see below).

Urinary stasis. Any condition predisposing to chronic urinary stasis can be complicated by urinary calculi. Examples include medullary sponge kidney (Chapter 29) and congenital hydronephrosis (Chapter 31). In medullary sponge kidney disease the common concurrent presence of renal tubular acidosis accentuates this predisposition (see above).

Hyperoxaluria. Though oxalate is a common component of calcium stones, excessive urinary oxalate excretion is rarely a cause of stone formation. Normal excretion is <0.6 mmol/24 hours. Dietary oxalate is derived from such foods as rhubarb and green leafy vegetables but is rarely more than a contributory factor to stone formation, though excessive ingestion should be avoided in calcium oxalate stone formers.

There are very rare genetic causes of hyperoxaluria (primary oxalosis) which are associated with renal stones, nephrocalcinosis and even renal failure.

Hyperexcretion of oxalate can also occur with ileal disease and gastrointestinal blind loops due to increased oxalate absorption from the gut. Oxalate stones can complicate these conditions.

Rarely, poisons such as radiator antifreeze (polyethyleneglycol) and methoxyfluorane anaesthesia can cause massive hyperoxaluria and renal failure due to interstitial oxalate deposition. Stones do not occur since these are acute conditions.

**Triple phosphate
(infection) stones**

Ten to 15% of stones are composed of calcium-magnesium-ammonium phosphate (Ca, Mg, NH_4^+, PO_4^{2-}) — struvite. Since urinary infection with an ammonium-splitting organism, usually *Proteus*, is invariably present, these are often called renal infection stones.

These stones are relatively soft, and grow to fill the renal pelvis, forming a radiopaque 'staghorn' calculus (Fig. 25.3). Because infection persists in any retained fragments rapid recurrence is the rule, unless special precautions are taken (see below). Bilateral staghorn calculi can cause chronic renal failure.

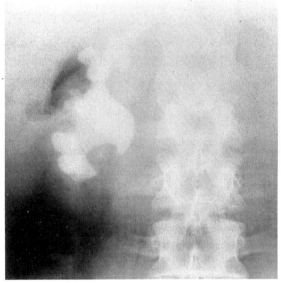

a

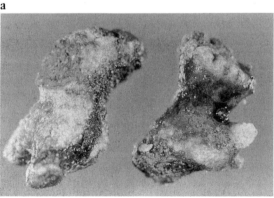

b

Fig. 25.3 Renal infection (triple phosphate) stones form a 'staghorn' shape in the renal pelvis. (a) Plain radiograph showing a fully developed staghorn calculus in the right kidney, and a smaller stone in the lower pole of left kidney. (b) Renal infection stone specimens

Pathogenesis

Urine infection with ammonium-splitting organisms, usually *Proteus mirabilis* (but occasionally *Klebsiella*, *Pseudomonas*, or *Staphylococcus* spp), is responsible for stone formation. *Escherichia coli* never splits urea, and if found is coincidental.

The reactions:

$$Urea \rightarrow NH_3 + H_2O + CO_2$$
$$\rightarrow NH_4^+ \text{ and } HCO_3^-$$

result in alkalinization of the urine and a high NH_4^+ concentration, with subsequent crystallisation of NH_4^+ with Ca, Mg, and phosphate.

An anatomical abnormality predisposing to chronic urine infection, such as ileal conduit, indwelling catheter or neurogenic bladder, is often present.

Uric acid stones

Five to 15% of stones are comprised of uric acid. They occur in patients with acid urine and usually excessive uric acid excretion. The stones are radiolucent, since they contain no dense atoms like calcium or sulphur (Fig. 25.4). Since they cannot be seen on plain X-ray unless there is some calcium content they are easily missed. They are, however, easily seen in a CT scan.

Pathogenesis

The cause is high excretion and concentration of urate in acid urine. Overexcretion of urate (greater then 3.6 mmol/24 hours) is usually genetically determined but can be worsened by over ingestion of high purine foods (organ meats), or chronic overproduction when there is high cell turnover (Chapter 24).

Most patients with uric acid stores constantly excrete urine of pH less than 5.5, for reasons which are poorly understood. The solubility of uric acid increases six-fold between pH 5 and 6, hence this is regarded as a major contributing factor to stone formation.

Cystine stones

Though cystinuria causes only 1–3% of stones, the propensity of this disease to cause recurrent stones commencing in childhood or adolescence, and to result in calculi filling the renal pelvis makes it a particularly important cause of stone-induced chronic renal failure.

The stones are usually multiple, and faintly radiopaque ('ground-glass' appearance) because of the sulphur content. They are usually smooth and fill the contours of the renal pelvis (Fig. 25.5).

Pathogenesis

Cystinuria is a genetically determined biochemical abnormality not to be confused with the completely different disease 'cystinosis' where cystine is deposited throughout the body.

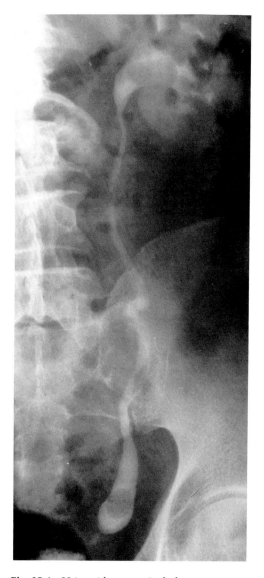

Fig. 25.4 Uric acid stones. Radiolucent stones are seen in the pelvis and lower ureter causing mild obstruction (IVP)

Cystinurics excrete large amounts of cystine in the urine. The normal upper limit of urinary cystine excretion is 0.63 mmol/24 hours. Cystine is a very insoluble amino acid, forming hexagonal ('benzene ring') crystals in neutral or acid urine (Fig. 8.8).

Gastrointestinal and renal tubular absorption of all dibasic amino acids (cystine, ornithine, arginine and lysine) is usually

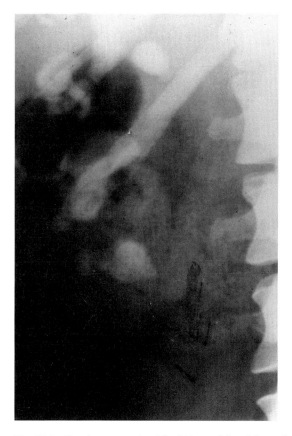

Fig. 25.5 Cystine stones in right kidney. Often bilateral, the stones are only moderately radiopaque (ground glass). They are multiple or conform to the shape of the renal pelvis (plain radiograph)

reduced. Patients with cystine stones are homozygous and usually excrete over 2 mmol/24 hours of cystine; heterozygotes excrete lower but still abnormal amounts but do not form cystine stones. Cystine stone formation therefore usually follows an autosomal recessive inheritance pattern.

CLINICAL FEATURES OF RENAL CALCULI

The common presenting complaints are:
- Renal or ureteric colic.
- Haematuria.
- Renal failure.
- Urine infection.
- Incidental radiological finding.

Renal or ureteric colic

Pain is the presenting complaint in over 75% of patients. Stones can produce pain from acute obstruction anywhere from the pelvi-ureteric junction to the distal urethra. Renal or ureteric colic is characterised by the abrupt onset of constant almost unbearable pain in the loin or flank, radiating to the groin, testicle or vulva. Patients are often pale, nauseated and perspire freely. They are usually unable to lie still, but instead roll about with the legs drawn up. Macroscopic haematuria occurs in about 10% of cases.

Haematuria

Macroscopic or microscopic haematuria can occur with colic, or as an isolated finding especially with calyceal stones.

Urine infection

Recurrent infection with the same organism is an occasional presentation, due to infection of the stone.

Renal failure

Renal infection stones and cystinuric stones are particularly liable to cause obstructive renal failure if both kidneys are involved or the obstruction affects a single functioning kidney. About 1% of end-stage renal failure is attributed to renal calculi.

MANAGEMENT OF RENAL CALCULI

The steps in the management of a patient presenting with renal colic are:
1 Management of the attack of renal colic.
2 Relief of obstruction.
3 Removal of the stone.
4 Determination of the cause.
5 Prevention of recurrence.

Management of the attack of renal colic

The diagnosis is usually obvious — few diseases cause such severe loin or abdominal pain without abdominal rigidity or rebound tenderness. The presence of haematuria on dipstick testing, and lower tract red cells (Chapter 8) with urine microscopy is supportive. Pyuria and infection must be excluded since pyelonephritis can cause similar symptoms, and also because the presence of an infected obstructed kidney constitutes an emergency as pyonephrosis and septicaemia can occur.

Pain relief with pethidine or morphine is required. Should this need to be repeated consideration should be given to admitting the patient to hospital.

Immediate investigation includes renal function testing, urinary microscopy and culture, and renal imaging to confirm the diagnosis and determine the site of the stone and degree of renal obstruction.

A plain X-ray of the abdomen, followed by injection of radio-contrast and sufficient films to determine the degree and site of obstruction (a 'limited IVP') should be performed as soon as practicable. If performed during colic this will usually be abnormal. Most stones are radiopaque, and unless very small will be seen in the pelvis or the line of the ureter. Obstruction will result in dilatation of the renal pelvis and ureter down to the site of the stone (Fig. 25.6). In early obstruction there may be a dense nephrogram, due to hold up of contrast in the tubules, but if there is persistent complete obstruction, or an already damaged kidney on that side, there may be no nephrogram or contrast excretion. In these cases renal ultrasound is invaluable, firstly to demonstrate the dilatation of the renal pelvis (Fig. 23.2) and secondly, to guide percutaneous antegrade pyelography (see below).

If it is suspected that there is a radiolucent uric acid stone in the renal pelvis, a CT scan of the kidney can be very helpful, as these stones are clearly seen with this technique.

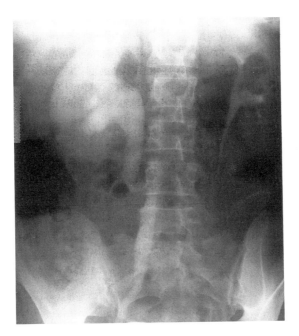

Fig. 25.6 Acute severe right ureteric obstruction by a radiolucent urate stone at the vesicoureteric junction. The nephrogram is denser and persistent when compared with the left kidney, and the renal pelvis and ureter are dilated down to the site of obstruction

Other causes of renal colic and obstruction include renal papillary necrosis with detachment of papillae (Chapter 22), intraluminal neoplasm such as transitional cell carcinoma (Chapter 30), and obstruction by blood clot from bleeding cysts, trauma or neoplasms. Occasionally acute pyelonephritis will cause severe loin pain (Chapter 13). Renal colic is also one of the commonest diseases simulated by addicts seeking injections of narcotics.

Relief of obstruction

If there is complete obstruction or urine infection (fever, pyuria or bacteriuria), free urinary drainage must be obtained as soon as possible, and with suspected urine infection the patient should also be given an appropriate parenteral antibiotic (Chapter 13). The simplest method to relieve obstruction is by percutaneous nephrostomy. In this procedure, under ultrasound or radiological control, a thin needle, guidewire and then catheter are introduced percutaneously into the renal pelvis, leaving the nephrostomy catheter to drain the obstructed organ until stone removal can be achieved.

Removal of the stone

Over 60% of ureteric stones will pass spontaneously, particularly those whose diameter is less than 0.5 cm. These are managed by encouraging a high urine output, analgesia and observation with repeated X-rays.

90% of renal stones and over 50% of ureteric stones whose diameter is greater than 10 mm will not be passed spontaneously. Nearly all such stones can now be removed by a wide range of minimally invasive techniques which require only a few days in hospital.

The procedures available include:
• Extracorporeal shock wave lithotripsy (ESWL) in which the stone is fragmented by shock waves.
• Percutaneous techniques, where percutaneous nephrostomy is used as access for disintegrating the stone or pulling it up to and out of the kidney.
• Cystoscopic techniques, with disintegration or removal of the stone via the bladder.
• Open surgical lithotomy, now required in only about 2% of cases of renal or ureteric stone.

Complete stone removal should be the aim, since any retained fragments can provide a nidus for infection and future stone formation and growth.

In all cases an important step is to retrieve any stone fragments passed or removed for chemical analysis as this is the most important step in determining the cause and hence the steps to be taken to prevent recurrence.

Determination of the cause

The single most important step is chemical analysis of any stone passed or removed. Accordingly all patients with renal colic should pass all urine into a container and examine or strain it for calculi until the stone is passed.

Important clues can be obtained from the history:
- Onset in childhood suggests cystinuria, or another major metabolic or anatomical abnormality.
- A strong family history is common with idiopathic hypercalciuria, cystinuria and urate stones.
- A history of recurrent urine infection occurs with infection stones and anatomical abnormalities.
- Family or past history of gout is common with uric acid stones.
- Analgesic abuse and diabetes can cause renal papillary necrosis.

Basic investigations to determine the cause are listed in Table 25.3. These include measurement of plasma and urinary crystalloids, determination of renal anatomy and function, and exclusion of urinary infection.

Table 25.3 Investigations for the cause of renal stones

The stone
Biochemical stone analysis
X-ray appearance

The patient
Urinalysis
  blood
  glucose
  pH
Urine microscopy and culture
  pyuria
  crystals
  bacteria
IVP
  stone(s)
  urinary tract abnormalities
Blood
  calcium
  uric acid
  electrolytes
  creatinine
24-hour urine collections
  calcium
  uric acid
  creatinine
  volume
In recurrent or young stone formers
  24-hour cystine, oxalate
  urinary acidification test

Dipstick testing of urine for blood, protein, glucose and pH should be performed. Persistently acidic urine suggests urate stones.

Urine microscopy and culture is important. Crystals may be seen in a concentrated first morning specimen of urine. The hexagonal plates of cystinuria (Fig. 8.5) and coffin-lids of triple phosphate stones (Fig. 8.8) are the most useful, since others are often seen in normal urine. Pyuria is commonly present with infection stones, and non-glomerular haematuria in all calculous disease. Plasma creatinine, electrolytes, calcium and uric acid are measured.

With the patient on a normal diet three 24–hour urine specimens are collected for:
- Assessment of urine volume.
- Creatinine excretion (to assess completeness of the collection).
- Calcium excretion — normal less than 6.3 mmol/24 hours.
- Urate excretion — normal less than 3.6 mmol/24 hours.

In young patients, or those with recurrent stone disease assessment of the following is performed:
- Cystine excretion — normal less than 0.63 mmol/24 hours.
- Oxalate excretion — normal less than 0.6 mmol/24 hours.
- Urinary acidification (Chapter 4).

An IVP is done in all patients, to give a clear picture of the stones as well as to show relevant renal abnormalities (such as papillary necrosis or medullary sponge kidney).

In most patients the cause will be apparent, though in a small number, perhaps 10–20%, no biochemical or anatomical abnormality can be found.

Non-specific treatment to prevent stone recurrence

Patients should be advised to increase their fluid intake, aiming for a urine output of 2–3 litre/day. This can be checked by noting the volume of 24-hour urine collections sent for review biochemistry. In particular nocturnal diuresis should be encouraged by a drink before going to bed.

Specific therapy to prevent stone recurrence

Calcium stones

The choice of therapy to prevent stone recurrence depends on the type and cause of stone formation.

Specific causes of hypercalciuria (Table 25.2) are treated appropriately.

Idiopathic hypercalciuria. Calcium excretion can be reduced by:
- Reduction of excessive calcium intake. Very low calcium diets

are not realistic, however, if the patient has a very high dairy product intake it should be reduced.

- Thiazide diuretics. These cause a reduction in urinary calcium excretion. This is less effective if the sodium intake is high, since it depends on low sodium delivery to the tubules. Chlorothiazide 500 mg twice daily or hydrochlorothiazide 25–50 mg twice daily will reduce urinary calcium excretion, often by as much as 50%, and reduce stone recurrence.

- A variety of agents, including cellulose phosphate and oral potassium citrate are being assessed but are not in widespread use.

Calcium stone formers with hyperuricosuria. Calcium stone formers with elevated uric acid excretion will benefit from allopurinol therapy (see below) which has been shown to reduce recurrence.

Calcium stone formers with normal calcium and urate excretion. Up to 20% of calcium stone formers have neither hypercalciuria nor hyperuricosuria. Other than adequate hydration no therapy is of proven benefit.

Renal infection stones	These are treated by stone removal and specific antibiotic therapy to eradicate or control infection. Because complete surgical removal is difficult, irrigation of the renal pelvis with a stone dissolving agent (Renacidin) may be used to eradicate retained fragments. Many patients will need lifetime treatment with antibiotics to suppress the infection associated with their stone.
Uric acid stones	The main aims of treatment are to increase urine pH and to reduce urine uric acid excretion.

Allopurinol. 100–300 mg orally daily will reduce urinary urate excretion (Chapter 24).

Urinary alkalinisation. Urine pH should be increased to 6.0–6.5 by oral alkali ingestion, as sodium bicarbonate or one of the potassium citrate mixtures. Usually 0.5–1.5 mmol/kg/day of alkali is required. This is difficult to achieve on a long term basis and can be monitored by dipstick. |
| *Cystine stones* | There are three steps in the treatment of cystinuria:
- *Hydration.* Adequate urine volumes are particularly important, and volumes of urine as large as 4 litre/24 hours should be encouraged. |

- *Urinary alkalinization* sufficient to prevent stone formation is difficult to achieve, since the pH needs to be raised to above 7.5, requiring 2−4 mmol/kg/day of alkali.
- *Oral penicillamine.* Penicillamine forms soluble complexes with cystine and accordingly increases urinary solubility. Commencing with 250 mg daily the dose is very gradually increased to as much as 2 g daily in divided doses. Nausea is frequent, and a variety of allergic side effects including skin rashes, loss of taste and membranous glomerulonephritis may limit the treatment.

26: *Diabetes and the Kidney*

Renal disease is one of the important causes of death in long-standing diabetes. It has been estimated that about 50% of Type I (insulin-dependent) diabetics develop chronic renal failure, usually between 10 and 30 years after the onset of diabetes. In Australia and the UK diabetic renal disease accounts for approximately 10% of patients on end-stage renal failure programmes, while in the USA the figure is closer to 25%.

RENAL COMPLICATIONS OF DIABETES

There are several processes which can cause renal damage or symptoms in diabetes (Table 26.1). The most prominent of these is diabetic glomerulosclerosis.

Diabetic glomerulosclerosis

Diabetic glomerulosclerosis is characterised by diffuse increase in mesangial matrix and focal glomerular sclerosis and is thought to be a result of prolonged hyperglycaemia.

Pathogenesis of diabetic glomerulosclerosis

The pathogenesis of this glomerular lesion seems to involve:
• Glycosylation of glomerular structural proteins.
• Hyperfiltration and hypertrophy of glomeruli.

Glycosylation of glomerular structural proteins. Non-enzymatic reactions of glucose with circulating and structural proteins occurs in hyperglycaemia (e.g. the glycosylation of haemoglobin produces haemoglobin A_1c). Glycosylation of basement membrane and

Table 26.1 Renal tract abnormalities in diabetes

Diabetic glomerulosclerosis
Vascular disease
Renal papillary necrosis
Urine infection
Radiocontrast nephrotoxicity
Hyporeninaemic hypoaldosteronism
Glycosuric polyuria
Autonomic neuropathy

mesangial proteins may be responsible for alterations in membrane permeability and increase in mesangial matrix.

Hyperfiltration and hypertrophy. In early uncontrolled diabetes an elevation of GFR commonly occurs, up to 40% above normal. This elevation is multifactorial in origin, with contributing factors including high blood glucose levels and abnormalities of glucagon, growth hormone, renin, angiotensin II and prostaglandin concentration or effect. The kidneys exhibiting increased GFR are larger than normal, and individual glomeruli are larger with increased area of GBM. As discussed in Chapter 6 it is believed that this may lead, by as yet undetermined pathways, to focal glomerulosclerosis (FGS).

Pathology of diabetic glomerulosclerosis

The glomerular lesions seen are:

Diffuse diabetic glomerulosclerosis. Diffuse thickening of mesangial matrix with eosinophilic material occurs in all glomeruli and is the basic lesion (Fig. 26.1).

Segmental (nodular) glomerular sclerosis. This less common lesion (the Kimmelstiel–Wilson lesion), is superimposed and consists of segmental nodular accretions of similar material (Fig. 26.2).

Capillary drops and fibrin caps. These two eosinophilic glassy lesions occur either just inside the Bowman's capsule or in the peripheral capillaries. Fibrin cap lesions are the same as the hyalinosis seen in focal glomerulosclerosis (Chapter 6).

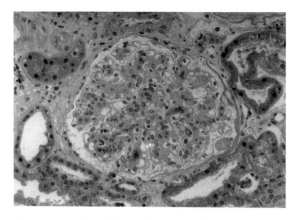

Fig. 26.1 Diffuse diabetic glomerulosclerosis

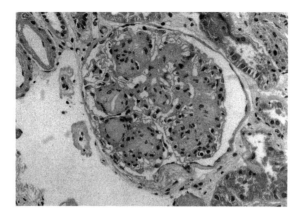

Fig. 26.2 Nodular diabetic glomerulosclerosis (Kimmelstiel–Wilson lesion)

Non-glomerular abnormalities commonly associated include hyalinosis of the afferent and efferent arterioles and chronic tubulointerstitial nephritis (Chapter 20) presumably secondary to glomerular loss, ischaemia, papillary necrosis and perhaps infection (see below).

Clinical features of diabetic glomerulosclerosis

Diabetic glomerulosclerosis usually occurs in patients with other manifestations of diabetic microvascular disease (retinopathy, neuropathy, peripheral vascular insufficiency). It is usually diagnosed 10–20 years after the onset of Type 1 (insulin-dependent) diabetes but in Type II (non-insulin dependent) diabetes the nephropathy may (uncommonly) be evident soon after the diagnosis of diabetes, or in exceptional cases before diabetes is clinically apparent.

The clinical manifestations have been best studied in Type I diabetes. The phases include:

Preclinical phase. In early or uncontrolled diabetes an increased GFR and enlarged kidneys are common. Microalbuminuria (i.e. of the order of 40–300 mg/day of urinary albumin) has been suggested to presage subsequent development of glomerulopathy.

Proteinuric phase. Moderate proteinuria occurs about 10–15 years after the onset of insulin dependency. Protein excretion is usually 1–3 g/day. Nephrotic syndrome (Chapter 9) can occur, and if so the prognosis is particularly poor, with a mean renal survival of around 3 years from onset of nephrosis. Diabetes is the cause of about 5% of cases of nephrotic syndrome in the adult. It is quite rare for proteinuria to first appear more than 30 years after the onset of diabetes. It therefore seems that about 50% of insulin-dependent diabetics do not develop diabetic glomerulosclerosis.

In about 20% of cases mild glomerular haematuria accompanies the proteinuria. Diabetic nephropathy is one of the diseases in which proteinuria is often out of proportion to haematuria (Table 9.3). If heavy haematuria is present other lesions should be suspected. Hypertension almost invariably occurs, and can be difficult to control.

Renal failure phase. The period of time from detection of proteinuria to end-stage renal failure varies considerably, but is usually between 5 and 15 years, and shortest in patients with heavy proteinuria and severe or poorly controlled hypertension.

Diabetic renal papillary necrosis

Infarction of the papilla may occur as a consequence of vascular disease affecting the papillary microcirculation. It is usually associated with infection in the urine. The clinical picture is often dramatic, with acute loin pain, fever and often septicaemia. Treatment consists of relief of obstruction and eradication of the infection. In other cases the necrosis is insidious and only diagnosed radiographically (Chapter 22), or as papillary necrosis *in situ* at postmortem.

Renovascular disease in diabetes

Accelerated atheroma and diabetic microvascular disease affect intrarenal and extrarenal vessels and contribute to hypertension and ischaemic renal damage.

Urine infection in diabetes

Urine infection has long been considered a particular risk in diabetes. Previously its incidence has probably been overemphassised, since the tubulointerstitial changes commonly seen in diabetic kidneys were once erroneously attributed to infection, while it is now clear that glomerular loss, renal papillary necrosis and renal ischaemia probably are more important causes. While urine infection is frequently found in hospitalised patients, it is likely that well diabetics have little greater risk of acquiring bacterial urine infections than non-diabetics. Urinary catheterisation and bladder neuropathy increase the risk significantly. The consequences of urine infection are much more serious in diabetics. Papillary necrosis, perirenal and intrarenal abscess and septicaemia all may occur. Fungal infection, especially with *Candida*, is more common in diabetics than non-diabetics.

Radiocontrast nephrotoxicity

Diabetics are particularly prone to radiocontrast induced nephrotoxicity (Chapter 34). It is wise to prehydrate these patients and use low ionic strength contrast media.

Hyporeninaemic hypoaldosteronism

Hyporeninaemic hypoaldosteronism is a syndrome in which hyperkalaemia occurs early in the progress of diabetic nephropathy, with associated metabolic alkalosis and mild renal functional impairment. The mechanism is unclear.

Glycosuric polyuria

With hyperglycaemia polyuria is due to the osmotic diuretic effect of glucose. If there is inadequate fluid intake, as is commonly the case in diabetic ketoacidosis, acute prerenal renal failure can occur (Chapter 10).

Autonomic neuropathy

Autonomic neuropathy can affect the bladder, leading to poor urine stream, hesitancy or a lack of feeling of bladder fullness. Chronic outflow obstruction and urine infection may follow. Severe postural hypotension can occur with autonomic neuropathy, resulting in difficulty in managing hypertension.

MANAGEMENT OF DIABETIC RENAL DISEASE

In patients with long standing diabetes, proteinuria and other signs of diabetic microvascular disease such as retinopathy and neuropathy, the diagnosis of diabetic glomerulosclerosis can be made on clinical grounds. Renal biopsy is usually unnecessary but should be considered if there are atypical features (early onset, rapid progression, severe nephrosis, haematuria, absence of non-renal manifestations of diabetic microvascular disease).

The important steps to be taken are:

Control diabetes. There is little clinical evidence that such control is able to stabilise nephropathy, perhaps because ideal control cannot be achieved. None the less, control should be as tight as possible. Insulin requirements usually fall in end-stage renal failure, as the result of reduced renal metabolism of glucose (Chapter 6).

Control hypertension. Poor blood pressure control is a major factor in accelerating both renal and retinal disease. There are reports suggesting that angiotensin-converting enzyme inhibitors might slow progression both by controlling hypertension and limiting hyperfiltration.

Prevent and control urine infection. The passage of urinary catheters to help in the management of diabetic coma should be discouraged. In patients with urine infection, effective treatment should be followed by investigation to determine whether papillary necrosis or bladder neuropathy is present.

Treat other diabetic complications. Treatment of retinopathy and vascular disease is important.

Avoid radiocontrast agents and dehydration
Prehydration and the use of low ionic strength contrast media has already been mentioned.

Early dialysis and transplantation. Renal replacement therapy should be introduced at a much earlier stage than in non-diabetics, usually when the plasma creatinine concentration is above 0.6 mmol/litre, and GFR below 20 ml/min. This is because uraemia is associated with acceleration of other diabetic complications e.g. retinopathy, ischaemic cardiomyopathy.

Continuous ambulatory peritoneal dialysis (Chapter 35) is the recommended method of dialysis, and preferably in such patients insulin is given intraperitoneally rather than subcutaneously, resulting in delivery through the portal system as is more appropriate physiologically. Early transplantation is the treatment of choice. Generally survival is worse than in non-diabetics. Combined pancreatic and renal transplantation is being performed in some centres.

27: *Multiple Myeloma, Amyloidosis and Paraproteinaemias (including Mixed Cryoglobulinaemia)*

MULTIPLE MYELOMA

Multiple myeloma is a particularly important cause of proteinuria and renal failure in elderly people. A variety of renal complications can occur (Table 27.1). Renal manifestations occur at some time in over half of patients, and are the cause of death in about 25%, making renal failure the second commonest cause of death after infection.

Pathogenesis of renal damage in myeloma

Renal damage can be due to the paraprotein, or to the tumour itself.

Nephrotoxic effects of circulating paraproteins

Different myelomas may produce a wide range of immuno-globulins or fragments such as heavy chains, light chains and fragments of light chains. The size and charge of the light chain paraprotein dictates whether it will be filtered by the glomerulus, or not filtered but deposited in the kidney substance.

Filtered light chains, which reach the urine as Bence-Jones proteins (see below), are directly toxic to renal tubular cells, hence early in the course of disease renal tubular dysfunction may occur. They are also likely to aggregate with Tamm–Horsfall urinary glycoproteins to form the obstructing casts typical of the myeloma kidney — the commonest pathological finding in severe renal failure. This is particularly likely if there is dehydration, or there are radiocontrast agents in the glomerular filtrate. Unfiltered light chains, particularly lambda light chains, may deposit in the kidney as amyloid.

Rare complications include hyperviscosity, light chain deposition in glomeruli and cryoglobulinaemia, all of which are discussed later in this chapter.

Tumour-related renal complications of myeloma

Hypercalcaemia. This occurs in 25% of cases and is attributed to bone resorption. Hypercalcaemia causes nausea and vomiting as well as a tubular concentrating defect and polyuria. The combination of effects can result in profound dehydration, which in turn can directly cause renal failure or aggravate myeloma kidney disease.

315

Table 27.1 Renal effects of myeloma

Common	Uncommon
Myeloma kidney (80% of renal failure)	Renal infiltration
Renal amyloid	Hyperviscosity
Renal tubular dysfunction	Light chain deposition disease
Hypercalcaemic nephropathy	Cryoglobulinaemic nephropathy
Acute urate nephropathy	

Hyperuricaemia. Acute urate nephropathy can occur, usually with treatment of the myeloma (Chapter 24).

Tumour involvement. Infiltrating plasmocytoma can (rarely) involve the kidney or ureters.

Renal pathology in myeloma

The common pathological entities are myeloma kidney and renal amyloidosis.

Myeloma kidney

This is the usual lesion seen in patients with renal failure. Dense eosinophilic casts fill the tubular lumen (Fig. 27.1) and there is severe chronic tubulointerstitial nephritis (Chapter 20), with tubular cell degeneration, interstitial mononuclear cell infiltrates and collagenous fibrosis.

Renal amyloid

10% of myelomas are associated with renal amyloid, which will be discussed later in this chapter. Light-chain derived (AL) renal amyloid occurs, in which light chains constitute the amyloid fibrils, as in primary amyloid.

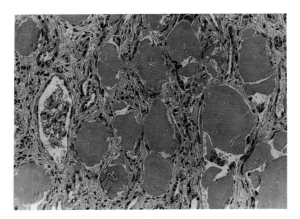

Fig. 27.1 Myeloma kidney. Cast filled tubules and severe chronic tubulointerstitial nephritis

Clinical features of myeloma kidney

The majority of patients are over 40 years of age (median 60 years), and present with insidious weight loss and anaemia, culminating in bone pain, vertebral collapse or pathological fractures. Over half the patients will develop renal failure at some time, usually only months before their death. Some patients present with symptoms of hypercalcaemia, with polyuria, thirst, and nausea, and a proportion present with proteinuria or renal failure.

Renal failure

Acute or chronic renal failure can be the presenting complaint in myeloma. Precipitating factors may include:
- Dehydration.
- Hypercalcaemia.
- Radiocontrast studies.
- Cytotoxic therapy with consequent dehydration or acute urate nephropathy.

Renal tubular dysfunction

In early myeloma, tubular dysfunction with Fanconi's syndrome, aminoaciduria, glycosuria, hypophosphataemia, hypokalaemia, renal tubular acidosis or renal concentrating defects (Chapter 28) is common though usually subclinical.

Laboratory investigation in myeloma

Bence-Jones proteins are found in the urine of 70–80% of myeloma patients. These light chains or fragments are not detected by dipsticks for albumin, but are recognised by:
- Heating. Bence-Jones proteins precipitate at 40–60°C. The sensitivity is only 300 mg/litre and false positive results can occur.
- Immunoelectrophoresis of concentrated urine. This is a much more reliable test than heating and allows classification into light chain subtype (kappa or lambda).

Plasma protein electrophoresis is used to demonstrate the immunoglobulin peak. Other immunoglobulins are generally depressed. The immunoglobulin type can be determined by immunoelectrophoresis.

Bone marrow biopsy confirms the diagnosis of myeloma by demonstrating excessive and malignant plasma cells.

Plasma calcium is often elevated, often without concurrent elevation of the plasma alkaline phosphatase.

Renal biopsy is recommended in patients with renal failure, since there are several renal pathologies which could be present (Table 27.1).

Treatment of myeloma kidney

The important steps are to prevent dehydration and to treat the myeloma.

Maintenance of hydration and diuresis

Because so many of the renal complications (myeloma kidney, urate nephropathy, hypercalcaemia) are aggravated by dehydration or poor urine flow it is very important that a good urine output is maintained at all times. This may require intravenous saline loading, particularly prior to treatment of the myeloma.

Treatment of the myeloma

Adequate treatment of the tumour will reduce the production of paraproteins and control tumour-related complications. Prednisolone and melphalan is usually given. The dose of melphalan should be reduced by about 50% in patients with renal functional impairment, since it is partially renally excreted and severe marrow depression will follow if normal doses are given in renal failure. Allopurinol is given prior to treatment (see below).

Other features of management

Consideration of plasma exchange. In patients with an exceptionally high light chain load and moderate renal failure, or patients with hyperviscosity, plasma exchange has been used to decrease the plasma concentration of paraprotein.

Avoidance of radiological contrast agents. These can precipitate renal failure in myeloma kidney. If they must be given, diuresis should be ensured by prior intravenous hydration.

Prevention of acute urate nephropathy. Allopurinol and adequate hydration should prevent this complication. Alkalinisation of the urine is also helpful.

Dialysis. Though survival is dramatically reduced, myeloma renal failure is not in itself regarded as a contraindication to maintenance dialysis.

RENAL AMYLOIDOSIS

Amyloid is eosinophilic material which can be found infiltrating tissues. There are several proteins that can form amyloid, since this is a common structure adopted by aggregations of globulins. The two important types of renal amyloid are amyloid AL (primary type), where immunoglobulin light chain is the main protein, and amyloid AA (secondary type), where the main protein is the plasma protein serum amyloid associated protein (SAA). Amyloid AL occurs as a primary disease or secondary to multiple myeloma. Amyloid AA is usually secondary to chronic inflammatory diseases (Table 27.2).

Table 27.2 Causes of renal amyloidosis

Amyloid AL (i.e. immunoglobulin light chain containing)
Primary amyloid
Malignant paraproteinaemia
   multiple myeloma
   Waldenström's macroglobulinaemia

Amyloid AA (i.e. acute phase reactant SAA containing)
Chronic infections
   tuberculosis
   bronchiectasis
   osteomyelitis
Chronic inflammation
   rheumatoid arthritis
   ulcerative colitis
   Crohn's disease
Neoplasms

Pathology of renal amyloidosis

In both forms of amyloidosis the renal histology is similar, with replacement and expansion of the glomerular mesangium by pink homogenous material in sections stained with haematoxylin and eosin stains (Fig. 27.2). Electron microscopy shows pleated bundles of fibrils. Other special techniques can also be helpful (Table 27.3).

Clinical features

AL (primary type) amyloid usually occurs in patients over 50 years of age and presents as a diffuse infiltrative disease affecting kidneys, heart, liver, spleen, tongue and gastrointestinal tract. Carpal tunnel syndrome, autonomic neuropathy and easy skin bruising are common. Over 75% will have proteinuria and commonly this will be in the nephrotic range. 50% have free urinary light chains, but no myeloma in marrow biopsy. About 10% of patients with multiple myeloma develop AL amyloidosis.

AA (secondary type) occurs in a wide variety of chronic inflammatory and neoplastic disorders (Table 27.2). Renal, hepatic and splenic involvement are common.

Renal features

The renal features of the two forms of amyloid are indistinguishable. Most patients have proteinuria, and this can be in the nephrotic range (>3.5 g/day) with consequent severe oedema. This is one of the diseases where urinary protein is often out of proportion to urinary red cell excretion (Table 9.3), and is one of the more common causes of nephrotic syndrome in elderly people. Hypertension is rarely an impressive feature; indeed, because of autonomic neuropathy and cardiomyopathy, mild hypotension is often seen. Renal failure is common at presentation.

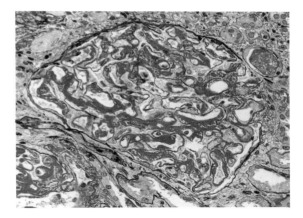

Fig. 27.2 Amyloid glomerulopathy

Course and management of renal amyloidosis

In patients with heavy proteinuria progress is usually rapid. Three-year survival for patients with nephrotic syndrome is only about 10%. Patients with mild proteinuria and normal renal function at the time of diagnosis have a highly variable course, however, death due to renal or other manifestations is usually inevitable. Recurrence in renal transplants occurs in about 10% of cases, usually quite rapidly.

A search for a treatable underlying condition is important. Even in patients without myeloma there appears to be a greater survival if patients with AA (primary) amyloid are treated as for myeloma with melphalan and prednisolone. In amyloidosis secondary to inflammatory disease, control of the underlying disease is important.

WALDENSTRÖM'S MACROGLOBULINAEMIA

Waldenström's macroglobulinaemia is characterised by monoclonal IgM overproduction from proliferative lymphoid cells. Renal involvement is rarely of major clinical importance but includes:
- Bence-Jones proteinuria (30%).

Table 27.3 Staining characteristics of amyloid

Homogeneous pink with eosin
Fluoresces when stained with Thioflavin T
Beta-pleating on electron microscopy
Positive green birefringence in polarised light
Red with Congo red
Immunostaining for immunoglobulin light chain or SAA

- Renal amyloid (20%).
- Acute renal failure due to hyperviscosity.
- Cryoglobulinaemic glomerulopathy.

Hyperviscosity renal failure

In Waldenström's macroglobulinaemia, multiple myeloma, and other diseases characterised by increased blood viscosity, there can be acute renal failure of the prerenal type (Chapter 10) secondary to the hyperviscosity. Invariably systemic effects of hyperviscosity, such as depressed conscious state and retinal haemorrhages, are also present. Plasma exchange is effective in reducing plasma viscosity.

LIGHT CHAIN DEPOSITION DISEASE

This very rare condition is secondary to monoclonal gammopathies in which light chains are produced. The tubular and glomerular basement membranes are thickened by homogeneous non-amyloid protein. This causes proteinuria, haematuria and renal failure.

CRYOGLOBULINAEMIC NEPHROPATHY

Cryoglobulins are proteins which precipitate at low temperatures. There are three types:

Type I. The cryoglobulins are monoclonal immunoglobulins produced by neoplastic overgrowth of lymphoid or plasma cells as in myeloma, macroglobulinaemia, lymphoma or monoclonal gammopathy.

Type II. The cryoglobulins are complexes of a monoclonal immunoglobulin and rheumatoid factor directed against it.

Type III — the most common form. The cryoglobulins are IgG—IgM complexes of mixed polyclonal immunoglobulin and rheumatoid factor directed against them. They can be associated with a wide variety of infections, connective tissue and lymphoproliferative disorders. In 30–40% no underlying disease is found and the condition is termed 'essential mixed cryoglobulinaemia'.

Clinical features of essential mixed cryoglobulinaemia

In both pathogenesis and some clinical features essential mixed cryoglobulinaemia resembles SLE, with features attributable to circulation of immune complexes.

The usual features are:

- Polyarthralgia (75%).
- Purpuric skin lesions (100%).
- Glomerulonephritis (55%).

Other manifestations include hepatomegaly, leg ulcers, and Raynaud's phenomenon.

Cryoglobinaemic nephropathy

There is usually an acute nephritic syndrome, although a more chronic glomerular illness can occur. There is often severe hypo-complementaemia and cryoglobulins are found in the plasma (the sample must be kept at 37°C until assayed). Renal biopsy shows a diffuse proliferative glomerulonephritis with prominent deposits of protein in the capillary loops. Treatment is with plasma exchange and immunosuppressive therapy (prednisolone, cyclophosphamide) to decrease cryoglobulin production.

28: *Disorders of Renal Tubular Function*

These are diseases characterised by specific or generalised deficiencies of tubular cell function. Glomerular dysfunction is either minimal or occurs secondarily to the tubular disorder. The most common are listed in Table 28.1.

DISORDERS OF WATER AND ELECTROLYTE RESORPTION

Nephrogenic diabetes insipidus

In this condition the tubules are unresponsive to the actions of antidiuretic hormone (ADH) resulting in an inability to concentrate the urine, even if ADH (vasopressin) is given parenterally. The clinical problem is polyuria with polydipsia and a predisposition to rapid dehydration and hypernatraemia (Chapter 14) should water intake be inadequate. The disease can be congenital or acquired; the commonest causes being lithium therapy and chronic tubulointerstitial nephritis (Table 28.2) where other abnormalities of tubular function commonly coexist.

Diagnosis and treatment

Diagnosis involves the demonstration that the urine does not concentrate with water restriction (care must be taken that severe

Table 28.1 Renal tubular disorders

Single resorption defects
Water
  nephrogenic diabetes insipidus
Phosphate
  familial hypophosphataemia
Calcium
  idiopathic hypercalciuria
Glucose
  renal glycosuria
Amino acids
  cystinuria
  Hartnup's disease

Multiple defects
Renal tubular acidosis
Fanconi's syndrome

323

Table 28.2 Causes of nephrogenic diabetes insipidus

Congenital
Sex-linked recessive

Acquired
Lithium therapy
Hypercalcaemia
Hypokalaemia
Diseases affecting tubules
   chronic tubulointerstitial nephritis
   recovering and partial tubular obstruction
   recovering and partial acute tubular necrosis
   multiple myeloma

dehydration is not provoked) or administration of ADH analogues (Chapter 5). Any underlying disease should be treated, and adequate water provided at all times.

Familial hypophosphataemia (hereditary vitamin D resistant rickets)

Phosphate resorption is impaired in this condition, which is inherited in a sex-linked dominant fashion, thereby affecting daughters of male sufferers, and half the sons and daughters of females with the disease. Persistent hypophosphataemia and rickets are characteristic.

Idiopathic hypercalciuria

Inadequate tubular resorption of calcium is believed to be one of the causes of idiopathic hypercalciuria — the commonest cause of renal stones (Chapter 25).

RENAL GLYCOSURIA

In up to 2% of the population the tubular resorption of glucose is inadequate to cope with the normal filtered load. This can be congenital or acquired, and may be associated with other proximal tubular defects in the Fanconi's syndrome (see below) or chronic tubulointerstitial nephritis. When present as an isolated phenomenon it is distinguished from glycosuria due to diabetes mellitus by a normal glucose tolerance test.

AMINOACIDURIAS

In these diseases there is defective resorption of amino acids by the tubule.

Cystinuria

This autosomal recessive disease is characterised by defective proximal tubular resorption of the dibasic amino acids — cystine, ornithine, arginine and lysine. The defect is also present in the small intestine. It causes recurrent renal stones (Chapter 25).

RENAL TUBULAR ACIDOSIS

In renal tubular acidosis (RTA) there is a defect in urinary acidi-fication. There are two main types: Type I or distal RTA, and Type II or proximal RTA (Table 28.3).

Distal (Type I) RTA

Distal RTA is more common than proximal RTA. It results from distal tubular .inability to maintain an adequate pH gradient between the tubular lumen and the blood. The consequence is excretion of inadequate amounts of H^+, and instead Na^+ and K^+ accompany the acid anions in the urine. Volume contraction results in secondary aldosteronism with consequent further K^+ loss.

Chronic metabolic acidosis stimulates skeletal buffering mechanisms resulting in bone dissolution and hypercalciuria. Tubular cell citrate production decreases in acidosis. The combi-nation of low urine citrate, high urine pH, and persistent hyper-calciuria leads to the formation of calcium containing renal stones (Chapter 25) and nephrocalcinosis.

Causes of distal (Type I) RTA

Type I RTA is often secondary to tubulointerstitial diseases such as analgesic nephropathy, transplant rejection, obstructive nephro-pathy, medullary sponge kidney, and hypercalcaemic nephropathy (Table 28.4). The disease can also complicate a variety of auto-immune diseases, such as Sjögren's syndrome and other hyper-globulinaemic states. Nephrotoxic causes include amphotericin and lithium therapy. Primary distal RTA may also occur as a genetic disorder or an isolated acquired defect of unknown cause.

Table 28.3 Distinction of type I and II renal tubular acidosis

	Distal Type I	Proximal Type II
Incidence	Common	Uncommon
Plasma HCO_3^- (mmol/litre)	12–18	16–20
Plasma K	Low	Very low
Nephrocalcinosis and renal stones	Common	Rare
Response to alkali	Good	Poor
Response to K repletion	Good	Poor

Table 28.4   Causes of distal (Type I) renal tubular acidosis

Primary
Genetic
Idiopathic acquired

Secondary
Tubulointerstitial disease
    medullary sponge kidney
    analgesic nephropathy
    obstructive nephropathy
    transplant rejection
    hypercalciuria
    sickle cell nephropathy
Autoimmune diseases
    Sjögren's syndrome
    primary biliary cirrhosis
    systemic lupus erythematosus
Drug toxicity
    amphotericin B
    lithium

Clinical features of distal RTA

These are:
- Chronic acidosis, with polyuria and polydipsia.
- Hypokalaemia, which may be life-threatening.
- Nephrocalcinosis or renal stones.
- Osteomalacia or rickets.
- Renal failure, due to nephrocalcinosis or stones.

Proximal (Type II) RTA

In this uncommon condition a defect in the proximal tubule results in less hydrogen ion excretion and inadequate bicarbonate resorption; bicarbonate is thus lost into the urine. As the plasma bicarbonate concentration falls there is less bicarbonate filtered and eventually distal tubular bicarbonate resorption is capable of handling the filtered load. A new steady state is achieved, where the plasma bicarbonate remains low but there is no loss of bicarbonate in the urine, i.e. the condition is self-limiting. Once this steady state is achieved wastage of potassium and calcium into the urine is also minimised. Administration of bicarbonate to attempt to improve the acidosis can result in renewed and potentially dangerous kaliuresis.

Causes of proximal (Type II) RTA

The disorder can be part of diffuse proximal tubular dysfunction (Fanconi's syndrome) or a specific isolated abnormality (Table 28.5). Uncommonly Type II RTA occurs as a primary condition, most commonly in male infants but occasionally in adults. It tends to improve with age.

Table 28.5 Causes of proximal (Type II) renal tubular acidosis

---

Primary
Genetically acquired Fanconi's syndrome
Isolated Type II RTA

Secondary to proximal tubular injury
Metabolic disorders
  cystinosis
  Wilson's disease
  glycogen-storage disease
Multiple myeloma and paraproteinaemias
Hyperparathyroidism
Transplant rejection
(Acetazolamide therapy)

Laboratory diagnosis of RTA

RTA should be suspected in any patient with chronic hyperchloraemic metabolic acidosis (a normal anion gap — Chapter 14). Hypokalaemia is usually present. RTA is then diagnosed by demonstrating an inability to appropriately acidify the urine in the face of acidosis.

Random urine pH in acidosis

In the presence of systemic acidosis the urine pH should be less than 5.5. If urine pH is less than 5.5, Type I RTA is excluded but Type II RTA could still be present. If urine pH is above about 5.8 RTA is quite likely.

Acid-load test

Ammonium chloride, 100 mg/kg, is given orally over about 30−60 min. Urine specimens are collected initially and every half hour and plasma bicarbonate measured initially and at 3 hours. Plasma bicarbonate should fall by at least 4 mmol/litre, and urine pH should decrease to 5.3 or less. The test should be avoided in incipient hepatic failure when the ammonium load can lead to encephalopathy and in renal failure when all patients have difficulty excreting acid loads.

In proximal RTA, patients can often adequately acidify their urine in response to an acid load, but there is a very poor response to attempted bicarbonate repletion due to urinary bicarbonate wastage.

Treatment of RTA
Treatment of distal (Type I) RTA

Oral potassium is given, as bicarbonate and citrate salts, to replace the potassium deficit, and oral bicarbonate (usually 40−70 mmol/day to repair the acidosis. The renal stones and osteomalacia may require additional specific treatment.

Table 28.6 Causes of Fanconi's syndrome

Genetic
Cystinosis — Lignac–Fanconi

Acquired
Multiple myeloma
Heavy metal poisoning — lead, cadmium, mercury
Wilson's disease (copper)
Glycogen storage disease
Idiopathic

Treatment of proximal (Type II) RTA

Treatment is difficult since oral bicarbonate cannot keep up with the renal losses unless huge doses are given and this may provoke worsening of the hypokalaemia. As the disease is self-limiting (see above), it is therefore usual to not treat the acidosis.

FANCONI'S SYNDROME

Fanconi's syndrome is a diffuse defect of proximal tubular function. The characteristic features are:
- Glycosuria.
- Aminoaciduria.
- Phosphaturia.
- Type II renal tubular acidosis.
- Low molecular weight (tubular) proteinuria.
- Nephrogenic diabetes insipidus.

Causes of Fanconi's syndrome

The disorder can be congenital or acquired (Table 28.6)

Cystinosis. This is an autosomal recessive condition characterised by a 'swan neck' deformity of the proximal tubule, Fanconi's syndrome, and deposits of cystine crystals in many organs, including the kidneys, cornea, liver, bone marrow and lymph nodes. Polyuria, polydipsia, renal bone disease with dwarfism and death from renal failure before adulthood is usual.

Acquired adult Fanconi's syndrome. This is usually secondary to nephrotoxic damage to the proximal tubule (Table 28.6). The presenting features are bone pain (osteomalacia), polyuria and polydipsia. The prognosis is generally good with appropriate treatment, including correction of the hypokalaemic acidosis with sodium bicarbonate and potassium citrate, vitamin D for the osteomalacia and, if possible, treatment of the cause.

29: Cystic Diseases of the Kidney

The important cystic diseases of the kidney are:
- Adult polycystic kidney disease — (APCK).
- Medullary sponge kidney disease — (MSK).
- Medullary cystic kidney disease — (MCK).
- Simple cysts of the kidney.
- Dysplastic cystic kidney disease.
- Juvenile polycystic kidney disease.
- Aquired uremic cystic kidney disease.

ADULT POLYCYSTIC KIDNEY DISEASE

This condition is characterised by cysts throughout the cortex and medulla of both kidneys (Fig. 29.1), and gradual deterioration into renal failure in mid or late adult life.

Aetiology

Adult polycystic kidney disease (APCK) is an autosomal dominant condition, in most cases due to an abnormality of a gene on the short arm of chromosome 16. APCK disease is found in all races. About 20% of patients have no family history of APCK. It seems likely that other genes on different chromosomes can produce an identical clinical picture.

Incidence

The disease is fairly common. The gene is found in about 1 in 1000 people. APCK is responsible for about 10% of patients entering end-stage renal failure (ESRF) programmes in Australasia, Europe and the USA.

Pathology

In early life, cysts begin forming in both kidneys. By adult life the kidneys are usually huge, with multiple cysts throughout the renal substance (Fig. 29.1). These cysts arise from the tubule at any level of the nephron, and contain fluid resembling either serum or urine. The pathogenesis of the cysts is unknown. Theories include:
- Obstruction by hyperplastic tubular cells.
- Defective tubular basement membrane with consequent 'blow-out'. This is consistent with some of the associated developmental abnormalities (Table 29.1).

329

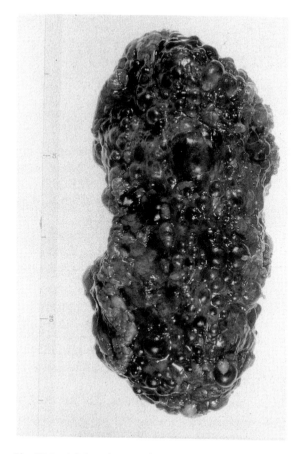

Fig. 29.1 Adult polycystic kidney disease. Note the large size (over 23 cm long) and multiple cysts filled with serous and serosanguinous fluid

Clinical features

Polycystic kidneys are almost invariably palpable bilaterally, though one kidney can be smaller than the other. They can be so large that they extend into the iliac fossa. When polycystic liver disease is also present it can fill the right abdomen and extend across the left hypochondrium, leaving only the lower pole of the left kidney to be felt. The kidneys are usually firm and their surface is very irregular, being comprised of inumerable cysts. Large kidneys will displace the bowel anteriorly, and thus though usually resonant, they may be dull to percussion over much of their anterolateral surface. They move vertically with respiration and can be ballotted from the loin.

Symptoms and signs can relate to:
- Family history.
- Progressive renal disease.

Table 29.1 Developmental abnormalities associated with polycystic kidney disease

Abnormality	Incidence (%)
Polycystic liver	40
Cystic pancreas	5
Cerebral arterial aneurysm	10

Cardiac valve abnormalities
  mitral valve prolapse
  aortic regurgitation
	10

- Complications of cysts.
- Associated developmental abnormalities.

Family history

A history suggesting renal disease or APCK is found in about 80% of cases. Typically an autosomal dominant pattern can be seen in the family tree.

Features of progressive renal disease

Hypertension occurs in about 50% of cases, with onset at about 20–30 years of age. Progressive renal failure usually follows, with ESRF between 30 and 60 years of age. Mild proteinuria is occasionally found. The anaemia of chronic renal failure is often less severe in patients with APCK, because of sustained erythropoietin production.

Complications of renal cysts

Complications directly attributable to the cysts include:
- Abdominal distention.
- Cyst haemorrhage.
- Cyst infection.
- Renal stones.

Abdominal distention can be severe, particularly if polycystic liver is associated. The patient often complains of a feeling of fullness or weight in the abdomen.

Cyst haemorrhage can occur sporadically or with minor trauma. Severe loin pain is common, due to cyst distention or clot colic, and macroscopic haematuria may be present.

Cyst infection is one of the more dangerous complications of renal cysts. Often multiple cysts are affected. Flank or abdominal pain and fever are usual and sometimes an area of extreme tenderness will be found over one kidney. Pyuria and usually bacteriuria is found. Aminoglycosides and penicillins penetrate cysts poorly, whereas chloramphenicol, quinolones, trimethoprim-sulphameth-oxazole, tetracycline, and erythromycin may penetrate quite well. In resistant cases percutaneous cyst puncture and aspiration, surgical cyst drainage or even nephrectomy may be required.

Renal stones occur with increased frequency, and are often seen nestling in cysts. They are often associated with urine infection. Stasis and infection are probably responsible for stone formation. They rarely cause renal or ureteric colic.

Associated developmental conditions

A variety of other developmental abnormalities are associated with APCK disease (Table 29.1).

About 40% of patients with APCK have a polycystic liver. This seems to occur in various family members with APCK with no apparent pattern. Polycystic liver disease can express itself clinically by causing:
- Gross abdominal distention.
- Abdominal pain due to cyst bleeding or infection.
- Portal hypertension or biliary obstruction, both rarely.

Liver failure does not occur. Occasionally cysts in the pancreas, which occur in 5−10% of patients, are associated with recurrent pancreatitis.

Saccular aneurysms of the cerebral arteries occur in about 10% of patients with APCK disease, and can cause subarachnoid haemorrhage.

Diagnosis of APCK

Usually the diagnosis is easily made by renal ultrasound, which shows multiple bilateral renal cysts (Fig. 29.2) Hepatic and pancreatic cysts can also be demonstrated. CT scanning will give a clearer picture, but it is rarely necessary (Fig. 29.3) though in a patient with no family history and proven renal cysts a CT scan may help differentiate between multiple simple cysts of the kidney and APCK disease. The IVP is not uniformly reliable as a diagnostic method, but the appearance can be quite characteristic, with large kidneys and 'spidery' stretched calyces (Fig. 29.4). As the cysts are usually not well developed before late adolescence, imaging before this time is not worthwhile in screening family members. Genetic screening is now possible in appropriate families. Recently magnetic resonance imaging (MRI) has been used to determine the nature of the cyst contents, however, its role has not been established (Fig. 29.5).

Treatment of APCK

There is no treatment available to prevent cyst growth and the progression of renal failure. Rarely cyst drainage is required for

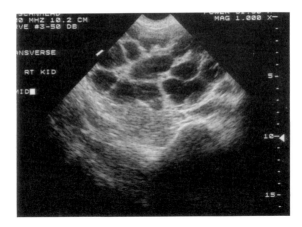

Fig. 29.2 Renal ultrasound showing multiple intrarenal cysts in adult polycystic kidney disease

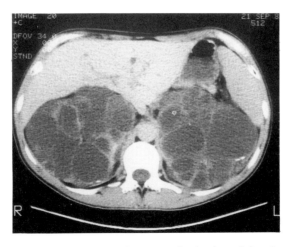

Fig. 29.3 Computerised tomography (CT) in adult polycystic kidney disease shows multiple cysts in both kidneys, and in this case no cysts in the liver

local infection or pressure related symptoms. Treatment is that of chronic renal failure (Chapter 11).

MEDULLARY SPONGE KIDNEY DISEASE

This condition is characterised by cystic dilatation of medullary and papillary collecting ducts. These may be seen as 1–3 mm linear dye-filled opacities in the medulla and papillae in the IVP (Fig. 29.6). There may be associated multiple small radiopaque

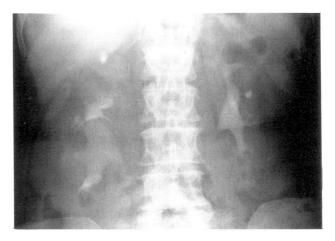

Fig. 29.4 IVP in adult polycystic kidney disease. Large (here over 23 cm) kidneys with 'spidery' calyces stretched over cysts

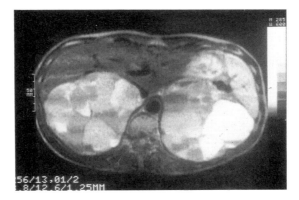

Fig. 29.5 Magnetic resonance imaging (MRI) shows kidneys with multiple cysts, darker when filled with urine, which appear white when filled with blood or pus

calcium stones. The aetiology is unknown, though it may be familial.

Usually the condition presents in middle age with recurrent passage of renal stones. About 20% also have 'distal' type I renal tubular acidosis (Chapter 28), which may be relevant to stone formation.

The disease does not cause renal failure and therefore management usually is aimed at prevention of stones by diuresis and vigorous treatment of UTI.

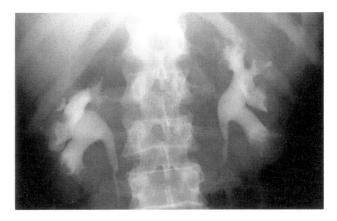

Fig. 29.6 Medullary sponge kidney. The IVP shows multiple elongated cysts in renal papillae, best seen in the left upper lobe

URAEMIC MEDULLARY CYSTIC DISEASE
(juvenile nephronopthisis)

This rare condition is an inheritable cause of chronic renal failure in children and young adults. There may be several subtypes, both clinically and genetically, with recessive, sporadic and even dominant inheritance.

The kidneys are small, with multiple small 1–20 mm cysts throughout, particularly at the corticomedullary junction. Renal failure in childhood or early adult life is usual, commonly with pronounced features of distal tubular dysfunction, including polyuria, salt-wasting, acidosis and early development of bone disease. The cysts are often not detectable by imaging techniques, though they are sometimes seen with careful ultrasound or CT scanning. Diagnosis is often based on the clinical picture, and a renal biopsy showing severe chronic tubulointerstitial nephritis (Chapter 20). There is no specific treatment though salt and bicarbonate supplementation is often required, and the eventual outcome is ESRF, often complicated by severe anaemia, growth retardation and renal bone disease.

CYSTIC RENAL DYSPLASIA

Sporadic cases occur in which one kidney is grossly deformed with cysts, primitive ducts and metaplastic cartilage. If unilateral the kidney is often not connected to the ureter and may be asymptomatic. In bilateral cases varying degrees of renal failure follow. Occasionally the disease is familial, and in infants multiple other organ abnormalities may be found.

Juvenile polycistic kidney disease

Infantile PKD is a subtype of cystic renal dysplasia where bilateral cystic dysplasia leads to oligohydramnios, can obstruct labour, and results in early death due to CRF. Autosomal recessive inheritance is usual.

SIMPLE RENAL CYSTS

One or more thin fluid-filled cysts are found in nearly half of the population over 50 years of age. With ultrasound and CT scanning they are more commonly being diagnosed.

They may be unilateral or bilateral, and single or multiple when they may be difficult to distinguish from polycystic kidney disease. Clinically they are usually silent, although infection, haemorrhage, pain and hypertension can occur. Most need no treatment but cyst aspiration with sclerosis by alcohol injection is occasionally successful in relieving local pain.

ACQUIRED URAEMIC CYSTIC DISEASE

In many dialysis patients multiple renal cysts develop over periods of years. The reason is unknown, and usually they are not clinically apparent.

Occasionally they cause:
- Cyst bleeding:
  (a) haematuria, or
  (b) retroperitoneal haemorrhage.
- Development of tumors — in as many as 13% of cases.
- Erythropoietin production with improvement of anaemia.

30: *Primary Renal Neoplasms*

ADENOCARCINOMA OF THE KIDNEY
(renal cell carcinoma, hypernephroma, Grawitz tumour)

This is by far the most common primary malignancy of the kidney in adults, forming a solid or mixed solid and haemorrhagic tumour of the renal substance. It spreads directly, by lymphatics, and by early blood borne metastasis, particularly to the lungs, bone and brain.

Clinical features

Renal cell carcinoma is a disease of adults, usually over 55 years of age. There are a variety of presenting complaints:
- *Haematuria*, sometimes with flank discomfort and a palpable mass in the loin, is the most common presenting complaint.
- *Paraneoplastic syndromes.* Renal carcinoma is one of the neoplasms characteristically presenting with unexplained fever. Abnormal liver function tests often accompany this syndrome, which resolves on removal of the tumour. Hypercalcaemia and peripheral neuropathy are other less common non-metastatic manifestations of renal carcinoma.
- *Renal vein thrombosis.* Characteristically the carcinoma grows into the renal vein, sometimes resulting in signs of inferior vena caval obstruction or pulmonary embolism.
- *Pulmonary metastases.* Single or multiple 'cannon ball' lung metastases can occur, particularly with renal vein involvement.
- *Polycythaemia.* A very rare complication, this is due to secretion of erythropoietin, either by the tumour or adjacent compressed renal tissue.

Diagnosis

A solid rounded space-occupying lesion projecting outward from the kidney is usually obvious on renal ultrasound or CT scanning. Calcification or patchy haemorrhage in the tumour may be found, as may cystic change. Urinary cytology is not helpful.

Treatment

Total nephrectomy is indicated, and may result in regression of metastases. Single lung metastases are also sometimes removed. Surgery should be preceded by careful investigation for local spread and renal vein involvement, often requiring both CT scanning and renal venography. Five year survival is about 30% and depends on histological grading and degree of spread at presentation.

TRANSITIONAL CELL CARCINOMA
(papillary carcinoma, uroepithelioma)

Transitional cell carcinoma of the uroepithelium can affect the renal pelvis, ureters or bladder, usually in older patients (55 to 70 years). Not uncommonly these are multiple or recurrent, occurring at different levels of the urinary system. Known carcinogens include cigarette smoke and aniline dyes. Transitional cell carcinoma of the renal pelvis is a late complication of analgesic nephropathy (Chapter 22).

Haematuria is almost always the presenting feature, with a radiolucent space lesion visible within the urinary tract on IVP. Occasionally urinary obstruction can occur. Urinary cytology is helpful in diagnosis. Treatment is usually by nephroureterectomy.

NEPHROBLASTOMA (Wilm's tumour)

This is one of the more common malignancies in children, and is rare in children older than 7 years of age. It may be bilateral. Haematuria, flank pain and signs of local metastasis are common presenting features. Treatment is nephrectomy and intensive chemotherapy.

RENIN-SECRETING TUMOUR

These are exceptionally rare, usually solitary and benign, tumours of the renal substance. The characteristic feature is the secretion of renin, leading to hypertension and hypokalaemia, often in younger patients. Diagnosis involves renal vein renin studies (Chapter 12) and renal CT scanning or arteriography. Partial nephrectomy is usually curative.

RENAL ONCOCYTOMA

These are benign rounded adenomata of the renal tubules. Their main importance is their distinction from malignant lesions. This is usually possible with arteriography since they demonstrate a 'cartwheel' pattern of vasculature. Local excision (partial nephrectomy) is usually adequate treatment.

31: *Miscellaneous Renal Conditions*

ANATOMICAL ABNORMALITIES

Duplication of kidney, pelvis or ureter

Duplication of part or all of the urinary tract on one or both sides is not uncommon. Most commonly there is partial or complete duplication of the pelvis and ureter from the kidney downward (Fig. 31.1). In partial duplication the ureters meet in a Y-junction before entering the bladder; in complete duplex ureter there are separate insertions. Occasionally the upper part drains through a ureter that terminates in an ectopic position (vagina, urethral) while the ureter from the lower part ends in the normal place.

Ureteric reflux, hydronephrosis and recurrent urinary tract infection are commonly associated, particularly in the case of ureters with an ectopic insertion. Partial duplex is also associated with urine infection, attributed to relative stasis as urine may flow from one ureter back up the other when their peristaltic waves are not coordinated.

Horseshoe kidney

In this condition the lower poles (rarely the upper) of the kidneys are fused across the midline, while the two pelves remain separate. The two ureters then pass anteriorly over the surface of the isthmus joining the two poles. Characteristically the calyces of the lower poles point laterally (Fig. 31.2). Usually this abnormality is asymptomatic.

Renal agenesis

Rarely one or both kidneys are absent. Usually the relevant ureter is rudimentary or missing. Bilateral agenesis is incompatible with life, and may cause oligohydramnios during pregnancy. Unilateral agenesis may be associated with failure of development of the ureter and trigone of the bladder on the same side. The remaining kidney is hypertrophied. Other congenital abnormalities, particularly of the female genital tract, are commonly associated.

Ectopic kidneys

Kidneys may develop lower in the iliac fossa or pelvis, or rarely on the opposite side, with the ureter crossing the midline to the bladder (crossed renal ectopia). Renal infection, hydronephrosis and abdominal pain may occur. Often there are other congenital abnormalities.

339

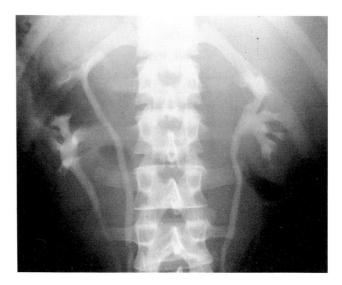

Fig. 31.1 Right-sided bifid system (IVP)

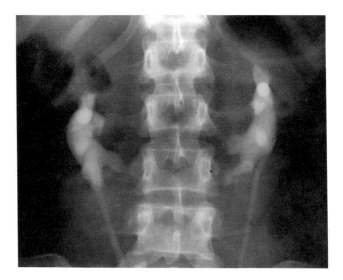

Fig. 31.2 Horseshoe kidney. The IVP shows lower polar fusion, with lower polar calyces directed toward the vertebrae

Congenital hydronephrosis

In this condition there is dilatation of the pelvis and calyces of one or both kidneys (Fig. 31.3). The cause is incomplete obstruction at the pelviureteric junction, probably due to neuromuscular incoordination, though fibrous bands or aberrant vessels may play a role. Usually asymptomatic, the condition may cause mild loin

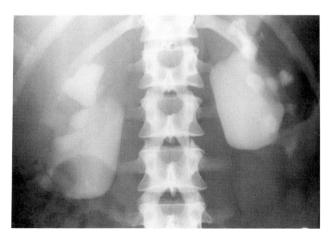

Fig. 31.3 Congenital hydronephrosis with functional pelviureteral junction obstruction (IVP). Despite the gross dilatation of the pelvicalyceal system, renal function is often excellent

pain, particularly after a large fluid intake, and is sometimes complicated by hypertension or renal stones. Treatment is by pyeloplasty.

URINARY DIVERSIONS

A variety of surgical procedures have been developed where diversion of the urine from the bladder is required to deal with abnormalities such as spina bifida with neurogenic bladder and ectopia vesicae. Unfortunately none of these is free from complications.

Uretero-sigmoidostomy

If the ureters are implanted into the lower bowel there is reflux of faecal material up the ureter, and absorption of urine by the bowel.

Sequelae include:
- Recurrent urine infection.
- Ureteral obstruction.
- Electrolyte disturbance — hyperchloraemic acidosis.

Hyperchloraemic acidosis is characterised by acidosis with a low plasma bicarbonate, high chloride and low potassium concentration. The plasma urea is also usually raised. The condition is attributed to:
- Resorption of chloride, hydrogen ions and urea from the urine by the bowel.
- Loss of potassium and bicarbonate from the irritated bowel mucosa into the faeces.

The electrolyte pattern is similar to that of renal tubular acidosis (Chapter 28). Treatment is with sodium bicarbonate, or a mixture of oral potassium and sodium citrate to correct the acidosis and hypokalaemia.

Ileal conduit

Here the ureters are implanted into a length of isolated ileum which in turn opens onto the skin. Initially the results are good, but with the passage of time urine infection, ureteric obstruction, and conduit obstruction often occur. Renal infection stones are common. Rarely hyperchloraemic acidosis is also seen in this condition.

HEREDITARY DISEASES

Glomerular diseases

There are many congenital or hereditary diseases affecting the glomeruli. The best characterised are Alport's syndrome and Fabry's disease.

Alport's syndrome and thin basement membrane disease

Alport's syndrome is an autosomal dominant condition which is much more severe in males. The features are glomerular disease, sensorineural deafness and often abnormality of the ocular lens. The glomerular disease usually presents as haematuria, frequently as recurrent macroscopic haematuria in childhood. Proteinuria is variable. Renal biopsy shows characteristic thinning and fragmentation of the glomerular basement membrane on electron microscopy. Light microscopy may be normal or show focal glomerulosclerosis. Males deteriorate to end-stage renal failure in the second or third decade, while females rarely develop renal failure.

In other patients with haematuria, there may be only mild abnormalities seen with light microscopy, but EM reveals thinning of the basement membranes. This has led to the introduction of the term 'thin basement membrane disease' for this entity, which commonly presents as persistent microscopic haematuria. Familial incidence can occur, and the prognosis seems to be usually good.

Fabry's disease

This is an X-linked deficiency of the enzyme cerumide trihexosidase, resulting in deposition of glycosphingolipid in many organs including vessels of the skin, nerves and the kidney. The main features are renal disease resembling chronic glomerulonephritis, red spots (angiokeratoma) on the scrotum, lower abdomen, axillae and buttocks, painful peripheral neuropathy and vascular occlusions (strokes and infarcts). Rarely females may be mildy affected.

The renal disease presents as mild haematuria and proteinuria with hypertension and progressive renal failure, resulting in end-stage renal failure in the third or fourth decade. Renal biopsy shows vacuolated foam cells in glomerular epithelial cells, and the disease is confirmed by demonstration of the enzyme deficiency. There is no effective treatment.

Tubulointerstitial diseases
Oxalosis

This is a very rare metabolic disorder resulting in deposition of oxalate in many organs, particularly the kidney where nephro-calcinosis, oxalate renal stones and renal failure occur. There are a variety of genetic causes, the most common being autosomal recessive, and the clinical onset is usually before 20 years of age. Urinary oxalate excretion is raised (normal <0.63 mmol/day) and oxalate crystals can be seen in the kidney, and blood vessels. There is little effective treatment, though high dose pyridoxine may be helpful. The renal disease progresses rapidly if acute tubular necrosis occurs, and also recurs quickly in renal transplants. Recently combined liver and renal transplantation has been effective in replacing the enzyme deficiency and treating the renal failure.

INFLAMMATORY DISEASES

Sarcoidosis and the kidney

Sarcoidosis, a systemic granulomatous disease of unknown origin, can affect the kidney in several ways.

The most common is acute or chronic renal failure secondary to hypercalcaemia. In the acute form there is usually severe hypercalcaemia, and good recovery of renal function with treatment of the sarcoidosis. In chronic hypercalcaemia nephrocalcinosis, interstitial fibrosis and renal calculi can cause irreversible damage.

Direct sarcoid involvement with severe interstitial nephritis and granulomata is less common, and responds, at least in part, to treatment with corticosteroids.

Rarely this inflammatory disease is complicated by membranous glomerulonephritis.

Subacute bacterial endocarditis

Proteinuria and microscopic glomerular haematuria are often found in patients with SBE. This can be due to an immune complex nephritis, with a focal and segmental proliferative glomerulonephritis. In the worst form, rapidly progressive disease with diffuse crescentic nephritis can occur. Hypocomplementaemia is usually found, and there are heavy deposits of immunoglobulins and C_3 in glomeruli.

Haematuria can also be due to renal infarcts, which are often multiple and small.

Renal tuberculosis

The kidney is the second most common organ affected by *Mycobacterium tuberculosis*. It produces caseating granulomatous lesions particularly in the renal medulla and papillae. This often produces papillary cavitics and the infection spreads down the ureters. There are often strictures in the ureters or within the pelvicalyceal system (infundibular stenoses).

Renal tuberculosis is often clinically silent, though fever and weight loss are usual and dysuria may occur if the bladder is involved. Usually there is constant pyuria — renal tuberculosis is one of the most important causes of a so-called 'sterile pyuria' (Table 13.4) since the organism has fastidious growth requirements.

The radiological appearance is characteristic (Fig. 31.4) with ulcerated papillae and ureteric strictures. Sometimes a whole kidney will be destroyed by caseation (autonephrectomy). Treatment is as for other forms of active tuberculosis. Currently a combination of isoniazid, rifampicin and ethambutol is recommended.

RENAL INVOLVEMENT IN LIVER DISEASE

The kidneys are affected in two major ways by liver disease; commonly with circulatory abnormalities leading to renal failure, and less commonly, at least clinically, with glomerular disease.

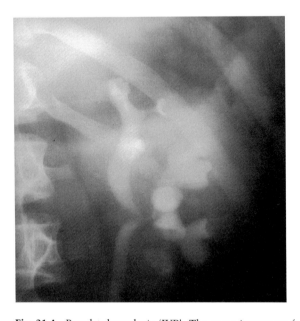

Fig. 31.4 Renal tuberculosis (IVP). The most important feature is development of strictures. Here a tight stricture of the lower pelvicalyceal system has occurred. Calyces may show ragged ulceration

Circulatory abnormalities

There are many factors reducing effective plasma volume in severe liver disease. Hypoalbuminaemia results in fluid loss to oedema and ascites, portal hypertension increases the ascites and may cause variceal bleeding, and there is generalised vasodilatation. In addition there appear to be abnormalities of intrarenal circulation related to neurohumoral or toxic stimuli. In jaundiced patients tubular necrosis can occur with minor insults, for reasons not well understood.

These circulatory abnormalities can be reflected in two major syndromes (Table 31.1).

Hepatorenal failure

In this syndrome a persistent 'prerenal' abnormality seems to exist. Invariably the patient has severe liver failure. The main features are persistent oliguria and acute renal failure, in which the plasma creatinine rises and often plateaus at about 0.6 to 0.8 mmol/litre. The urine is highly concentrated, with a very low (<10 mmol/litre) sodium concentration and high urine to plasma creatinine and urea ratios. The prognosis is poor, since the liver disease is usually terminal; overall survival is less than 20%. The kidney itself is normal, and will function immediately if transplanted into a patient with normal liver function.

Acute tubular necrosis

Acute tubular necrosis often occurs, particularly because of septicaemia or shock secondary to variceal bleeding or pancreatitis. It can be distinguished from hepatorenal failure because the urine is poorly concentrated, with a high sodium concentration (Table 31.1).

Glomerular abnormalities

The body's largest collection of macrophages are the Kupffer cells in the liver, and the gut contains a vast reservoir of organisms and antigens which could gain access via the portal vein to the systemic circulation. Not surprisingly a wide range of glomerular changes have been described in liver disease, particularly mesangial IgA deposition (Chapter 15).

Table 31.1 Distinction of hepatorenal failure from acute tubular necrosis

	Hepatorenal syndrome	Acute tubular necrosis
Urine volume (ml/day)	50–1000	50–3000
Urine specific gravity	High	Low
Urine sodium (mmol/litre)	<10–20	>20
Urine sediment	Normal	Tubular cells and casts

Management of renal failure in liver disease

1 Establish whether ATN or hepatorenal failure is present (Table 31.1):

    (a) urine osmolality or specific gravity,

    (b) urine sodium concentration, and

    (c) urine sediment.

2 Correct any prerenal factors (Chapter 10).

3 In ATN treat as for acute renal failure (Chapter 10).

4 In hepatorenal syndrome:

    (a) treat hepatic disease and hepatic failure,

    (b) slowly expand plasma volume with albumin, and

    (c) give diuretics with great care.

Septicaemia and bleeding secondary to the liver failure are common fatal complications. A Levine shunt (peritoneum to right atrium) may avert the condition in patients with severe ascites. Liver transplantation may be indicated, since the renal failure will recover with improved liver function. Exchange blood transfusion, plasma exchange, dialysis and a range of experimental procedures have not been shown to influence the mortality, which basically depends on recovery of liver function.

NON-RENAL CANCER AND THE KIDNEY

The commonest renal complication of cancer is metastatic involvement, which is usually focal with carcinomas, and diffuse with lymphomas and leukaemias.

Glomerulonephritis is a rare complication of carcinoma or lymphoma. Membranous glomerulonephritis may be found in association with a wide range of carcinomas, particularly bronchial, pancreatic, gastrointestinal and ovarian. Tumour-related immune complexes are believed responsible. Minimal change glomerulonephritis can occur with Hodgkin's disease. A disorder of lymphocyte function is postulated. Very rarely vasculitis complicates carcinoma or lymphoma.

Other complications include the effects of hypercalcaemia, hyperuricaemia and paraproteinaemia on the kidney (Chapters 14, 24 & 27).

32: *Thrombotic Microangiopathy*

Two closely related diseases, haemolytic uraemic syndrome and thrombotic thrombocytopenic purpura, are characterised by thrombotic microangiopathy — the formation of microthrombi in arterioles and glomerular vessels (Fig. 32.1). This process can also occur as a complication of a variety of other microvascular diseases (Table 32.1).

HAEMOLYTIC URAEMIC SYNDROME

Haemolytic uraemic syndrome (HUS) is a disease of children usually under 3 years of age. Often there is a prodromal acute febrile illness (frequently severe gastroenteritis) followed by a sudden onset of:
- *Acute microangiopathic haemolytic anaemia*, often with jaundice.
- *Acute oliguric renal failure*, often with severe hypertension.
Varying features include circulating fibrin degradation products, thrombocytopenia and rarely central nervous system involvement as in thrombotic thrombocytopenic purpura (see below).

The blood film shows distorted fragmented red cells (microangiopathic haemolytic anaemia). In the renal biopsy there are

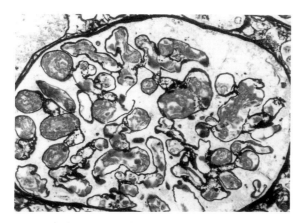

Fig. 32.1 Thrombotic thrombocytopenic purpura (TTP). Glomerular microangiopathy, with platelet and fibrin thrombi in glomerular capillaries

347

Table 32.1 Diseases causing thrombotic microangiopathy

Primary
Haemolytic uraemic syndrome
Thrombotic thrombocytopenic purpura

Secondary
Scleroderma
Malignant hypertension
Renal transplant rejection
Disseminated intravascular coagulation
Renal cortical necrosis
Idiopathic postpartum renal failure
Radiation nephritis

---

microscopic intracapillary thrombi in the glomeruli (Fig. 32.1) and sometimes in larger vessels, with associated cortical infarction.

Specific therapy is controversial, though antioxidant therapy with vitamin E and lipid infusions, prostaglandin treatment and plasma exchange may be effective if commenced in the first few days of the illness. Supportive therapy (dialysis, antihypertensive therapy) is important. About 70% of children recover spontaneously, 25% are left with varying degrees of renal failure (often with severe hypertension) and about 5% die during the illness.

THROMBOTIC THROMBOCYTOPENIC PURPURA

TTP is a disease of adults in which widespread thrombotic microangiopathy, often following a mild gastrointestinal or respiratory illness, is associated with:

1 *Thrombocytopenic purpura.*
2 *Fluctuating central nervous system abnormalities*, particularly brainstem lesions, confusion and coma.
3 *Renal failure*, often with microscopic haematuria.

All features vary considerably between patients, and in some a severe microangiopathic anaemia is also prominent as in HUS. The blood film shows thrombocytopenia and distorted, fragmented red cells. The disease course also varies, from an acute overwhelming illness to a more chronic illness with remissions and exacerbations.

Renal biopsy usually shows arteriolar and glomerular capillary thrombi. Treatment is controversial, with plasma exchange, infusion of pooled gamma globulin or fresh frozen plasma, and occasionally splenectomy.

33: *Pregnancy and the Kidney*

EFFECTS OF PREGNANCY ON THE NORMAL
URINARY SYSTEM

In normal pregnancy the following changes occur.

Dilatation of the upper urinary tract

Dilatation of the calyces, renal pelvis and ureter above the brim of the pelvis occurs from the end of the first trimester until term. Contributing factors include hormone induced relaxation of smooth muscles (relaxin, progesterone) and some degree of obstruction at the pelvic brim by the enlarging uterus. The main consequence is stasis of urine, hence an increased risk of acute pyelonephritis in women with bacteriuria.

Increase in glomerular filtration rate

GFR increases by 30–50% during pregnancy. The GFR is significantly elevated by 1 month after conception, rises rapidly during the first trimester, and remains above normal until delivery, although a slight decline may occur in the last month.

The result is a fall in plasma creatinine concentration, hence the normal upper limit for plasma creatinine in mid and later pregnancy is about 0.08 mmol/litre compared with 0.11 mmol/litre in non-pregnant women.

The increase in GFR, and probably alterations in tubular resorption and secretion, lead to a fall in the maximal tubular resorption of a variety of substances. Renal glycosuria is the most clinically relevant consequence of this, occurring in 10–40% of pregnant women. Aminoaciduria, and lactosuria are other common abnormalities in pregnancy.

Fall in blood pressure

The blood pressure falls about 10 mmHg mainly due to peripheral vasodilatation. Plasma volume rises, as does total body water.

Renal hypertrophy

An increase in renal length by about 1 cm occurs during pregnancy.

RENAL COMPLICATIONS OF PREGNANCY

Pre-eclampsia

About 10% of primigravidae experience a syndrome characterised by hypertension, proteinuria and oedema; usually after the 20th week of gestation. GFR falls, plasma uric acid increases and non-selective heavy proteinuria is common. There are no long term renal sequelae. The pathogenesis is obscure, although hyper-coagulability has been demonstrated.

The syndrome is more likely in patients with:

- Underlying renal disease.
- Twin or multiple pregnancies.
- First pregnancies to a given father.

The glomerular abnormalities consist of a decrease in the capillary lumen by fibrinoid subendothelial deposits and swollen endothelial and mesangial cells, which resolve quickly after delivery. Treatment consists of bed rest, antihypertensive therapy and early delivery if the syndrome does not abate. Diuretics should be avoided. There is some evidence that various anti-thrombotics and anticoagulants, (aspirin, heparin) are effective in prevention and control.

Pregnancy-induced hypertension

Patients in whom blood pressure rises rather than falls with pregnancy include women:

- With prior hypertension.
- With incipient pre-eclampsia.
- With renal disease.
- Who presumably are in the preclinical phase of essential hypertension, which they later go on to develop.

Acute tubular and cortical necrosis

Pregnant women are particularly prone to acute tubular and cortical necrosis (Chapter 10). Common precipitants include antepartum and postpartum haemorrhage, and disseminated intravascular coagulation (DIC), often associated with eclampsia. Treatment includes replacement of blood loss, repletion of coagulation factors lost due to DIC, and dialysis as required.

Idiopathic postpartum renal failure

This rare condition is characterised by acute oliguric renal failure in the early puerperium, often with evidence of microangiopathic haemolytic anaemia or consumptive coagulopathy akin to the haemolytic–uraemic syndrome or thrombotic thrombocytopenic purpura (Chapter 31). There may be severe hypertension. Treatment consists of control of hypertension and renal failure. Intensive plasma exchange may be helpful.

HAT syndrome

An uncommon syndrome of hepatosis (acute fatty liver with jaundice), acute renal failure and disseminated intravascular coagulation with thrombocytopenia occurs in late pregnancy and the early puerperium. The aetiology is unknown, and fetal and maternal mortality is high.

PREGNANCY IN RENAL DISEASE

While there is some dispute as to the exact risk of pregnancy in renal disease there are some facts that seem beyond dispute.

Urine infection

About 6−8% of pregnant women have asymptomatic bacteriuria, and of these about 30−40% will go on to develop acute pyelonephritis, with consequent hospitalisation and risk of fetal loss. All pregnant women should be screened for bacteriuria and treated, preferably by single dose therapy with a safe drug such as amoxycillin 3 g orally. If bacteriuria recurs, renal ultrasound should be performed to diagnose renal stones, hydronephrosis and other gross abnormalities. Prophylaxis throughout pregnancy with low dose nitrofurantoin (50−100 mg *nocte*) should then continue until after delivery. About 6 months postpartum most of the pregnancy-induced anatomical changes should have resolved and an IVP should be performed.

Worsening of pre-existing hypertension

Both essential and renal hypertension are likely to worsen with pregnancy. The risks are of placental insufficiency, with fetal loss, and maternal vascular complications. Good blood pressure control is important, bearing in mind that most women in the mid-trimester have a blood pressure around 10 mmHg less than in non-pregnant women.

Increase in proteinuria

In patients with renal disease the increase in GFR with pregnancy may lead to an increase in glomerular proteinuria. This persists for up to 6 months after pregnancy in many patients.

Impaired renal function

The presence of significantly impaired renal function, with an elevated plasma creatinine, increases the risks of hypertension, fetal loss, and deterioration in maternal renal function during pregnancy. While women with a plasma creatinine above 0.2 mmol/litre rarely become pregnant, in the vast majority of women in whom this has occurred deterioration occurs during pregnancy and the postpartum period. The mechanism may involve hyperfiltration (Chapter 6), pregnancy-induced hypertension or hypercoagulability. Focal glomerulosclerosis, both primary and secondary (Chapter 6 & 15), appears to be accelerated by pregnancy.

We therefore strongly advise women whose plasma creatinine

exceeds 0.2 mmol/litre not to become pregnant, and advise women with plasma creatinine 0.12–0.2 mmol/litre of the risks of pregnancy.

SLE and scleroderma These two diseases are particularly likely to be aggravated by pregnancy, especially if they are poorly controlled prior to conception.

34: Drugs and the Kidney

RENAL EXCRETION OF DRUGS

The kidneys are one of the most important pathways for the excretion of drugs and their metabolites. The main mechanisms of renal excretion are glomerular filtration and tubular secretion, though some are metabolised by tubular cells. For example gentamicin is excreted by glomerular filtration, para-aminohippurate and many acidic drugs like penicillin by glomerular filtration plus tubular secretion, and insulin is handled by glomerular filtration plus tubular catabolism.

Some drugs with predominantly renal excretion are listed in Table 34.1.

DRUG USE IN RENAL FAILURE

Care is required with drug use in renal failure because:
• Many drugs or their metabolites are renally excreted; accordingly dose adjustments often need to be made. This is particularly important if there is a narrow range from the therapeutic to the toxic plasma concentration (e.g. aminoglycosides, digoxin).
• Some drugs are more toxic in uraemic patients because of additive effects to the effects of uraemia (e.g. anticoagulants and salicylates can increase the already present risk of bleeding, particularly from the gastrointestinal tract, and sedatives can heighten uraemic cerebral depression).
• Altered bioavailability due to alteration in protein binding or volume distribution can affect drug effects and toxicity (e.g. phenytoin can cause cerebral toxicity despite normal total plasma drug levels due to decreased protein binding).
The safest practice in patients in renal failure is to:
• Reduce the number and dosage of drugs to the minimum.
• Use only drugs whose handling and safety in renal failure is known.
• Monitor plasma levels of potentially dangerous drugs.
• Avoid nephrotoxic drugs, since these can lead to a cycle of drug accumulation, impairment of function and then further drug accumulation.

Table 34.1 Renally excreted drugs

Anti-infective agents
Aminoglycoside antibiotics** (e.g. gentamicin, kanamycin, streptomycin)
Nitrofurantoin***
Tetracyclines***, particularly oxytetracycline, tetracycline
Vancomycin**
Penicillins and cephalosporins (varies)*
Trimethoprim-sulphamethoxazole**

*Diuretics***

*Digoxin***

Hypoglycaemic agents
Tolbutamide*, glibenclamide* (active metabolites)
Insulin*

Beta-adrenergic blocking drugs (varies)
Atenolol**

*Captopril***

In renal failure:
* Minor dose adjustments usually required.
** Major dose adjustments required.
*** Avoid

Dose adjustments in renal failure

Many drugs require major dose adjustments in renal failure. The loading dose is usually the same, and the options are to decrease the maintenance doses, or to increase the interval between them (Fig. 34.1). In practice a combination of these approaches is usually

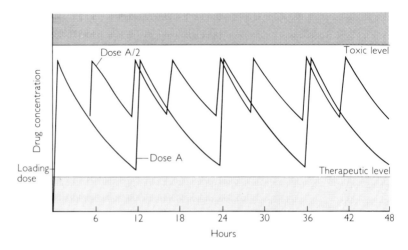

Fig. 34.1 Options for dose alterations for renally excreted drugs (e.g. gentamicin) in renal failure: either the same dose (A) less frequently or reduced dose (A/2) at the same frequency

employed to produce a sensible regimen. For example if a dose of 80 mg 8-hourly, i.e. 240 mg total daily dose, is to be reduced by 75%, as would occur with gentamicin in a person whose GFR is 25% of normal, a sensible regimen might be 60 mg every 24 hours, with close monitoring of the resultant drug concentrations.

Aminoglycoside antibiotics	Gentamicin, kanamycin, streptomycin and other aminoglycoside antibiotics are almost entirely renally excreted, and are both nephrotoxic and ototoxic. It is our practice to give the usual loading dose and then to adjust the dosage according to peak and trough blood levels. As a rough guide, since excretion is proportional to GFR, the dose is reduced proportionally to GFR, or inversely with plasma creatinine, e.g. if plasma creatinine is 0.16 mmol/litre in a patient in whom normal plasma creatinine would be expected to be 0.08 mmol/litre the daily dose is reduced by 50%, usually mainly by increasing dose interval.
Digoxin	Digoxin is predominantly renally excreted, with a normal half-life of 0.5 day increasing to 4.4 days in anuric patients. The drug is not removed by dialysis since it is heavily protein bound. Commonly the loading dose is reduced by 25% and the dose reduced to 0.0625 mg daily or less in anuric patients, according to plasma levels.
Vancomycin	This drug is mainly renally excreted and very protein bound, hence not dialysable. Dosage is very reduced in CRF, and dose intervals of up to 7 days have been shown to be necessary in dialysis-dependent patients.
Oral hypoglycaemics	Chlorpropamide, tolbutamide, and glibenclamide are all partially renally excreted or have active renally excreted metabolites. Their dose often needs to be reduced in renal failure and blood glucose should be monitored. Gliclazide may be safer.
Insulin	Insulin resistance is usually outweighed by the increased half-life of insulin due to decreased renal catabolism. Therefore, doses are usually less, and are monitored according to blood glucose levels.
Allopurinol	Toxic metabolites of this drug are renally excreted. A syndrome of skin rash, hepatitis and nephrotoxicity can occur in renal failure if it is used in excessive dosage. The dose should be reduced to 100 mg daily once the plasma creatinine is elevated (GFR < 50 ml/min) and to 100 mg on alternate days in ESRF patients on dialysis. The plasma uric acid should be monitored.

Nitrofurantoin　　Nitrofurantoin should be avoided in renal failure. It is ineffective in treating urine infection in renal failure, and accumulation can cause peripheral neuropathy.

Tetracyclines　　Tetracyclines other than doxycycline are all at least partially renally excreted. Their use in renal failure can result in drug accumulation which causes a catabolic and acidosis producing effect. The resultant nausea and vomiting can then lead to prerenal renal failure and further drug accumulation. Tetracyclines other than doxycycline should be avoided in renal failure.

NEPHROTOXICITY

There are a variety of ways in which drugs can alter or decrease renal function (Table 34.2). Mechanisms include:
- Prerenal effects.
- Allergic disease:
  (a) glomerular, and
  (b) tubulointerstitial.
- Tubular toxicity.

Extrarenal or prerenal effects　　Diuretics, by decreasing blood volume, can lead to dehydration, while drugs containing a high sodium content (e.g. Resonium A, urinary alkalinisers, effervescent calcium and phosphate pre-

---

Table 34.2　Drugs which may cause renal damage

Prerenal effects
Diuretics (dehydration)
Sodium-containing drugs (cardiac failure)

Allergic reactions
Glomerular disease
　　membranous glomerulonephritis (gold, penicillamine, captopril,
　　　mercury,tolbutamide, probenecid)
　　minimal change nephritis (NSAIDs)
　　drug-induced SLE (hydrallazine, procainamide)
Allergic tubulointerstitial nephritis (penicillins, sulphonamides, allopurinol)
(see Table 20.1)

Tubular toxicity
Directly toxic causing acute tubular necrosis — see Table 19.1
　　(aminoglycosides, amphotericin polymyxin, colystin)
Crystalluria or crystal deposition
　　(sulphonamides, ethacrynic acid fluothane oxalate crystals)
Renal papillary necrosis — causing analgesic nephropathy
　　(aspirin, phenacetin, NSAIDs)

---

parations) can precipitate cardiac failure. Increased catabolism, as with corticosteroids and tetracyclines, increases plasma urea and the resultant nausea and osmotic diuresis can cause dehydration.

Allergic drug-induced renal disease
Drug-induced glomerular disease

There are several glomerular abnormalities induced by various drugs:

Drug-induced membranous glomerulonephritis. Nephrotic syndrome, with a typical membranous picture in the renal biopsy (Chapter 15), can occur with gold, penicillamine, captopril and a variety of other agents. Most evidence suggests that the drugs themselves are not implanted in the glomeruli, rather that they affect other tissues, e.g. by causing release of renal tubular brush-border antigens which then deposit in glomeruli.

Drug-induced minimal change glomerulonephritis. Non-steroidal anti-inflammatory drugs (NSAIDs) are associated with the nephrotic syndrome, due to usually minimal change nephritis (Chapter 15), often in association with acute allergic interstitial nephritis (see below).

Drug-induced SLE. Several drugs, particularly procainamide and hydralazine, are associated with production of an SLE-like syndrome, with positive ANF and anti-DNA binding antibodies (Chapter 17). Predispositions include high dosage, female sex, slow acetylator status and DRw4. In some cases severe glomerular involvement can occur, particularly with hydralazine.

Drug-induced allergic tubulo-interstitial nephritis

Acute allergic interstitial nephritis (Chapter 20) is an important cause of acute renal failure. Common causes include trimethoprim-sulphamethoxazole and amoxycillin (Table 20.1).

Tubular nephrotoxicity

Tubular cell toxins. Some drugs are directly toxic to renal tubular cells, and may cause acute tubular necrosis (Chapter 19) The toxicity depends on renal tubular luminal drug concentrations, and is increased by:
- High dose or duration of treatment.
- Old age.
- Poor renal function.
- Salt and water depletion.
- The presence of other nephrotoxins.

The commonest direct nephrotoxins are aminoglycoside antibiotics and radiocontrast agents, but many other drugs and industrial toxins can also cause acute tubular necrosis (Table 19.1).

Crystalluria and tubular damage. Some drugs can cause renal failure by obstruction of the lumen by crystals of the drug. Modern sulphonamides rarely cause sulphonamide crystal deposition, but ethacrynic acid can cause this problem.

Crystal formation and tubular obstruction occurs with uric acid crystals when treating myeloproliferative disorders (Chapter 24), and tubular obstruction perhaps contributes to radiocontrast nephrotoxicity especially in myeloma patients. Crystal deposition in tubular cells and the lumen with oxalate crystals probably plays a major role in acute renal failure in fluothane and ethylene glycol nephrotoxicity.

SPECIFIC DRUGS AND THE KIDNEY

NSAIDs

The NSAIDs have a wide variety of effects on the kidney. These include:

• *Acute reduction in GFR* in the presence of dehydration or other prerenal factors. This is believed to be an effect of reduction in vasodilatory intrarenal prostanoids. Occasionally acute tubular necrosis can occur.

• *Acute allergic tubulointerstitial nephritis* (TIN), which may in some cases be associated with a concurrent nephrotic syndrome (see below). The acute TIN can present as ARF and is commonly:

(a) in elderly patients;
(b) months after commencing the drug;
(c) not associated with any other evidence of allergy.

• *Acute nephrotic syndrome*, with a glomerular picture of minimal change disease (Chapter 15).

• *Analgesic nephropathy* with renal papillary necrosis (Chapter 22).

• *Acute hyperkalaemia*, particularly in patients with impaired function.

Aminoglycoside antibiotics

Aminoglycoside antibiotics (gentamicin, kanamycin, tobramycin, netilmycin, streptomycin, neomycin, etc.) are currently the most common causes of drug-induced renal failure. Aminoglycoside-induced ARF is typically:

• Associated with prolonged and higher doses.

• Non-oliguric.

• Slow to recover.

• Seen in older patients and those with other factors such as sepsis and renal failure from other causes.

Amphotericin B

Amphotericin B exerts its main toxic effect on the distal tubule. The syndrome includes:
- Use of over 600−1000 mg of amphotericin.
- Preceded by renal potassium wasting, nephrogenic diabetes insipidus and distal renal tubular acidosis.
- Incomplete recovery if amphotericin is continued.

Radiographic contrast agents

Renal damage due to radiocontrast agents is becoming increasingly common, particularly with the large volumes of dye used in arteriography and contrast-enhanced CT scanning.

Mechanisms seem to include direct tubular toxicity, tubular obstruction, and occasional allergic reaction. Nephrotoxicity with radiographic contrast agents is most likely in patients with:
- Multiple myeloma.
- Diabetes mellitus.
- Pre-existing renal failure.
- Dehydration or salt depletion.
- Old age.

Cyclosporin A

The nephrotoxicity of this immunosuppressive agent is particularly important as it is commonly used in renal transplantation, where acute tubular necrosis, acute allograft rejection and other causes of ARF are also common.

The drug is nephrotoxic in two main ways. First it is a tubular nephrotoxin, in that it seems to reduce blood supply to the medulla, predisposing to acute tubular necrosis if there is also hypotension or dehydration. The effect is partly dose dependent and often an improvement in function will occur with dose reduction. Second, in bone-marrow transplant recipients especially, a severe thrombotic microangiopathy can occur. Both effects may relate to modification of intrarenal prostaglandins.

Lithium

Lithium carbonate treatment, as given for manic-depressive illness, induces in most patients a mild syndrome of polyuria−polydipsia, and in a small minority severe vasopressin resistant diabetes insipidus, particularly if toxic plasma levels occur. This is usually reversible with cessation of the drug. There is evidence that prolonged use may cause irreversible tubulointerstitial nephritis.

35: *Dialysis and Transplantation*

With the advent of dialysis and transplantation very few patients now die from renal failure alone. In chronic renal failure, integrated programmes, where patients are managed by various forms of dialysis or transplantation as their medical condition and treatment availability dictates, have resulted in survival rates of over 90% at 1 year and 70% at 5 years. In most cases the quality of life is very acceptable, with 60% of dialysis patients and 95% of transplant patients able to work.

DIALYSIS

In dialysis the patient's blood is separated by a semipermeable membrane from dialysis fluid (dialysate), and waste solutes (e.g. urea, creatinine, potassium) diffuse from the blood into the fluid.

There are two major methods of dialysis: haemodialysis and peritoneal dialysis. Both can readily be performed by the patient in the home.

Haemodialysis

In this procedure the blood is passed outside the body (extracorporeal) through an artificial kidney (dialyser). The membrane in the dialyser is a cellulose or synthetic material with pores which allow the passage of small molecules (up to about 1000 Da), but not of larger molecules and cells. The equipment is seen in Fig. 35.1.

Blood access devices

Access to the circulation, through which about 300–500 ml/min of blood can be removed and replaced, is required. Access devices include:

- Arteriovenous fistulas constructed by joining a peripheral artery to a subcutaneous vein. Usually the brachial artery and cephalic vein are joined at the wrist. The vein, carrying a large volume (about 500 ml/min) of arterial blood, becomes dilated, thick-walled and easy to needle. Two large bore needles (to and from the dialyser) are inserted for each dialysis. This is the access of choice for chronic renal failure.
- Artificial conduits which are inserted under the skin to join an artery and vein.

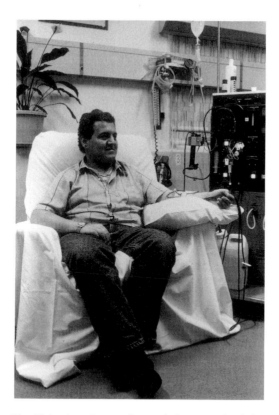

Fig. 35.1 A patient on haemodialysis. On his left can be seen the dialysis machine with the dialyser in a clamp on the side

- Arteriovenous shunts. A Teflon cannula is placed in a large artery and a large vein and between dialyses the cannulas are joined by silastic tubing. Disadvantages include clotting, infection and the problems of a plastic tube permanently outside the body. Shunts are now rarely used, and usually only for acute access.
- Subclavian or femoral vein or artery catheters for acute access.

Dialysers

Three major forms of dialyser — parallel plate, coil and hollow fibre dialysers are available. Most common are hollow fibre dialysers (Fig. 35.2).

Dialysate

A typical formula for haemodialysate is given in Table 35.1. Urea, creatinine, potassium, phosphate, uric acid, and a wide variety of other blood constituents diffuse from the patient along a concentration gradient, while acetate or bicarbonate diffuse in, correcting acidosis. The dialysate is prepared by machines which mix a fixed proportion of a dialysate concentrate with water (proportioning machines).

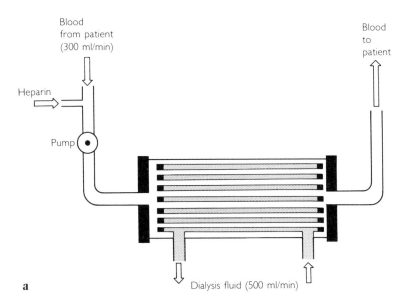

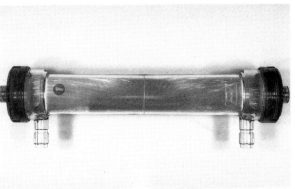

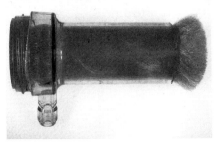

Fig. 35.2 (a) Haemodialysis circuit in a hollow fibre dialyser — blood and dialysate pass in a countercurrent fashion separated by a semipermeable membrane. (b) Hollow fibre dialyser — blood passes through the end and dialysate through side ports. (c) Hollow fibre dialyser cut to demonstrate the capillary fibres of semipermeable membrane (e.g. cuprophane)

Table 35.1 Composition of haemodialysate and plasma compared

	Dialysate* (mmol/litre)	Plasma (mmol/litre)
Sodium	138 (130–140)	135–145
Potassium	2 (0–3)	3.5–54
Acetate or bicarbonate	40	20–30
Calcium	1.5–2.5	2.1–2.6
Magnesium	0.25	0.7–1.3

* With added clean (not sterile) water in which contaminants are negligible; heated to 37°C and deaerated. Usual flow 500 ml/min.

The water is usually pretreated to remove organic contaminants (e.g. insecticides), deliberately added contaminants normally found in our water supplies (e.g. aluminium, fluoride, chlorine) and other particulate and ionic contaminants (e.g. solids, calcium in hard water).

Dialysis machine

The dialysis machine has a proportioning machine, a blood pump and monitoring devices. Blood flow rates are usually 100–300 ml/min. Modern dialysis machines have a large number of monitors and alarms to ensure patient safety. Whenever any of these alarms is activated the patient is isolated from the machine by occlusion clamps on the arterial and venous tubing.

Anticoagulation

Heparin is added to the blood as it enters the system to prevent coagulation in the blood circuit; consequently patients are also anticoagulated during the procedure.

Haemodialysis regimen

Most patients haemodialyse for 3 to 5 hours three times per week. Since the clearances of creatinine and urea are around 100–150 ml/min during the dialysis this still achieves only overall clearances of about 5–10 ml/min when calculated for the whole week. Accordingly predialysis plasma creatinine and urea concentrations are usually above 0.8 mmol/litre and 20 mmol/litre respectively, i.e. the patient is held in a state of chronic uraemia of near end-stage severity. During the procedure water is removed from the patient by exerting negative pressure on the dialysate compartment of the dialyser (ultrafiltration). The patient gains fluid volume and weight between dialyses (usually 0 to 3 kg), and must restrict fluid and salt intake to prevent fluid overload and hypertension. The usual restriction is to a daily intake of 60 g of protein, 60 mmol of sodium, 60 mmol of potassium and a fluid intake of 500 ml plus urine output.

Peritoneal dialysis

In peritoneal dialysis the peritoneal membrane is the semi-permeable dialysing membrane. Dialysate is similar to haemo-dialysis dialysate except that the fluid must be sterile and it contains glucose (1–4 g/dl) to provide osmotic forces to remove fluid from the patient. The basic procedure is infusion of 2 litre of peritoneal dialysate into the peritoneal cavity where it is left to equilibrate, then drained. This can be repeated continuously, as is commonly the case in acute PD, or with variable 'dwell times', as is usual in chronic PD. With chronic intermittent peritoneal dialysis about 10 cycles, each of 2 litre, are performed on three occasions per week, usually overnight.

Continuous ambulatory peritoneal dialysis (CAPD) is a useful method for home dialysis. A permanent peritoneal catheter (Tenchkoff catheter) is inserted, and the patient performs four to five exchanges of 2 litre of fluid (less in children) each day. Creatinine clearances of about 10 ml/min are achieved, i.e. patient biochemistry is similar to that in haemodialysis. The procedure provides continuous dialysis and is generally preferred over haemo-dialysis in children, diabetics, and patients with cardiovascular disease in whom vascular access may be difficult and the tolerance of the fluctuations associated with haemodialysis poorly tolerated.

HAEMOFILTRATION

This procedure is particularly useful in the management of acute renal failure where continuous arteriovenous haemofiltration (CAVH) has special advantages.

Ultrafiltration, where hydrostatic pressure causes filtration of plasma through a semipermeable membrane, is the basis of this technique. Large volumes of an ultrafiltrate of plasma are removed and replaced with infusion of electrolyte-containing fluid. The process thus resembles glomerular filtration, and the clearance is equal to the ultrafiltration rate. Larger molecules, i.e. of MW above 1000–10 000 Da are better removed by this procedure than with haemodialysis.

Haemofiltration can be performed intermittently (e.g. 20 litre three times a week) but is most often used continuously in CAVH where a very simple circuit without a blood pump is all that is required (Fig. 35.3). In CAVH ultrafiltration rates of 300–1200 ml/hour may be achieved, providing continuous removal of both toxins and fluid, with clearances of 5 to 20 ml/min. A further modification uses a pump to provide veno–venous hemofiltration (CVVH), and even greater clearances can be achieved by a slow (1–2 litre/hour) flow of dialysate in the outer compartment

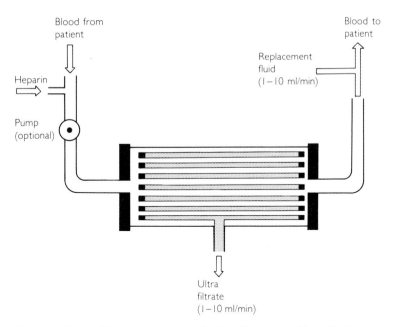

Fig. 35.3 Haemofiltration circuit in a hollow fibre haemofilter. Fluid passes across the membrane from the blood to drain. The rate of fluid removal equals the 'clearance' of small molecules

(CVVHD). CVVHD is now the usual method of managing acute renal failure in our intensive care unit.

MEDICAL PROBLEMS OF CHRONIC DIALYSIS

The medical problems of chronic dialysis may be divided into:
1 Complications of chronic renal failure.
2 Complications of the procedure — haemodialysis or peritoneal dialysis.

Complications of renal failure

Haemodialysis and peritoneal dialysis achieve clearances of only 5–10 ml/min when calculated across a whole week. The patient is thus held in a suspended state of chronic uraemia. Dialysis does nothing to replace erythropoietin and vitamin D nor to correct other hormonal deficiencies.

Major problems are anaemia, bone disease, cardiovascular disease, infection and the two more recently described complications of chronic dialysis, aluminium toxicity and dialysis-related amyloid osteodystrophy.

Anaemia in dialysis patients

Persistent anaemia is a problem affecting most dialysis patients — haemoglobin concentrations range from about 4 to 15 g/dl, and average about 8 g/dl. It is mainly due to erythropoietin deficiency, uraemic marrow depression and reduced red-cell life-span. It is aggravated by:

- Blood loss, as occurs in chronic haemodialysis.
- Bilateral nephrectomy.
- Aluminium toxicity (see below).
- Severe hyperparathyroidism, with marrow fibrosis.

Frequent transfusion will make the problem worse, as it tends to depress erythropoietin production and induce anti-red cell antibodies. Iron and folate supplements are usually given. Human erythropoietin (rHEpo) is now available for injection and has proven very effective in controlling anaemia in dialysis patients. The main disadvantage is its expense.

Bone disease in dialysis patients

Long-term dialysis patients have a high incidence of all forms of renal bone disease including aluminium-related bone disease.

Cardiovascular

The most common cause of death in dialysis and transplant patients is vascular disease. Cardiac failure secondary to fluid overload, hypertension and anaemia is common, and can be aggravated by the 300 to 500 ml/min of blood passing through the AV fistula. Hypertension occurs unless fluid volume is kept low. In about 5% of patients blood pressure cannot be controlled by limiting body fluid, very high plasma renin concentrations are found, and the elevated blood pressure responds to nephrectomy or angiotensin-converting enzyme inhibitors. Hyperlipidaemia and hypercholesteraemia are commonly found in dialysis patients.

Infection

The second most common cause of death is infection, including septicaemia related to fistula needling or peritonitis. Hepatitis B and AIDS are potential risks to both patients and the staff, and all patients should be screened for these diseases and immunised against hepatitis B.

Psychosocial aspects of chronic dialysis

The psychosocial problems of maintenance dialysis patients cannot be overstated. The interference with normal work, home, social and sexual life can be devastating in a minority of patients, and continuous medical and social worker surveillance is essential.

Aluminium toxicity

Aluminium in dialysis water and in aluminium hydroxide used as an oral phosphate binder is responsible for a syndrome characterised by:

- Osteomalacic bone disease.
- Dementia.
- Anaemia.

Aluminium-related osteomalacia, caused by deposition at the ossification front is characterised by bone pain, multiple fractures, soft tissue calcification and an elevated plasma calcium.

Aluminium-related encephalopathy is characterised by ataxia, dysarthria and dementia with a rapidly progressive and fatal course.

Aluminium-related anaemia is hypochromic and microcytic, resembling iron deficiency anaemia.

Prevention of aluminium toxicity includes treatment of water to remove aluminium (it is deliberately added in dams as 'alum' to sediment suspended materials), and avoidance, as far as possible, of aluminium hydroxide as a phosphate binder. Treatment involves intravenous desferrioxamine, 1 g i.v. three times per week, which will remove aluminium from the circulation and tissues. The best treatment is transplantation.

Dialysis-related amyloid

Carpal tunnel syndrome and wrist joint arthritis occurs because of deposition of β_2-microglobulin as amyloid in synovia and bone cysts. It occurs usually after 10 years of haemodialysis. In all dialysis patients there are high plasma concentrations of β_2-microglobulin, which is normally a renally excreted plasma protein. This appears to relate to poor removal of β_2-microglobulin by dialysis. At present no effective prevention is proven, and the only treatment is successful renal transplantation.

Procedure related problems
Haemodialysis

Bleeding. Patients are heparinised with each treatment, as well as having uraemic platelet disorders. Haemarthrosis, gastrointestinal, retroperitoneal, cerebral and access site bleeding can occur.

Infection. Access needling can introduce organisms. Staphylococcal septicaemia is a frequent result.

Cardiovascular collapse. Rapid fluid removal, poor acetate metabolism and the rapid fall in plasma potassium concentration inducing arrythmia all contribute to a common syndrome of cardiovascular collapse on dialysis.

Hypoxaemia. During haemodialysis, especially with first use of cellophane based membranes, a fall in PO_2 of 5–10% regularly occurs. Non-cellulose dialysers should be used in intensive care, since this hypoxaemia appears to be a result of poor biocompatibility, perhaps via complement activation and polymorph margination in the lungs.

Dialysis disequilibrium. This acute postdialysis confusional state particularly occurs in older patients subjected to rapid dialysis. It is due to blood to brain osmotic, pH and other gradients. Cerebral oedema can occur.

Peritoneal dialysis

Peritoneal infection is the main bugbear of peritoneal dialysis. There is about one episode per patient per year. Improved techniques may reduce this but it remains a limitation, and occasional cause of death.

Tenchoff catheter obstruction occurs due to omental wrapping, fibrin deposition and other causes. The catheter usually requires replacement.

Peritoneal membrane failure can occur in patients with multiple peritonitis or operations and can result in failure of the technique.

RENAL TRANSPLANTATION

Renal transplants can be from live donors (living donor transplants) or from cerebrally dead donors (cadaver donors).

Donors

Best results are achieved with identical twin donors since they are immunologically identical. Otherwise a high degree of compatibility for the human leukocyte antigens (HLA), especially HLA-B and HLA-Dr antigens which are carried on chromosome 6, is preferred.

Donors are screened for
- Blood and HLA compatibility.
- Renal function and anatomy.
- Hypertension.
- Infections including hepatitis B and HTLV III antibodies (AIDS).
- Carcinoma.

Recipients

Transplantation should be performed only in patients who are physically well other than from the chronic renal failure. Patients are screened for:
- HLA and blood group.
- Infections especially pulmonary tuberculosis.
- Cardiac and other general medical complaints.
- Hepatitis B and HIV antibodies.
- Peptic ulcer disease.

Operation

The donor kidney is usually placed in an extraperitoneal position in the iliac fossa. The artery is anastomosed to the internal or common iliac artery and the vein to the external iliac vein. The ureter is inserted into the bladder with an antireflux procedure.

Drugs

Immunosuppressant drugs are given to prevent loss of the kidney due to immune rejection by the recipient. Most centres use a combination of corticosteroids, azathioprine and cyclosporin. High doses of steroids and antilymphocyte antibodies are also used to combat acute rejection (see below).

Corticosteroids

Prednisolone and other corticosteroids are important drugs both in chronic immunosuppression and treatment of acute rejection (see below). Usually a maintenance dose of 10 mg orally daily is given. In the first 6 months higher doses are usual. Common steroid-induced complications are listed in Table 35.2.

Azathioprine

This mercaptopurine (alkylating agent) precursor interferes with immune cell numbers and activity. Its major side effects are bone marrow depression and predisposition to infection. Usual doses are 75−150 mg/day (1−3 mg/kg/day).

Cyclosporin

Cyclosporin is a very lipid soluble agent which interferes with T-lymphocyte mediated immune responses. Side effects include dose-related nephrotoxicity (Chapter 34), hepatotoxicity, hypertension, hirsutism and gingival hypertrophy. Usual doses are 5−15 mg/kg/day, with blood level monitoring.

Antilymphocyte antibodies

Antilymphocyte globulin (ALG), antithymocyte globulin (ATG) and monoclonal antilymphocyte antibodies (e.g. OKT_3) are often used to treat acute rejection. They are injected intravenously and cause a rapid fall in circulating lymphocyte count. Common reactions include fever, pulmonary oedema and infections, particularly with cytomegalovirus.

Complications of transplantation
Renal complications

Acute tubular necrosis. About 10−20% of cadaver kidneys do not immediately function but go through a conventional ATN course (Chapter 19). This interferes with graft monitoring since rejection is more difficult to detect.

Table 35.2 Common side-effects of corticosteroids

Facial obesity, acne and erythema
Truncal obesity with prominent striae
Peptic ulceration
Osteoporosis
Growth failure in children
Aseptic necrosis of the hips
Lens cataracts
Precipitation of diabetes
Predisposition to infection
Hypertension

Operative complications. Renal artery or vein occlusions, ureteric or bladder leaks, lymphocele and other surgical complications occur in less than 5% of patients.

Acute rejection is the cause of loss of about 5 to 10% of grafts in the first year after transplantation. Most patients experience one or more acute rejection episodes. These are characterised by:
• Deterioration in renal function.
• Swelling and tenderness of the graft kidney.
• Fever.
• Oliguria, fluid gain and sometimes hypertension.
   Diagnosis is confirmed by renal biopsy which shows mononuclear cell infiltrates, and vessel changes of intimal hyperplasia. Endothelial cell injury and thromboses are bad prognostic features.
   Treatment involves:
• Short courses of high dose prednisolone.
• Courses of ATG, ALG or OKT$_3$.

Chronic rejection. A slow process of gradual graft loss commonly occurs. Renal biopsy shows a chronic tubulointerstitial nephritis with marked vessel intimal hyperplasia. No therapy is available and this is the commonest cause of graft loss after 12 months.

Renal artery stenosis. A stenosis develops at the site of arterial anastomosis in a small percentage of patients. Increasing blood pressure and falling function are usual. A renal artery bruit is common, but bruits over grafts are commonly heard in the absence of stenosis. If thrombosis occurs the graft dies since it has no collateral supply.

Non-renal complications

Common complications are drug related (see above) and include:
• *Infection.* This is the commonest cause of early patient death. Bacterial (pneumonia, sepsis, reactivation of tuberculosis), viral (cytomegalovirus, herpes simplex and zoster), protozoal (*Pneumocystis*) and fungal (*Candida, Cryptococcus*) infections all can occur in these highly immunosuppressed patients.
• *Vascular disease* (myocardial, cerebral) is the commonest cause of late patient death. Multiple factors, including predialysis chronic renal failure and posttransplant hypertension and chronic renal failure, all play a role.
• *Tumours.* In Australia over 50% of patients 10 years posttransplant have skin cancers. Non-skin cancers (lymphoma particularly) are also increased in frequency by about 100-fold. Immunosuppression is generally blamed, although oncogenic viruses are possibly involved.

Further Reading

MAJOR TEXTS

Brenner B.M. & Rector F.C. (eds) (1986) *The Kidney* (3rd edition). W.B. Saunders Co., Philadelphia.
Massry S.G. & Glassock R.J. (eds) (1983) *Textbook of Nephrology*. Williams & Wilkins, Baltimore.
Schrier R.W. & Gottschalk C.W. (eds) (1988) *Diseases of the Kidney* (4th edition). Little, Brown & Co., Boston.

CHAPTER 1

Renal Anatomy

Coupland R.E. (1972) The anatomy of the human kidney. In Black, Sir Douglas (ed.), *Renal Disease* (3rd edition), pp. 1–52. Blackwell Scientific Publications, Oxford.
Gosling J.A., Dixon, J.S. & Humpherson J.R. (1983) *Functional Anatomy of the Urinary Tract*. Churchill Livingstone, London.
Heptinstall R.H. (1983) *Pathology of the Kidney*, pp. 1–60. Little, Brown & Co., Boston.
Kincaid-Smith P. & Whitworth J.A.W. (1987) *The Kidney, A Clinicopathological Study* (2nd edition), pp. 3–16. Blackwell Scientific Publications, Oxford.
Moffat D.B. (1979) The anatomy of the renal circulation. In Black, Sir Douglas & Jones F.N. (eds), *Renal Disease* (4th edition), pp. 3–29. Blackwell Scientific Publications, Oxford.

CHAPTER 2

Renal Imaging

Asscher A.W., Moffat D.B. & Sanders E. (1982) *Nephrology Illustrated, An Integrated Text and Colour Atlas*. Pergamon Medical Publications, Oxford.
Britton K.E. (1979) Radionuclides in the investigation of renal disease. In Black, Sir Douglas & Jones F.N. (eds), *Renal Disease* (4th edition), pp. 270–304. Blackwell Scientific Publications, Oxford.
Doyle T., Hare T., Thomson K. & Tress B. (1989) *Procedures in Diagnostic Radiology* (2nd edition). Churchill Livingstone, Edinburgh.
Fitzgerald-Finch O.P. (1981) *Renal Radiology and Imaging*. MTP Press Limited, Lancaster.
Pollack H.M. (ed.) (1990) *Clinical Urography*. W.B. Saunders Co., Philadelphia.
Resnick M.I. & Sanders R.C. (eds) (1984) *Ultrasound in Urology* (2nd edition). Williams & Wilkins, Baltimore.
Weill F.S., Bihr E., Rohmer P. & Zeltner F. (eds) (1986) *Renal Sonography* (2nd edition). Springer-Verlag, Berlin.

Renal Biopsy and Pathology

Brun C. & Olsen S. (1981) *Atlas of Renal Biopsy*. W.B. Saunders Co., Munksgaard.
Churg J. & Sobin L.H. (1982) *Renal Disease, Classification and Atlas of Glomerular Disease*. Igaku-Shoin Ltd, Tokyo.

371

Dunhill M.S. (1984) *Pathological Basis of Renal Disease* (2nd edition). Baillière Tindall, London.

Heptinstall R.H. (1983) *Pathology of the Kidney* (3rd edition). Little, Brown & Co., Boston.

Kincaid-Smith P., Dowling J. & Mathews D. (1985) *Diagnostic Atlas of Kidney Pathology. Morphological and Clinical Correlations.* ADIS Health Science Press, Sydney.

Kincaid-Smith P. & Whitworth J.A.W. (1987) *The Kidney. A Clinicopathological Study* (2nd edition). Blackwell Scientific Publications, Oxford.

Mandel A.K. (1979) *Electron Microscopy of the Kidney in Renal Disease and Hypertension.* Plenum Medical Book Co., New York.

CHAPTERS 3 & 4

Renal Physiology

Ballermann B.J., Levenson D.J. & Brenner B.M. (1986) Renin, angiotensin, kinins, prostaglandins, and leukotrienes. In Brenner B.M. & Rector F.C. (eds), *The Kidney*, pp. 281–342. W.B. Saunders Co., Philadelphia.

Brenner B.M., Hostetter T.H. & Humes H.D. (1978) Molecular basis of proteinuria of glomerular origin. *New Eng J Med* **298**, 826–833.

Dunn M.J. (ed.) (1983) *Renal Endocrinology.* William & Wilkins, Baltimore.

Norris S.H. (1990) Renal eicosanoids. *Sem Nephrol* **10**, 64–88.

Renkin E.M. & Robinson R.R. (1974) Glomerular filtration. *New Eng J Med* **290**, 785–792.

Ryan G.B. (1986) The glomerular filtration barrier. In Lote C.J. (ed.), *Advances in Renal Physiology* pp. 1–32. Croom Helm, London.

Seldin D.W. & Giebisch G. (eds) (1985) *The Kidney, Physiology and Pathophysiology.* Raven Press, New York.

CHAPTER 5

Assessment of Renal Function

Cockcroft D.W. & Gault M.H. (1976) Prediction of creatinine clearance from serum creatinine. *Nephron* **16**, 31–41.

Gabriel R. (1986) Time to scrap creatinine clearance? *Br Med J* **293**, 1119–1120.

Kassirer J.P. & Harrington J.J. (1988) Laboratory evaluation of renal function. In Schrier R.W. & Gottschalk C.W. (eds), *Diseases of the Kidney* (4th edition), pp. 393–441. Little, Brown & Co., Boston.

Levey A.S. (1990) Measurement of renal function in chronic renal disease. *Kidney Int* **38**, 167–184.

Mitch W.E., Walser M., Buffington G.A. & Lehman J. Jr (1976) A simple method of estimating progression of chronic renal failure. *Lancet* **ii**, 1326–1328.

CHAPTER 6

Pathophysiology of Renal Failure

Anderson S. & Brenner B.M. (1989) Progressive renal disease, a disorder of adaptation. *Quart J Med* **263**, 185–189.

Diamond J.R. & Karnovsky M.J. (1988) Focal and segmental glomerulosclerosis, analogies to atherosclerosis. *Kidney Int* **33**, 917–924.

Eschbach J.W. (1989) The anemia of chronic renal failure, pathophysiology and the effect of recombinant erythropoietin. *Kidney Int* **35**, 134–148.

Fine L. (1986) The biology of renal hypertrophy. *Kidney Int* **29**, 619–634.

Klahr S., Schreiner G. & Ichikawa I. (1988) The progression of renal disease. *New Eng J Med* **318**, 1657–1666.

Schrier R.W., Harris D.C.H., Chan L. *et al.* (1988) Tubular metabolism as a factor in the progression of chronic renal failure. *Am J Kid Dis* **12**, 243−249.

Scmitz P.G., Kasiske B.L., O'Donnell M.P. & Keane W.F. (1989) Lipids and progressive renal injury. *Semin Nephrol* **9**, 354−369.

Walser M. (1990) Progression of chronic renal failure in man. *Kidney Int* **37**, 1195−1210.

Wesson L.G. (1989) Compensatory growth and other growth responses of the kidney. *Nephron* **51**, 149−184.

CHAPTER 7

Clinical Approach

Schrier R.W. (ed.) (1990) *Manual of Nephrology, Diagnosis and Therapy.* Little, Brown & Co., Boston.

CHAPTER 8

Urinalysis

Birch D.F. & Fairley K.F. (1982) A simplified method of identifying glomerular bleeding. *Kidney Int* **2**, 105−108.

Fairley K.F. (1988) Urinalysis. In Schrier R.W. & Gottschalk C.W. (eds), *Diseases of the Kidney* (4th edition), pp. 359−391. Little, Brown & Co., Boston.

Gibbs D.D. & Lynn K.L. (1990) Red cell volume distribution curves in the diagnosis of glomerular and non-glomerular haematuria. *Clin Nephrol* **33**, 143−147.

Piccoli G., Varese D. & Rotuno M. (1984) *Atlas of Urinary Sediments, Diagnosis and Clinical Correlations in Nephrology.* Raven Press, New York.

CHAPTER 9

Syndromes of Glomerular Disease

Bernard D.B. (1988) Extrarenal complications of the nephrotic syndrome. *Kidney Int* **33**, 1184−1202.

Cameron J.S. (1979) The natural history of glomerulonephritis. In Black, Sir Douglas & Jones F.N. (eds), *The Kidney* (4th edition), pp. 329−383. Blackwell Scientific Press, Oxford.

Cameron J.S. (1984) Acute renal failure in glomerular disease. In Andreucci V.E. (ed.), *Acute Renal Failure*, pp. 271−295. Martinus Nijhoff, Boston.

Cameron J.S. (1987) The nephrotic syndrome and its complications. *Am J Kid Dis* **10**, 157−171.

Cameron J.S. & Glassock R.J. (1988) *The Nephrotic Syndrome.* Marcel Decker, New York.

Couser W.G. (1982) Idiopathic rapidly progressive glomerulonephritis. *Am J Nephrol* **2**, 57−69.

Couser W.G. (1988) Rapidly progressive glomerulonephritis, classification, pathogenetic mechanisms and therapy. *Am J Kid Dis* **11**, 449−464.

Glassock R.J. (1987) Clinical aspects of glomerular diseases. *Am J Kid Dis* **10**, 181−185.

Keane W.F. & Kasiske B.L. (1990) Hyperlipidemia in the nephrotic syndrome. *New Eng J Med* **323**, 603−604.

CHAPTER 10

Acute Renal Failure

Andreucci V.E. (ed.) (1984) *Acute Renal Failure.* Martinus Nijhoff, Boston.

Badr K.F. & Ichikawa I. (1988) Prerenal failure, a deleterious shift from renal compensation to decompensation. *New Eng J Med* **319**, 623−629.

Bihari D. & Nield G. (eds) (1990) *Acute Renal Failure in the Intensive Therapy Unit*. Springer-Verlag, Heidelberg.

Cameron J.S. (1986) Acute renal failure — the continuing challenge. *Quart J Med* **59**, 337–343.

Cameron J.S. (1990) Acute renal failure thirty years on. *Quart J Med* **273**, 1–2.

Chugh K.S., Sakhaja V., Malhotra H.S. & Pereira B. (1989) Changing trends in acute renal failure in third world countries, Chandigarh study. *Quart J Med* **272**, 1123–1173.

Hou S.H., Bushinsky D.A., Wish J.B. *et al.* (1983) Hospital acquired renal insufficiency, a prospective study. *Am J Med* **74**, 243–248.

Liano F., Garcia-Martin F., Gallego A. *et al.* (1989) Easy and early prognosis in acute tubular necrosis, a forward analysis of 228 cases. *Nephron* **51**, 307–313.

Myers B.D. & Moran S.M. (1986) Hemodynamically mediated acute renal failure. *New Eng J Med* **314**, 97–105.

Turney J.H., Marshall D.H., Brownjohn A.M. *et al.* (1990) The evolution of acute renal failure, 1955–1988. *Quart J Med* **273**, 83–104.

Whitworth J.A. (1989) Acute renal failure in surgical patients, prevention and recognition. *Aust NZ J Med* **59**, 835–836.

Wilkes B.M. & Mailloux L.U. (1986) Acute renal failure, pathogenesis and prevention. *Am J Med* **80**, 1129–1136.

CHAPTER 11

Chronic Renal Failure

Bennett W.M., Aroneff G.R., Morrison G. *et al.* (1983) Drug prescribing in renal failure, dosing guidelines for adults. *Am J Kid Dis* **3**, 155–193.

Curtis J.R. (1990) Intervention in chronic renal failure. Treatment may slow progression in severe cases. *Br J Med* **301**, 622–624.

Eggers, P.W. (1988) Effect of transplantation on the Medicare end-stage renal disease program. *New Engl J Med* **318**, 223–229.

Fine L.G. (1988) Preventing the progression of human renal disease. Have rational therapeutic principles emerged? *Kidney Int* **33**, 116–128.

Fraser C.L. & Arieff A.I. (1988) Nervous system complications in uraemia. *Annals Int Med* **109**, 143–153.

Kopple J.D., Winchester J., Massry S.G. & Heidland A. (eds) (1987) An update on nutrition and metabolism in kidney disease. *Kidney Int* (Supp 22).

Maher J.F. (ed.) (1989) *Replacement of Renal Function by Dialysis*. Kluwer Academic, Dordrecht.

Malluche H. & Faugere M-C. (1990) Renal bone disease 1990, an unmet challenge for the nephrologist. *Kidney Int* **38**, 193–211.

Remuzzi G. (1988) Bleeding in renal failure. *Lancet* **i**, 1205–1208.

Tufveson G., Geerlings W., Brunner F.P. *et al.* (1989) Combined report on regular dialysis and transplantation in Europe. *Nephrol Dial Transplant* **4** (Supp 2), 5–29.

CHAPTER 12

Hypertension

Calhoun D.A. & Oparil S. (1990) Treatment of hypertensive crisis. *New Eng J Med* **323**, 1177–1183.

Hunyor S. & Whitworth J.A.W. (eds) (1990) *Hypertension Management*. MacLennan & Petty, Sydney.

Kaplan N.M., Brenner B.M. & Laragh J.H. (eds) (1987) *The Kidney in Hypertension*. Raven Press, New York.

Kincaid-Smith P.S. & Whitworth J.A.W. (eds) (1982) *Hypertension, Mechanisms and Management*. ADIS Health Science Press, Sydney.

CHAPTER 13

Urinary Tract Infection

Asscher A.W. (1980) *The Challenge of Urinary Tract Infection*. Academic Press, London.

Bailey R.R. (1983) *Single Dose Therapy of Urinary Tract Infection*. ADIS Health Science Press, Sydney.

Editorial (1986) Urinary tract infection in the elderly. *Br Med J* **293**, 771–772.

Harber M.J. & Asscher A.W. (1985) Virulence of urinary pathogens. *Kidney Int* **28**, 717–721.

Kunin C.M. (1987) *Detection, Prevention and Management of Urinary Tract Infection* (4th Edition). Lea & Febiger, Philadelphia.

Lipsky B.A. (1989) Urinary tract infections in men. *Annals Int Med* **110**, 138–150.

McKerrow W., Davidson-Lamb N. & Jones P.F. (1984) Urinary tract infection in children. *Br Med J* **289**, 299–304.

Maskell R. (1988) *Urinary Tract Infection in Clinical and Laboratory Practice*. Edward Arnold, London.

Murphy B.F., Fairley K.F., Birch D.F. *et al.* (1984) Culture of a midcatheter specimen urine collected via an open-ended catheter, a reliable guide to bladder bacteriuria. *J Urol* **131**, 19–21.

Stamey T.A. (1980) *Urinary Infections*. Williams & Wilkins, Baltimore.

Stamm W.E., Counts G.W., Running K.R. *et al.* (1982) Diagnosis of coliform infection in acutely dysuric women. *New Eng J Med* **307**, 463–468.

Stamm W.E., Wagner K.F., Amsel R. *et al.* (1980) Causes of the urethral syndrome in women. *New Eng J Med* **303**, 409–415.

CHAPTER 14

Electrolyte and Acid–Base Disturbances

Goldberger E. (1986) *A Primer of Water, Electrolyte and Acid-Base Syndromes* (7th edition). Lea & Febiger, Philadelphia.

Schrier R.W. (ed.) (1986) *Renal and Electrolyte Disorders* (3rd edition). Little, Brown & Co., Boston.

Willatts S.M. (1986) *Lecture Notes on Fluid and Electrolyte Balance* (2nd edition). Blackwell Scientific Publications, Oxford.

Williams G.H. (1986) Hyporeninemic hypoaldosteronism. *New Eng J Med* **314**, 1041–1042.

CHAPTER 15

Primary Glomerular Diseases

Abuelo J.G., Esparza A.R., Matarese R.A. *et al.* (1984) Crescentic IgA nephropathy. *Quart J Med* **228**, 396–405.

Cameron J.S. (1979) The natural history of glomerulonephritis. In Black, Sir Douglas & Jones F.N. (eds), *The Kidney* (4th edition), pp. 329–383. Blackwell Scientific Press, Oxford.

Cameron J.S. (1984) The treatment of rapidly progressive crescentic glomerulonephritis and of Goodpasture's syndrome. In Suki W.N. & Massry S.G. (eds), *Therapy of Renal Diseases and Related Disorders*, pp. 210–219. Martinus Nijhoff, Boston.

Cameron J.S., Turner D.R., Heaton J. *et al.* (1983) Idiopathic mesangiocapillary glomerulonephritis, comparison of types I & II in children and adults and long-term prognosis. *Am J Med* **74**, 175–192.

Churg J. & Sobin L.H. (1982) *Renal Disease, Classification and Atlas of Glomerular Disease*. Igaku-Shoin Ltd, Tokyo.

Couser W.G. (1988) Rapidly progressive glomerulonephritis, classification, pathogenetic mechanisms and therapy. *Am J Kid Dis* **11**, 449–464.

D'Amico G. (1987) The commonest glomerulonephritis in the world, IgA nephropathy. *Quart J Med* **64**, 709–728.

D'Amico G., Minetti L., Ponticelli C. *et al.* (1986) Prognostic indicators in idiopathic IgA mesangial nephropathy. *Quart J Med* **59**, 363–378.

Heptinstall R.H. (1983) *Pathology of the Kidney* (3rd edition). Little, Brown & Co., Boston.

Kincaid-Smith P., D'Apice A.J.F. & Atkins R.C. (eds) (1979) *Progress in Glomerulonephritis*. Wiley Medical, New York.

Kincaid-Smith P., Dowling J. & Mathews D. (1985) *Diagnostic Atlas of Kidney Pathology. Morphological and Clinical Correlations*. ADIS Health Science Press, Sydney.

Kincaid-Smith P., Mathew T.H. & Becker E.L. (eds) (1973) *Glomerulonephritis, Morphology, Natural History and Treatment*. John Wiley & Sons, New York.

Kincaid-Smith P. & Whitworth J.A.W. (1987) *The Kidney, A Clinicopathological Study* (2nd edition). Blackwell Scientific Publications, Oxford.

Korbet S.M., Schwartz M.M. & Lewis E.J. (1986) The prognosis of focal glomerular sclerosis of adulthood. *Medicine* (Baltimore) **65**, 304–311.

Mallick N.P., Short C.D. & Manos J. (1983) Clinical membranous nephropathy. *Nephron* **34**, 209–219.

Nicholls K.M., Fairley K.F., Dowling J.P. & Kincaid-Smith P. (1984) The clinical course of mesangial IgA nephropathy. *Quart J Med* **53**, 227–250.

Nield G.H., Cameron J.S., Ogg C.S. *et al.* (1983) Rapidly progressive glomerulonephritis with extensive crescent formation. *Quart J Med* **52**, 395–416.

Rodicio J.L. (1984) Idiopathic IgA nephropathy. *Kidney Int* **25**, 717–729.

Rodriguez-Iturbe B. (1984) Epidemic poststreptococcal glomerulonephritis. *Kidney Int* **25**, 126–136.

Suki W.N. & Massry S.G. (eds) (1991) *Therapy of Renal Disease and Related Disorders* (2nd edition). Martinus Nijhoff, Boston.

Swainson C.P., Robson J.S., Thomson D. & MacDonald M.K. (1983) Mesangiocapillary glomerulonephritis. A long term study of 40 cases. *J Pathol* **141**, 449–468.

Zamurovic D. & Churg J. (1984) Idiopathic and secondary mesangiocapillary glomerulonephritis. *Nephron* **38**, 145–153.

CHAPTER 16

Goodpasture's Syndrome

Cameron J.S. (1984) The treatment of rapidly progressive crescentic glomerulonephritis and of Goodpasture's syndrome. In Suki W.N., Massry S.G. (eds), *Therapy of Renal Diseases and Related Disorders*, pp. 210–219. Martinus Nijhoff, Boston.

Leatherman J.W., Sibley R.K. & Davies S.F. (1982) Diffuse intrapulmonary haemorrhage and glomerulonephritis unrelated to anti-glomerular basement membrane antibody. *Am J Med* **72**, 401–410.

Walker R.G., Scheinkestel C., Becker G.J. *et al.* (1985) Clinical and morphological aspects of the management of crescentic anti-glomerular basement membrane antibody (anti-GBM) nephritis/Goodpasture's syndrome. *Quart J Med* **54**, 75–89.

CHAPTER 17

Systemic Lupus Erythematosus

Austin H.A., Muenz L.R., Joyce J.M. *et al.* (1983) Prognostic factors in lupus nephritis. Contribution of renal histologic data. *Am J Med* **75**, 382–391.

Editorial (1984) Antinuclear antibodies. *Lancet* **ii**, 611–613.

Hess E. (1988) Drug-related lupus. *New Eng J Med* **318**, 1460–1462.

Hughes G.R.V. (1984) Autoantibodies in lupus and its variants, experience in

1000 patients. *Br Med J* **289**, 339–342.

Ihle B.U., Whitworth J.A., Dowling J.P. & Kincaid-Smith P. (1984) Hydralazine and lupus nephritis. *Clin Nephrol* **22**, 230–238.

Leaker B., Becker G.J., Dowling J.P. & Kincaid-Smith P. (1986) Rapid improvement in lupus glomerular lesions following intensive plasma exchange. *Clin Nephrol* **25**, 236–244.

Leaker B., Fairley K.F. & Kincaid-Smith P. (1987) Lupus nephritis, clinical and pathological correlations. *Quart J Med* **62**, 123–179.

Rheumatoid Arthritis

Mutru O., Laasko M., Isomaki H. & Koota K. (1985) Ten year mortality and causes of death in patients with rheumatoid arthritis. *Br Med J* **290**, 1797–1799.

Ramirez G., Lambert R. & Bloomer H.A. (1981) Renal pathology in patients with rheumatoid arthritis. *Nephron* **29**, 124–126.

Sellars L., Siamopoulos K., Wilkinson R. *et al.* (1983) Renal biopsy appearances in rheumatoid arthritis. *Clin Nephrol* **20**, 114–120.

Scleroderma

Steen V.D., Medsger T.A., Osial T.A. *et al.* (1984) Factors predicting development of renal involvement in progressive systemic sclerosis. *Am J Med* **76**, 779–786.

Traub Y.M., Shapiro A.P., Rodnan G.P. *et al.* (1983) Hypertension and renal failure (scleroderma renal crisis) in progressive systemic sclerosis. *Medicine (Baltimore)* **62**, 335–352.

CHAPTER 18

Vasculitis

Editorial (1985) Systemic vasculitis. *Lancet* **i**, 1252–1253.

Editorial (1987) Renal micropolyarteritis. *Br Med J* **295**, 70–71.

Falk R.J. (1990) ANCA-associated renal disease. *Kidney Int* **38**, 998–1010.

Falk R.J. & Jennett J.C. (1988) Antineutrophil-cytoplasmic autoantibodies with specificity for myeloperoxidase in patients with systemic vasculitis and idiopathic necrotising and crescentic glomerulonephritis. *New Eng J Med* **318**, 1651–1657.

Fauci A.S., Haynes B.F., Katz P. & Wolff S.M. (1983) Wegener's granulomatosis, prospective clinical and therapeutic experience with 85 patients for 21 years. *Annals Int Med* **98**, 76–85.

Fuiano G., Cameron J.S., Raftery M. *et al.* (1988) Improved prognosis of renal microscopic polyarteritis in recent years. *Nephrol Dial Transplant* **3**, 383–391.

Haworth S.T., Savage C.O.S., Carr D. *et al.* (1985) Pulmonary haemorrhage complicating Wegener's granulomatosis and microscopic polyarteritis. *Br Med J* **290**, 1775–1778.

Jennett J.C. & Falk R.J. (1990) Antineutrophil cytoplasmic autoantibodies and associated diseases, a review. *Am J Kid Dis* **15**, 517–529.

Pinching A.J., Lockwood C.M., Pussell B.A. *et al.* (1983) Wegener's granulomatosis, observations on 18 patients with severe renal disease. *Quart J Med* **52**, 435–460.

Serra A., Cameron J.S., Turner D.R. *et al.* (1984) Vasculitis affecting the kidney, presentation, histopathology and long-term outcome. *Quart J Med* **53**, 181–207.

CHAPTER 19

Acute Tubular Necrosis

Better O.S. & Stein J.H. (1990) Early management of shock and prophylaxis of acute renal failure in traumatic rhabdomyolysis. *New Eng J Med* **322**, 825–829.

CHAPTER 20

Tubulointerstitial
Nephritis

Buysen J.G.M., Houhoff H.T., Krediet R.F. & Arisz L. (1990) Acute interstitial nephritis, a clinical and morphological study in 27 patients. *Nephrol Dial Transplant* **5**, 95–99.

Cameron J.S. (1988) Allergic interstitial nephritis. *Quart J Med* **66**, 97–115.

Eknoyan G., McDonald M.A., Appel D. & Truong L.D. (1990) Chronic tubulo-interstitial nephritis, correlation between structural and functional findings. *Kidney Int* **38**, 737–743.

Murray T. & Goldberg M. (1975) Chronic nephritis, etiologic factors. *Annals Int Med* **82**, 453–459.

Neilson E.G. (1989) Pathogenesis and therapy of interstitial nephritis. *Kidney Int* **35**, 1257–1270.

Pusey C.D., Saltissi D., Bloodworth L. *et al.* (1983) Drug associated acute interstitial nephritis, clinical and pathological features and the response to high dose steroid therapy. *Quart J Med* **52**, 194–214.

Sutton J.M. (1986) Urinary eosinophils. *Arch Intern Med* **146**, 2243–2244.

Ten R.M., Torres V.E., Milliner D.S. *et al.* (1987) Acute interstitial nephritis — immunologic and clinical aspects. *Mayo Clin Proc* **63**, 921–930.

CHAPTER 21

Reflux Nephropathy

Becker G.J. (1985) Reflux nephropathy. *Aust NZ J Med* **15**, 668–676.

Becker G.J., Ihle B.U., Fairley K.F. *et al.* (1986) Effect of pregnancy on moderate renal failure in reflux nephropathy. *Br Med J* **292**, 796–798.

Birmingham Reflux Study Group (1983) Prospective trial of operative versus non-operative treatment of severe vesicoureteric reflux, two years observation in 96 children. *Br Med J* **295**, 237–241.

Cotran R.S. (1982) Glomerulosclerosis in reflux nephropathy. *Kidney Int* **21**, 528–534.

El-Khatib M.T., Becker G.J. & Kincaid-Smith P. (1987) Morphometric aspects of reflux nephropathy. *Kidney Int* **32**, 261–266.

El-Khatib M.T., Becker G.J. & Kincaid-Smith P. (1990) Reflux nephropathy and primary vesicoureteric reflux in adults. *Quart J Med* **77**, 1241–1253.

Hodson C.J., Heptinstall R.J. & Winberg J. (eds) (1984) *Reflux Nephropathy Update, 1983*. Karger, Basel.

Hodson C.J. & Kincaid-Smith P. (eds) (1979) *Reflux Nephropathy*, Masson, New York.

Kincaid-Smith P. & Fairley K.F. (eds) (1970) *Renal Infection and Renal Scarring*. Mercedes, Melbourne.

Smellie J.M., Ransley P.G., Normand I.C.S. *et al.* (1985) Development of new renal scars, a collaborative study. *Br Med J* **290**, 1957–1960.

Zucchelli P. & Gaggi R. (1991) Reflux nephropathy in adults. *Nephron* **57**, 2–9.

CHAPTER 22

Analgesic Nephropathy

Duggin G.G. (1980) Mechanisms in the development of analgesic nephropathy. *Kidney Int* **18**, 553–561.

Editorial (1989) Analgesic nephropathy — a preventable renal disease. *New Eng J Med* **320**, 1269–1271.

Hare W.S.C. & Poynter J.D. (1974) The radiology of renal papillary necrosis as seen in analgesic nephropathy. *Clin Radiol* **25**, 423–443.

Kincaid-Smith P. (1988) Analgesic nephropathy. *Aust NZ J Med* **18**, 251–254.

Kincaid-Smith P. (1990) Analgesic nephropathy and the effect of non-steroidal anti-inflammatory drugs on the kidney. In Catto G.R.D. (ed.), *Drugs and the Kidney*, pp. 1–35. Kluwer Academic, Lancaster.

Nanra R.S. (1983) Renal effects of antipyretic analgesics. *Am J Med* **74**, 70–81.

CHAPTER 23

Obstructive Nephropathy

Bishop M.C. (1985) Diuresis and functional recovery after chronic retention. *Br J Urol* **57**, 1–5.

Editorial (1987) Hydronephrosis, renal obstruction and renography. *Lancet* **i**, 1301–1302.

Gillenwater J.Y. (1986) The pathophysiology of urinary obstruction. In Walsh P.C., Gittes R.F., Perlmutter A.D. & Stamey T.A. (eds), *Campbell's Urology* (5th edition), pp. 542–578. W.B. Saunders Co., Philadelphia.

O'Reilly P.H. (ed.) (1986) *Obstructive Nephropathy*. Springer-Verlag, Berlin.

Schleuter W. & Batlle D.C. (1988) Chronic obstructive nephropathy. *Sem Nephrol* **8**, 17–28.

CHAPTER 24

Gout, Uric Acid and the Kidney

Cameron J.S. & Simmonda H.A. (1987) Use and abuse of allopurinol. *Br Med J* **294**, 1504–1505.

Dykman D., Simon E.E. & Avioli L.V. (1987) Hyperuricemia and uric acid nephropathy. *Arch Intern Med* **147**, 1341–1348.

Reif M.C., Constantiner A. & Levitt M.F. (1981) Chronic gouty nephropathy, a vanishing syndrome? *New Eng J Med* **304**, 535–536.

CHAPTER 25

Renal Calculi

Coe F.L. & Parks J.H. (1986) Recurrent renal calculi, causes and management. *Hosp Practice* **21**, 49–86.

Coe F.L. & Parks J.H. (1988) *Nephrolithiasis, Pathogenesis and Treatment.* Year Book Medical Publishers, Chicago.

Drach G.W. (1986) Urinary lithiasis. In Walsh P.C., Gittes R.F., Perlmutter A.D. & Stamey T.A. (eds), *Campbell's Urology* (5th edition), pp. 1094–1191. W.B. Saunders Co., Philadelphia.

Kumar R. (ed.) (1990) Medical and surgical management of nephrolithiasis. *Sem Nephrol* **10**, 64–88.

Linari F., Marangella M. & Bruno M. (eds) (1981) *Pathogenesis and Treatment of Nephrolithiasis*. Karger, Basel.

Payne F.R. & Webb D.R. (eds) (1988) *Percutaneous Renal Surgery*. Churchill Livingstone, Edinburgh.

Singer A. & Das S. (1989) Cystinuria, a review of the pathophysiology and management. *J Urol* **142**, 669–673.

Wickham J.E.A. & Buck A.C. (eds) (1990) *Renal Tract Stone — Metabolic Basis and Clinical Practice*. Churchill Livingstone, Edinburgh.

CHAPTER 26

Diabetes Mellitus

Brownlee M., Cerami A. & Vlassara H. (1988) Advanced glycosylation end products in tissue and the biochemical basis of diabetic complications. *New Eng J Med* **318**, 1315–1321.

Brunner F.P., Brynger H., Challah W. *et al.* (1988) Renal replacement therapy in patients with diabetic nephropathy 1980–1985. *Nephrol Dial Transplant* **3**, 585–595.

De Fronzo R. (ed.) (1990) Diabetic nephropathy. *Sem Nephrol* **10**, 183–293.

Hostetter T.H. (1985) Diabetic nephropathy. *New Eng J Med* **315**, 642–644.

Mogensen C.E. (1987) Microalbuminuria as a predictor of clinical diabetic nephropathy. *Kidney Int* **31**, 673–689.

Mogensen C.E. (1988) Management of diabetic renal involvement and disease. *Lancet* **i**, 867–870.

Solders G., Wilczek H., Gunnarsen R. *et al.* (1987) Effects of combined pancreatic and renal transplantation on diabetic neuropathy, a two year follow up study. *Lancet* **ii**, 1232–1235.

Wardle E.N. (1987) Diabetic nephropathy. *Nephron* **45**, 177–181.

Zatz R. & Brenner B.M. (1986) Pathogenesis of diabetic nephropathy, the hemodynamic view. *Am J Med* **80**, 443–453.

CHAPTER 27

Multiple Myeloma and Paraproteinaemias

Ben-Bassat M., Boner G., Rosenfeld J. *et al.* (1983) The clinicopathological features of cryoglobulinemic nephropathy. *Am J Clin Path* **79**, 147–156.

Confalonieri R., Di Belgiojoso G.B., Banfi G. *et al.* (1988) Light chain nephropathy, histologic and clinical aspects in 15 cases. *Nephrol Dial Transplant* **2**, 150–156.

Cohen D.J., Sherman W.H., Osserman E.F. & Appel G.B. (1984) Acute renal failure in patients with multiple myeloma. *Am J Med* **76**, 247–256.

Iggo N. & Parsons V. (1990) Renal disease in multiple myeloma, current perspectives. *Nephrol Dial Transplant* **56**, 229–233.

MRC Working Party on Leukaemia in Adults (1984) Analysis and management of renal failure in the fourth MRC myelomatosis trial. *Br Med J* **288**, 1411–1415.

Rota S., Mougenot B., Baudouin B. *et al.* (1987) Multiple myeloma and severe renal failure, a clinicopathologic study of outcome and prognosis in 34 patients. *Medicine* (Baltimore) **66**, 126–137.

Zucchelli P., Pasquali S., Cagnoli L. & Ferrari G. (1988) Controlled plasma exchange trial in acute renal failure due to multiple myeloma. *Kidney Int* **33**, 1175–1180.

CHAPTER 29

Cystic Diseases

Gabow P.A. (1990) Autosomal dominant polycystic kidney disease, more than a renal disease. *Am J Kid Dis* **16**, 403–413.

Gardner K.D. & Bernstein J. (eds) (1990) *The Cystic Kidney.* Kluwer Academic, Dorderecht.

Parfrey P.S., Bear J.C., Morgan J. *et al.* (1990) The diagnosis and prognosis of autosomal dominant polycystic kidney disease. *New Eng J Med* **323**, 1085–1090.

Reeders S.T., Breuning M.H., Corney G. *et al.* (1986) Two genetic markers closely linked to adult polycystic kidney disease on chromosome 16. *Br J Med* **292**, 851–854.

Yenot E.R. (1982) Medullary sponge kidney and nephrolithiasis. *New Eng J Med* **306**, 1106–1107.

CHAPTER 30

Primary Renal Neoplasms

De Kernion J.B. (1986) Renal tumors. In Walsh P.C., Gittes R.F., Perlmutter A.D. & Stamey T.A. (eds), *Campbell's Urology* (5th edition), pp. 1294–1342. W.B. Saunders Co., Philadelphia.

Ritchie A.W.S. & Dekernion J.B. (1987) The natural history and clinical features of renal carcinoma. *Sem Nephrol* **7**, 131–139.

CHAPTER 31

Miscellaneous Renal Conditions

Dabbs D.J., Striker L. M-M. & Striker G. (1986) Glomerular lesions in lymphomas and leukemias. *Am J Med* **80**, 63–70.

Epstein M. (ed.) (1983) *The Kidney in Liver Disease*. Elsevier, New York.

Glassock R.J. (1989) Through thick and thin. *New Eng J Med* **320**, 51–53.

Glassock R.J., Cohen A.H., Danovich G. & Parsa K.P. (1990) Human immuno-deficiency virus (HIV) infection and the kidney. *Annals Int Med* **112**, 35–49.

Gubler M.C., Levy M., Broyer M. *et al.* (1981) Alport's syndrome, a report of 59 cases and a review of the literature. *Am J Med* **70**, 493–505.

Jeraj K., Kim Y., Vernier R.L. *et al.* (1983) Absence of Goodpasture's antigen in male patients with familial nephritis. *Am J Kid Dis* **11**, 626–629.

Kasiske J.T. (1986) Renal disease in patients with massive obesity. *Arch Intern Med* **146**, 1105–1112.

Kibukamusoke J.W. (ed.) (1984) *Tropical Nephrology*. Citforge, Canberra.

Neal D.E. (1985) Complications of ileal conduit. *Br Med J* **290**, 1695–1697.

Tiebusch A.T.M.G., Frederik P.M., Vriesman P.J.Cv.B. *et al.* (1989) Thin-basement-membrane nephropathy in adults with persistent hematuria. *New Eng J Med* **320**, 14–18.

Walsh P.C., Gittes R.F., Perlmutter A.D. & Stamey T.A. (eds) (1986) *Campbell's Urology* (5th edition). W.B. Saunders Co., Philadelphia.

Watts R.W.E. (1990) Treatment of renal failure in the primary hyperoxalurias. *Nephron* **56**, 1–5.

CHAPTER 32

Thrombotic Microangiopathy

Aster R.H. (1985) Plasma therapy for thrombotic thrombocytopenic purpura. *New Eng J Med* **312**, 985–987.

Drummond K.N. (1985) Hemolytic uremic syndrome — then and now. *New Eng J Med* **312**, 116–118.

Editorial (1984) Haemolytic uremic syndrome. *Lancet* **ii**, 1078–1079.

Eknoyan G. & Riggs S.A. (1986) Renal involvement in patients with thrombotic thrombocytopenic purpura. *Am J Nephrol* **6**, 117–131.

Jones H.W., Bowker C.A. & Diblasi R.J. (1983) Postpartum hemolytic uremic syndrome. *Am J Obstet Gynecol* **146**, 856–7.

Remuzzi G. (1987) HUS and TTP, variable expression of a single entity. *Kidney Int* **32**, 292–308.

CHAPTER 33

Pregnancy and the Kidney

Andreucci V.E. (ed.) (1986) *The Kidney in Pregnancy*. Martinus Nijhoff, Boston.

Becker G.J., Fairley K.F. & Whitworth J.A.W. (1985) Pregnancy exacerbates glomerular disease. *Am J Kid Dis* **6**, 266–272.

Becker G.J., Ihle B.U., Fairley, K.F. *et al.* (1986) Effect of pregnancy on moderate renal failure in reflux nephropathy. *Br Med J* **292**, 796–798.

Davison J.M. (1987) Overview, kidney function in pregnant women. *Am J Kid Dis* **9**, 248–252.

Editorial (1989) Pregnancy and glomerulonephritis. *Lancet* **ii**, 253–254.

Eisenbach G.B. & Brod J. (eds) (1981) *Kidney and Pregnancy*. Karger, Basel.

Hou S.H., Grossman S.D. & Madias N.E. (1985) Pregnancy in women with renal disease and moderate renal insufficiency. *Am J Med* **78**, 185–194.

Ihle B.U., Long P. & Oats J. (1987) Early onset preeclampsia, recognition of underlying renal disease. *Br Med J* **294**, 79–81.

Jones H.W., Bowker C.A. & Diblasi R.J. (1983) Postpartum hemolytic uremic syndrome. *Am J Obstet Gynecol* **146**, 856–7.

Kincaid-Smith P. (1987) The management of hypertensive disorders of pregnancy. *Aust NZ J Med* **17**, 187–188.

Kincaid-Smith P., North R.A., Becker G.J. & Fairley K.F. (1980) Proteinuria during pregnancy. In Andreucci VE (ed.), *The Kidney in Pregnancy*, pp. 133–164. Martinus Nijhoff, Boston.

Lindheimer M.D. & Katz A.I. (1985) Hypertension in pregnancy. *New Eng J Med* **313**, 675–679.

CHAPTER 34

Drugs and the Kidney

Appel G.B. & Neu H.C. (1977) The nephrotoxicity of antimicrobial agents. *New Eng J Med* **296**, 663–670, 722–728, 784–787.

Bennett W.M. (1986) *Drugs and Renal Disease* (2nd edition). Churchill Livingstone, New York.

Bennett W.M., Aroneff G.R., Morrison G. *et al.* (1983) Drug prescribing in renal failure, dosing guidelines for adults. *Am J Kid Dis* **3**, 155–193.

Brezis M. & Epstein F.H. (1989) A closer look at radiocontrast-induced nephropathy. *New Eng J Med* **320**, 179–181.

Hall C.L. (1988) Gold nephropathy. *Nephron* **50**, 265–272.

Hande K.R., Noone R.M. & Stone W.J. (1984) Severe allopurinol toxicity. Description and guidelines for prevention in patients with renal insufficiency. *Am J Med* **76**, 47–56.

Hou S.H., Bushinsky D.A., Wish J.B. *et al.* (1983) Hospital acquired renal insufficiency, a prospective study. *Am J Med* **74**, 243–248.

Paller M.S. (1990) Cyclosporine nephrotoxicity and the role of cyclosporine in living-related donor transplantation. *Am J Kid Dis* **16**, 414–416.

CHAPTER 35

Dialysis and Transplantation

Bennett W.M. (1986) *Drugs and Renal Disease* (2nd edition). Churchill Livingstone, New York.

Bennett W.M., Aroneff G.R., Morrison G. *et al.* (1983) Drug prescribing in renal failure, dosing guidelines for adults. *Am J Kid Dis* **3**, 155–193.

Fine R.N. & Gruskin A.B. (eds) (1984) *Endstage Renal Disease in Children*. W.B. Saunders Co., Philadelphia.

Kahan B.D. (1989) Cyclosporine. *New Eng J Med* **321**, 1725–1737.

Maher J.F. (ed.) (1989) *Replacement of Renal Function by Dialysis*. Kluwer Academic, Dordrecht.

Mathew T.H. (1988) Recurrence of disease following renal transplantation. *Am J Kid Dis* **12**, 85–96.

Moncrief J.W., Popovich R.P. & Nolph K.D. (1990) The history and current status of continuous ambulatory peritoneal dialysis. *Am J Kid Dis* **16**, 579–584.

Morris P.J. (ed.) (1988) *Kidney Transplantation, Principles and Practice* (3rd edition). W.B. Saunders Co., Philadelphia.

Paller M.S. (1990) Cyclosporine nephrotoxicity and the role of cyclosporine in living-related donor transplantation. *Am J Kid Dis* **16**, 414–416.

Sethi D., Morgan T.C.N., Brown E.A. *et al.* (1990) Dialysis arthropathy, a clinical, biochemical, radiological and histological study of 36 patients. *Quart J Med* **77**, 1061–1082.

Index

Page numbers in *italics* refer to figures, and numbers in **bold** refer to tables. Abbreviations used: GFR, glomerular filtration rate; GN, glomerulonephritis; FSHS, focal and segmental hyalinosis and sclerosis; SLE, systemic lupus erythematosus